SEIDEL'S Physical Examination Handbook

AN INTERPROFESSIONAL APPROACH

11TH EDITION

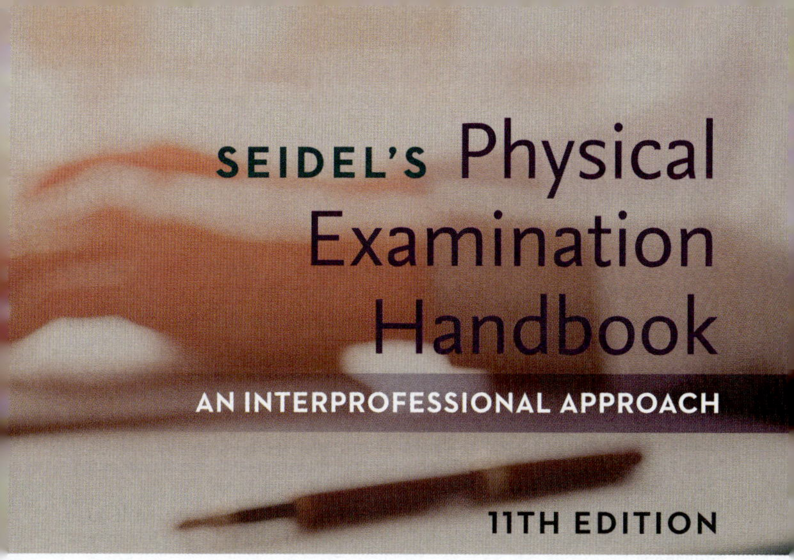

SEIDEL'S Physical Examination Handbook

AN INTERPROFESSIONAL APPROACH

11TH EDITION

Joyce E. Dains, DrPH, JD, APRN, FNP-BC, FNAP, FAANP, FAAN

Professor, The University of Texas MD Anderson Cancer Center, Houston, Texas

John A. Flynn, MD, MBA, MEd

Professor of Medicine, Baylor College of Medicine, Houston, Texas

JoAnne Silbert-Flagg, DNP, CPNP, IBCLC, CNE, FAAN, FAANP

Associate Dean for Clinical Practice, Johns Hopkins University School of Nursing, Baltimore, Maryland; Pediatric Nurse Practitioner, Columbia Medical Practice, Columbia, Maryland

Barry S. Solomon, MD, MPH

Professor of Pediatrics, Assistant Dean for Medical Student Affairs, Johns Hopkins University School of Medicine, Baltimore, Maryland

Rosalyn W. Stewart, MD, MS, MBA

Professor of Internal Medicine and Pediatrics, Johns Hopkins University School of Medicine, Baltimore, Maryland

ELSEVIER

Elsevier
3251 Riverport Lane
St. Louis, Missouri 63043

SEIDEL'S PHYSICAL EXAMINATION HANDBOOK: AN INTERPROFESSIONAL APPROACH, 11th EDITION ISBN: 978-0-443-40915-8

Content Strategist: Sonya Seigafuse
Senior Content Development Specialist: Elizabeth McCormac
Publishing Services Manager: Deepthi Unni
Project Manager: Arul Viveaun S
Design Direction: Brian Salisbury

Printed in India

Last digit is the print number: 9 8 7 6 5 4 3 2 1

Preface

Seidel's Physical Examination Handbook: An Interprofessional Approach, 11th edition, is a portable clinical reference on physical examination that is suitable for students of nursing, medicine, chiropractic, osteopathic, and other allied health disciplines, as well as for practicing clinicians. It offers brief descriptions of examination techniques and step-by-step guidelines on how the examination should proceed. This handbook is intended to be an aid for reviewing and recalling the procedures of physical examination. Because of its brevity, specific techniques of history taking by organ system are not described.

The handbook begins with an outline of what information should be obtained for the patient's medical history and review of systems, followed by essential guidance for recording in the medical record. Subsequent chapters for each of the body systems list equipment needed to perform the examination and present the techniques to be used. Expected and Unexpected Findings follow the description of each technique, presented in distinctive color type for easy recognition. Numerous illustrations interspersed throughout the text reinforce techniques and possible findings. Pediatric examination variations are highlighted in each body systems chapter.

Each chapter offers Aids to Differential Diagnosis. Subjective and Objective Data are clearly differentiated for each abnormality in the Aids to Differential Diagnosis section of each chapter.

As in previous editions, separate chapters give an overview of the entire examination for all adults; for infants, children, and adolescents; persons with disabilities; for transgender and gender-diverse patients; and for those participating in sports. The final chapter gives guidelines for emergency or life-threatening situations.

Joyce E. Dains
John A. Flynn
JoAnne Silbert-Flagg
Barry S. Solomon
Rosalyn W. Stewart

Acknowledgments

We want to acknowledge Henry M. Seidel, MD, William Benedict, MD, and Jane Ball PhD, RN, CPNP, three of our original authors, who served on seven, six and ten editions, respectively. Their commitment to the relationship with the patient and their appreciation of the importance of interprofessional collaboration helped shape this text.

We also want to acknowledge and thank Paula M. Neira, JD, MSN, RN, CEN, FAAN, Assistant Professor of Plastic and Reconstructive Surgery and Clinical Program Director of the Johns Hopkins Center for Transgender Health, for her review and previous contributions.

CHAPTER

1

The History and Interviewing Process

Building the History

The following patient history outline is a guideline and should not be considered a rigid structure. You are beginning your relationship with the patient at this point. Choose a comfortable setting and help the patient get settled. Maintain eye contact and use a conversational tone. Begin by introducing yourself and explaining your role. Help the patient understand why you are building the history and how it will help in their care. Start with open-ended questions and explore responses with additional questions: where, when, what, how, and why. Be sensitive to the patient's emotions. Avoid confrontation and leading questions.

Chief Concern

- Primary concern, problem, or symptom: reason for visit
- Duration of problem
- Other concerns: secondary issues, fears, what made patient seek care
- Always consider why this particular problem may be affecting this particular patient at this time. Why did this patient succumb to a risk or an exposure when others similarly exposed did not?

History of Present Illness

When more than one concern is identified, address each separately.

- Chronologic ordering: sequence of events patient experiences
- State of health just before onset of the concern
- Complete description of first symptom: time, date of onset, location, and characteristics
- Possible exposure to infection or toxic agents or risk to personal safety
- If symptoms are intermittent, describe typical episode: onset, duration, symptoms, variations, factors that incite, exacerbate, or relieve
- Effect of illness on: lifestyle, ability to function; or limitations imposed by illness
- "Stability" of problem: intensity, variations, improvement, worsening, staying the same

- Reason for seeking attention, particularly for long-standing problem
- Review of affected system when there is a disturbance of a particular organ or system
- Medications tried: current and recent, doses, nonprescription medications
- Use of complementary or alternative therapies and medications; home remedies
- At conclusion, review information gathered for each problem: patient's confirmations and corrections

Medical History

- Hospitalizations and/or surgeries: dates, hospital/location, diagnosis, complications, injuries, disabilities
- Childhood illnesses: asthma, autism, cerebral palsy, pneumonia, osteomyelitis
- Adult illnesses: tuberculosis, hepatitis, diabetes mellitus, hypertension, coronary artery disease/myocardial infarction, psychiatric, substance use disorders, tropical or parasitic infection, other infections
- Serious injuries: traumatic brain injury, liver laceration, spinal injury, fractures
- Immunizations: polio, diphtheria, pertussis, tetanus toxoid, hepatitis B, measles, mumps, rubella, *Haemophilus influenzae*, varicella, influenza, hepatitis A, meningococcal, human papillomavirus (HPV), pneumococcal, zoster, typhoid, anthrax, smallpox, bacille Calmette-Guérin, COVID-19, last tuberculin test, unusual reaction to immunizations
- Medications: past, current, and recent (dosage, nonprescription medications, vitamins); complementary and herbal therapies
- Allergies: drugs, foods, environmental allergens along with the allergic reaction (e.g., rash, anaphylaxis)
- Transfusions: reason, date, and number of units transfused; reaction, if any
- Mental health: mood disorders, psychiatric therapy or medications
- Recent laboratory tests: glucose, A1c, cholesterol, Pap smear/HPV, HIV, hepatitis screening, mammogram, bone density, colonoscopy, Cologuard, fecal immunochemical test or fecal occult blood test, prostate-specific antigen

Family History

The genetic basis for a patient's response to risk or exposure may determine whether the patient becomes ill when others do not.

- Relatives with similar illness
- Immediate family: ethnicity, health, cause of and age at death
- History of disease: heart disease, high blood pressure, hypercholesterolemia, vascular disease, cancer, tuberculosis, stroke, epilepsy, diabetes, gout, kidney disease, thyroid disease, asthma, arthritis, blood diseases, psychiatric illnesses, sexually transmitted infections, substance use disorders, other familial diseases
- Spouse and children: age, health, genetic relationship
- Hereditary disease: history of grandparents, aunts, uncles, siblings, cousins; consanguinity

Personal and Social History

- Cultural background and practices, birthplace, where raised, home environment as youth, education, family, marital status, gender identity and sexual orientation, general life satisfaction, hobbies, interests, sources of stress
- Home environment: number of individuals in household, relationship to patient, pets, economic situation
- Occupation: usual work and present work if different, list of job changes, work conditions and hours, physical or mental strain, duration of employment; present and past exposure to heat and cold, industrial toxins; protective devices required or used; military service
- Environment: home, school, work, structural barriers if physically disabled, community services utilized; travel and other exposure to contagious diseases, residence in tropics; water and milk supply, other potential sources of infection
- Current health habits and/or risk factors: exercise; smoking (pack years: packs per day × duration); salt intake; obesity/weight control; diet; alcohol intake (amount/day), duration; CAGE (Cutting down, Annoyance by criticism, Guilty feeling, Eye-openers) or TACE (Take, Annoyed, Cut down, Eye-opener) question responses (see Appendix on special histories); substance use and methods (e.g., injection, ingestion, sniffing, smoking, or use of shared needles)
- Exposure to chemicals, toxins, poisons, asbestos, lead, or radioactive material at home or work, and duration of exposure; caffeine use (amount/day)
- Sexual activity: partners, practices, contraceptive or barrier protection methods used; past sexually transmitted infections; treatment
- Screen for intimate partner violence: see Appendix on special histories

- Complementary and alternative health and medical systems: history and current use
- Religious preference: religious proscriptions concerning medical care
- Concerns about cost of care, health care and prescription coverage

Review of Systems

It is unlikely that all questions in each system will be asked on every occasion. The following questions are among those that should be asked, particularly at the first interview:

- General constitutional symptoms: fever, chills, malaise, excess fatigue, night sweats, weight (average, preferred, present, change over a specified period and whether change was intentional)
- Skin, hair, and nails: rash or eruption, itching, pigmentation or texture change; growths, excessive sweating, unusual nail or hair growth
- Head and neck: frequent or unusual headaches, location, dizziness, syncope; brain injuries, concussions, loss of consciousness (momentary or prolonged)
- Eyes: visual acuity, blurring, double vision, light sensitivity, pain, change in appearance or vision; use of glasses/contacts, eye drops, other medication; history of trauma, glaucoma, familial eye disease
- Ears: hearing loss, pain, discharge, tinnitus, vertigo
- Nose: sense of smell, frequency of colds, obstruction, nosebleeds, postnasal discharge, sinus pain
- Throat and mouth: hoarseness or change in voice; frequent sore throats, bleeding or swelling of gums; dental caries, recent tooth abscesses or extraction; dentures, implants, and devices; soreness of tongue or buccal mucosa, ulcers; disturbance of taste
- Lymphatic: enlargement, tenderness, suppuration
- Chest and lungs: pain related to respiration, dyspnea, cyanosis, wheezing, cough, sputum (frequency, character, and quantity), hemoptysis, night sweats, exposure to tuberculosis; most recent chest radiograph
- Breasts: development, pain, tenderness, discharge, lumps, galactorrhea, implants, mammograms (screening or diagnostic), breast biopsies
- Heart and coronary arteries: chest pain or distress, precipitating causes, timing and duration, relieving factors, palpitations, dyspnea, orthopnea (number of pillows), edema, hypertension, previous myocardial infarction, exercise tolerance (flights of steps, distance walking), past electrocardiogram and cardiac tests

- Peripheral vasculature: claudication (frequency, severity), evaluation, tendency to bruise or bleed, thromboses, thrombophlebitis
- Hematologic: anemia, any known blood disorder
- Gastrointestinal: appetite, digestion, intolerance of any foods, dysphagia, heartburn, nausea, vomiting, hematemesis, bowel regularity, constipation, diarrhea, change in stool color or contents (clay, tarry, fresh blood, mucus, undigested food), flatulence, hemorrhoids, hepatitis, jaundice, dark urine; history of ulcer, gallstones, polyps, tumor; previous radiographic studies, colon cancer screening (modality, where, when, findings), procedures; indication, what type, findings
- Diet: appetite, likes and dislikes, restrictions (because of religion, allergy, or other), vitamins and other supplements, food diary or daily recall of food and liquid intake
- Endocrine: thyroid enlargement or tenderness, heat or cold intolerance, unexplained weight change, polydipsia, polyuria, changes in facial or body hair, increased hat and glove size, skin striae
- Male patients: puberty onset, gender affirming surgery, erections, emissions, testicular pain, tucking, libido, infertility
- Female patients: gender affirming surgery; menses onset, regularity, duration, amount of flow; dysmenorrhea; last period; intermenstrual discharge or bleeding; itching; date of last Pap smear/HPV test; age at menopause; libido; frequency of intercourse; sexual difficulties
- Pregnancy: infertility; gravidity and parity (G = number of pregnancies, P = number of childbirths, A = number of abortions/miscarriages, L = number of living children); number and duration of each pregnancy, delivery method; complications during any pregnancy or postpartum period; use of oral or other contraceptives
- Genitourinary: dysuria, flank or suprapubic pain, urgency, frequency, nocturia, hematuria, polyuria, hesitancy, dribbling, loss in force of stream, passage of stone; edema of face, stress incontinence, hernias, sexually transmitted infection
- Musculoskeletal: joint stiffness, pain, restriction of motion, swelling, redness, heat, bony deformity, number and pattern of joint involvement
- Neurologic: syncope, seizures, weakness or paralysis, problems with sensation or coordination, tremors
- Mental health: depression, mania, mood changes, difficulty concentrating, nervousness, tension, suicidal thoughts, irritability, sleep disturbances

Concluding Questions

- Is there anything else that you think would be important for me to know?
- If there are several problems: Which issue concerns you the most?
- If the history is vague, complicated, or contradictory: What do you think is the matter with you, or what worries you the most?
- Do you have any questions or concerns that we have not addressed?

PEDIATRIC VARIATIONS

BUILDING THE HISTORY

These are guidelines; you are free to modify as the needs of your patients and your judgment dictate.

CHIEF CONCERN

A guardian or other responsible adult will generally be the major resource. When age permits, the child should be involved as much as possible. Remember that every chief concern has the potential of an underlying concern. What really led to your visit? Was it just the sore throat?

RELIABILITY

Note relationship to patient of person who is the resource for history, and record your impression of the reliability of that person as a historian.

HISTORY OF PRESENT ILLNESS

Be sure to give a clear chronologic sequence to the story.

MEDICAL HISTORY

In general, the age of the patient and the nature of the problem will guide your approach. In a continuing relationship, or with electronic health record sharing, much of what is to be known will already have been recorded. Different aspects of the history require varying emphasis depending on the nature of the immediate problem. Certain specifics will command attention, including the following:

- Pregnant person's health:
    - Infectious disease
    - Approximate gestational age

- Weight gain/edema
- Hypertension
- Proteinuria
- Bleeding; approximate time
- Eclampsia, threat of eclampsia
- Special or unusual diet or dietary practices
- Medications (hormones, vitamins)
- Quality of fetal movements, time of onset
- Radiation exposure
- Prenatal care/consistency

- Birth and perinatal experience:
  - Duration of pregnancy
  - Delivery site
  - Labor: spontaneous/induced, duration, anesthesia, complications
  - Delivery: presentation, forceps/spontaneous, complications
  - Condition at birth: time of onset of cry; Apgar scores, if available
  - Birth weight and, if available, length and head circumference
- Neonatal period:
  - Hospital experience: length of stay, feeding experience, oxygen needs, vigor, color (jaundice, cyanosis), cry. Did infant go home with mother?
  - First month of life: color (jaundice), feeding, vigor, any suggestion of illness or untoward event
- Feeding:
  - Bottle and/or breast: any changes and why; type of formula, amounts offered/taken, feeding frequency; weight gain
  - Present diet and appetite: introduction of solids, current routine and frequency, age weaned from bottle or breast, daily intake of milk, food preferences, ability to feed self; elaborate on any feeding problems

DEVELOPMENT

Guidelines suggested in Chapter 5 are complementary to the milestones detailed in the following lists. Those included in this section are commonly used. Photographs also may occasionally be of some help. *Note*: It is important to define the growth and developmental status of each child, regardless of the particular concern. That status will inform your understanding of the child and, if developmental abnormities are related to their principal problem, will facilitate the institution of a management plan.

- Age when:
  - Held head erect while held in sitting position

  - Sat alone, unsupported
  - Walked alone
  - Talked in sentences
  - Toilet trained
- School: grade, performance, learning and social problems
- Dentition: ages at first teeth, loss of deciduous teeth, first permanent teeth
- Growth: height and weight at different ages, changes in rate of growth or weight gain or loss
- Sexual: present status (e.g., in people assigned female at birth, time of breast development, nipples, pubic hair, description of menses; in people assigned male at birth, development of pubic hair, voice change, acne, emissions). Follow Tanner stages of physical sexual maturity development guides

FAMILY HISTORY

- Maternal gestational history: all pregnancies with status of each, including date, age, cause of death of all deceased siblings, and dates and duration of pregnancy in the case of miscarriages; mother's health during pregnancy
- Age of parents at birth of patient
- Are parents related to each other in any way?

PERSONAL AND SOCIAL HISTORY

- Personal status:
  - School adjustment
  - Nail biting
  - Thumb sucking
  - Breath-holding spells
  - Temper tantrums
  - Pica
  - Tics
  - Rituals
- Home conditions:
  - Parental occupation(s)
  - Principal caretaker(s) of patient
  - Food preparation, routine, family preferences (e.g., kosher, vegan, vegetarianism), person(s) in charge of preparation
  - Adequacy of clothing
  - Dependency on relief or social agencies
  - Number of persons and rooms in house or apartment
  - Sleeping routines and sleep arrangements for child

REVIEW OF SYSTEMS (SOME SUGGESTED ADDITIONAL QUESTIONS OR PARTICULAR CONCERNS)

- Ears: otitis media (frequency, laterality)
- Nose: snoring, mouth breathing
- Teeth: dental care, dentist visits
- Genitourinary: nature of urinary stream, forceful or a dribble
- Skin, hair, nails: eczema or seborrhea

OLDER ADULT VARIATIONS

FUNCTIONAL ASSESSMENT

- Activities of daily living (ADLs): ability to independently perform or amount of assistance needed with the following:
  - Bathing
  - Dressing
  - Toileting
  - Transfers
  - Grooming
  - Feeding
- Instrumental ADLs: ability to independently perform or amount of assistance needed with the following:
  - Administering own medication
  - Grocery shopping
  - Preparing meals
  - Using the telephone
  - Driving and transportation
  - Handling own finances
  - Housekeeping
  - Laundry
- Risk for falls: falls in the past 6 months or year; use of rugs at home
- Cognitive functioning: see Chapter 4.

CHAPTER

2 The Health Record

After performing the history and physical examination, the clinician must organize, synthesize, and record the data along with the concerns identified and the rationale for diagnostic evaluation and plan of care. This cognitive effort goes well beyond simply transcribing or importing data that may exist from other sources or completing prescribed templates. The information in the patient's health record must enable you and your colleagues to know and care for the patient by identifying health problems, listing diagnoses, and making judgments regarding the diagnostic testing needed, planning appropriate care, and monitoring the patient's responses to treatment. The patient's health record is only as good as the accuracy, pertinent depth and detail, and thoughtful synthesis provided by the documenting caregivers. With the transition to the electronic health record (EHR), it is even more critical to maintain standards of documentation excellence. Within the EHR environment, there is great risk in overwhelming the reader with volumes of insignificant or inaccurate data by importing preexisting and unverified information from other sources within the record. This phenomenon, sometimes referred to as "note bloat," must be guarded against.

The patient's health record is a legal document. All information contained in it may be used in court and in other legal proceedings. Your documentation will be read by many individuals; increasingly, and appropriately, this includes the patient and their family members. It is your responsibility to document the facts of the history and your physical examination findings accurately.

Subjective Data—The History

Subjective data are the positive and negative pieces of information that the patient offers. Record the patient's history, especially during an initial visit, to provide a comprehensive database. Arrange information appropriately in specific categories (usually in a particular sequence such as chronologic order) with most recent information first. Include both positive and negative data that contribute to the assessment. Use the following organized sequence as a guide.

Identifying information is typically gathered by your facility's registration department. This includes:

- Patient's name
- Identification number/social security number
- Age, gender
- Marital status
- Address (home and business)
- Phone numbers
- Occupation, employer
- Insurance plan, number
- Date of visit
- For children and dependent adults, names of parents or next of kin
- Document who is providing the history and their relationship to the patient
- Indicate which information is obtained from existing health records
- State judgment about reliability of information

CHIEF CONCERN/PRESENTING PROBLEM/REASON FOR SEEKING CARE

Record a description of the patient's main reasons for seeking health care, in the patient's own words, with quotation marks. Paraphrase only if this makes the patient's concern more clear. Include the duration of the concern.

HISTORY OF PRESENT PROBLEM

- In reverse chronological order, list and describe current symptoms of the chief concern and their appearance, dating events, and symptoms.
- List any expected symptoms that are absent.
- Identify anyone in household with same symptoms.
- Note pertinent information from review of systems, family history, and personal/social history along with findings.
- When more than one problem is identified, address each in a separate paragraph, including the following details of symptom occurrence:
  - Onset: when problem first started, chronologic order of events, setting and circumstances, and manner of onset (sudden versus gradual)
  - Location: exact location, localized or generalized, radiation patterns
  - Duration: how long problem has lasted, intermittent or continuous, duration of each episode

- Character: nature of symptom
- Aggravating/associated factors: food, activity, rest, certain movements; nausea, vomiting, diarrhea, fever, chills, etc.
- Relieving factors: prescribed treatments and/or self-remedies, alternative or complementary therapies, their effect on the problem; food, rest, heat, ice, activity, position, etc.
- Temporal factors: frequency; relation to other symptoms, problems, and functions; symptom improvement or worsening over time
- Severity of symptoms: quantify on a 0 (minimal) to 10 (severe) scale; effect on patient's lifestyle

MEDICAL HISTORY

- List and describe each of the following with dates of occurrence and any specific information available:
  - General health and strength over lifetime as patient perceives it; disabilities and functional limitations
  - Hospitalization and/or surgery: dates, hospital, diagnosis, complications
  - Injuries and disabilities
  - Major childhood illnesses
  - Adult illnesses and serious injuries
- Immunizations: COVID-19, polio, respiratory syncytial virus (RSV), diphtheria-pertussis-tetanus, tetanus toxoid, *Haemophilus influenza* type b, hepatitis A and B, measles, mumps, rubella, varicella, pneumococcal, influenza, anthrax, smallpox, cholera, typhus, typhoid, meningococcal, pneumococcal, *Bacillus* Calmette-Guérin (BCG), last purified protein derivative or other skin tests, unusual reaction to immunizations
- Medications: past, current, recent (prescribed, nonprescription, complementary therapies, home remedies); dosages
- Allergies: drugs, foods, environmental
- Transfusions: reason, date, number of units transfused, reactions
- Emotional status: history of mood disorders, psychiatric attention, or medications
- Recent laboratory tests (e.g., glucose, cholesterol, Pap smear, mammogram, prostate-specific antigen)

Family History

- Present information about age and health of family members in narrative or pedigree form, including at least three generations.

- Family members: Include parents, grandparents, aunts and uncles, siblings, spouse, and children. For deceased family members, note age at time of death and cause, if known.
- Major health or genetic disorders: Include hypertension; cancer; cardiac, respiratory, kidney, or thyroid disorders; strokes; asthma or other allergic manifestations; blood dyscrasia; psychiatric difficulties; tuberculosis; diabetes mellitus; hepatitis; or other familial disorders. Note spontaneous abortions and stillbirths.

PERSONAL/SOCIAL HISTORY

- Include information according to concerns of patient and influence of health problem on patient's and family's life:
  - Cultural background and practices, birthplace, position in family
  - Marital status
  - Religious preference, religious, or cultural proscriptions for medical care
- Home conditions: economic condition, number in household, pets, presence of smoke detectors, presence, and security of firearms
- Occupation: work conditions and hours; physical or mental strain; protective devices used; exposure to chemicals, toxins, poisons, fumes, smoke, asbestos, or radioactive material at home or work
- Environment: home, school, work; structural barriers if handicapped, community services utilized; travel; exposure to contagious diseases
- Current health habits and/or risk factors: exercise; smoking; salt intake; weight control; dental hygiene; diet, vitamins, and other supplements; caffeinated beverages; alcohol or recreational drug use; response to CAGE, TACE, or CRAFFT questions (see Appendix) related to alcohol use; participation in a drug or alcohol treatment program or support group
- Sexual activity: protection method, contraception
- General life satisfaction, hobbies, interests, sources of stress, adolescent's response to HEEADSSS questions (see Appendix)

REVIEW OF SYSTEMS

- Organize in general head-to-toe sequence, including an impression of each symptom.
- Record expected or negative findings as absence of symptoms or problems.
- When unexpected or positive findings are stated by patient, include details from further inquiry as you would in the present illness.

- Include the following categories of information (sequence may vary):
  - General constitutional symptoms
  - Diet
  - Skin, hair, nails
  - Head and neck
  - Eyes, ears, nose, mouth, throat
  - Endocrine
  - Breasts
  - Heart and blood vessels
  - Chest and lungs
  - Hematologic
  - Lymphatic and immunologic
  - Gastrointestinal
  - Genitourinary
  - Musculoskeletal
  - Neurologic
  - Psychiatric

Objective Data—Physical Findings

Objective data are the findings resulting from direct observation—what you see, hear, and touch.

GENERAL STATEMENT

- Age, race, sex, general appearance
- Nutritional status, weight, height, frame size, body mass index
- Vital signs: temperature, pulse rate, respiratory rate, blood pressure (two extremities, two positions)

MENTAL STATUS

- Physical appearance and behavior
- Cognitive: memory, reasoning, attention span, response to questions
- Speech and language: voice quality, articulation, content, coherence, comprehension
- Emotional stability: anxiety, depression, disturbance in thought content

SKIN

- Color, integrity, temperature, hydration, tattoos, scars
- Presence of edema, excessive perspiration, unusual odor
- Presence and description of lesions (size, shape, location, inflammation, tenderness, induration, discharge), parasites

- Hair texture and distribution
- Nail configuration, color, texture, condition, presence of clubbing, nail plate adherence, firmness

HEAD

- Size and contour of head, scalp appearance, and movement
- Facial features (characteristics, symmetry)
- Presence of edema or puffiness, tenderness
- Temporal arteries: characteristics

EYES

- Visual acuity, visual fields
- Appearance of orbits, conjunctivae, sclerae, eyelids, eyebrows
- Pupillary shape, consensual response to light and accommodation, extraocular movements, corneal light reflex, cover–uncover test
- Ophthalmoscopic findings of cornea, lens, retina, optic disc, macula, retinal vessel size, caliber, and arteriovenous crossings

EARS

- Configuration, position, and alignment of auricles
- Otoscopic findings of canals (cerumen, lesions, discharge, foreign body) and tympanic membranes (integrity, color, landmarks, mobility, perforation)
- Hearing: air and bone conduction tests, whispered voice, conversation

NOSE

- Appearance of external nose, nasal patency, flaring
- Nasal mucosa and septum, color, alignment, discharge, crusting, polyp
- Appearance of turbinates
- Presence of sinus tenderness or swelling
- Discrimination of odors

MOUTH AND THROAT

- Number, occlusion, and condition of teeth; presence of dental appliances
- Lips, tongue, buccal and oral mucosa, floor of mouth (color, moisture, surface characteristics, ulcerations, induration, symmetry)
- Oropharynx, tonsils, palate (color, symmetry, exudate)
- Symmetry and movement of tongue, soft palate, and uvula; gag reflex
- Discrimination of taste

NECK

- Mobility, suppleness, strength
- Position of trachea
- Thyroid size, shape, tenderness, nodules
- Presence of masses, webbing, skinfolds

CHEST

- Size and shape of chest, anteroposterior versus transverse diameter, symmetry of movement with respiration
- Presence of retractions, use of accessory muscles, diaphragmatic excursion

LUNGS

- Respiratory rate, depth, regularity, quietness, or ease of respiration
- Palpation findings: symmetry and quality of tactile fremitus, thoracic expansion
- Percussion findings: quality and symmetry of percussion notes, diaphragmatic excursion
- Auscultation findings: characteristics of breath sounds (pitch, duration, intensity, vesicular, bronchial, bronchovesicular), unexpected breath sounds
- Characteristics of cough
- Presence of friction rub, egophony, whispered pectoriloquy

BREASTS

- Size, contour, venous patterns
- Symmetry, texture; masses, scars, tenderness, thickening, nodules, discharge, retraction, or dimpling
- Characteristics of nipples and areolae

HEART

- Anatomic location of apical impulse
- Heart rate, rhythm, amplitude, contour
- Palpation findings: pulsations, thrills, heaves, or lifts
- Auscultation findings: characteristics of S1 and S2 (location, intensity, pitch, timing, splitting, systole, diastole)
- Presence of murmurs, clicks, snaps, S3, or S4 (timing, location, radiation intensity, pitch, quality)

BLOOD VESSELS

- Blood pressure: comparison between extremities with position change

- Jugular vein pulsations and distention, pressure measurement
- Presence of bruits over carotid, temporal, renal, and femoral arteries, abdominal aorta
- Pulses in distal extremities
- Temperature, color, hair distribution, skin texture, nail beds of lower extremities
- Presence of edema, swelling, vein distention, Homans sign, or tenderness of lower extremities

ABDOMEN

- Shape, contour, visible aorta pulsations, venous patterns, hernia
- Auscultation findings: bowel sounds in all quadrants, character
- Palpation findings: aorta, organs, feces, masses, location, size, contour, consistency, tenderness, muscle resistance
- Percussion findings: areas of different percussion notes, costovertebral angle tenderness
- Liver span

FEMALE GENITALIA

- Appearance of external genitalia and perineum, distribution of pubic hair, inflammation, excoriation, tenderness, scarring, discharge
- Internal examination findings: appearance of vaginal mucosa, cervix, discharge, odor, lesions
- Bimanual examination findings: size, position, tenderness of cervix, vaginal walls, uterus, adnexa, ovaries
- Rectovaginal examination findings
- Urinary incontinence with bearing down

MALE GENITALIA

- Appearance of external genitalia, circumcision status, location and size of urethral opening, discharge, lesions, distribution of pubic hair
- Palpation findings: penis, testes, epididymides, vasa deferentia, contour, consistency, tenderness
- Presence of hernia or scrotal swelling

ANUS AND RECTUM

- Sphincter control, presence of hemorrhoids, fissures, skin tags, polyps
- Rectal wall contour, tenderness, sphincter tone
- Prostate size, contour, consistency, mobility
- Color and consistency of stool

LYMPHATIC

- Presence of lymph nodes in head, neck, epitrochlear, axillary, or inguinal areas
- Size, shape, consistency, warmth, tenderness, mobility, discreteness of nodes

MUSCULOSKELETAL

- Posture: Alignment of extremities and spine, symmetry of body parts
- Symmetry of muscle mass, tone, and muscle strength; grading of strength, fasciculations, spasms
- Range of motion, passive and active; presence of pain with movement
- Appearance of joints; presence of deformities, effusions, warmth, tenderness, or crepitus

NEUROLOGIC

- Cranial nerves: specific findings for each or specify those tested, if findings are recorded in head and neck sections
- Cerebellar and motor function: gait, balance, coordination with rapid alternating motions
- Sensory function, symmetry (touch, pain, vibration, temperature, monofilament)
- Superficial and deep tendon reflexes: symmetry, grade

Assessment

The assessment section is composed of your interpretations and conclusions, their rationale, the diagnostic possibilities, and present and anticipated problems—what you think.

For each new and existing problem on the problem list, make a differential diagnosis list with rationale based on subjective and objective data. Describe disease progression or complication.

Plan

The plan describes the need to invoke diagnostic resources, therapeutic modalities, and other resources, and the rationale for these decisions—what you intend to do.

- Diagnostic tests ordered or performed
- Therapeutic treatment plan
- Patient education
- Referrals initiated
- Future visit to evaluate plan

CHAPTER 3

Vital Signs and Pain Assessment

Equipment

- Thermometer
- Sphygmomanometer
- Stethoscope
- Pain scales
- Pulse Oximeter (optional)

EXAMINATION

TECHNIQUES	FINDINGS

Vital Signs

Temperature

Take the temperature with an oral, tympanic, axillary, forehead, or rectal thermometer.

EXPECTED: Temperature range of 97.2°F to 99.9°F (36.2°C to 37.7°C).

UNEXPECTED: Fever, hypothermia.

Pulse rate

Palpate the radial or brachial pulse to count the heart rate for 30 seconds, then multiply by 2. Note the contour and amplitude of the pulsation. See Chapter 13 for rhythm assessment.

EXPECTED: Rate 60 to 90 bpm, average 70, regular rhythm.

UNEXPECTED: Bradycardia, tachycardia, irregular rhythm.

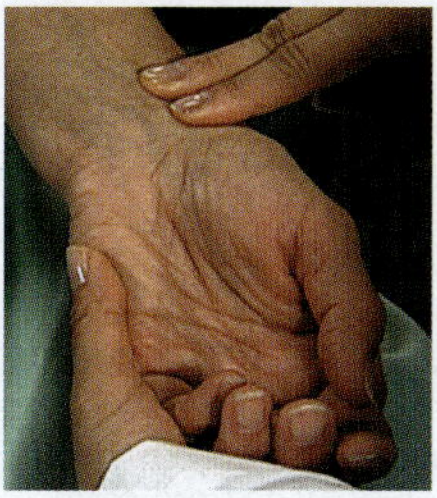

Palpate the radial pulse.

TECHNIQUES	FINDINGS
Respiratory rate	
Observe the chest rise and fall to count the respiratory rate for 30 seconds, then multiply by 2. See Chapter 11 to assess the pattern of respirations.	**EXPECTED:** Breathing easy, normally, without distress. Pattern even. Rate 12 to 20 respirations/min. Ratio of respirations to heartbeats about 1:4. **UNEXPECTED:** Tachypnea, bradypnea, dyspnea.
Blood pressure	
Measure in both arms at least once annually. Patient's arm should be slightly flexed and positioned or held at the level of the heart. Palpate the systolic blood pressure first to detect an auscultatory gap when using the stethoscope. Immediately deflate the cuff completely, pause 30 seconds, and then auscultate the systolic and diastolic blood pressure.	**EXPECTED:** Less than 120 mm Hg systolic and less than 80 mm Hg diastolic. Readings between arms may vary by 10 mm Hg. **UNEXPECTED:** An elevated blood pressure is now defined as a blood pressure between 120 and 129 mm Hg systolic and less than 80 mm Hg diastolic. Take several measurements before diagnosing hypertension (see the following table). Unusually low readings should be evaluated for clinical significance.

Classification of Blood Pressure for Adults Aged 18 Years and Older

CATEGORY	SYSTOLIC (MM HG)		DIASTOLIC (MM HG)
Optimal	<120	*and*	<80
Elevated	120–129	*and*	<80
Hypertension			
Stage 1	130–139	*or*	80–89
Stage 2	≥140	*or*	≥90
Hypertensive Crisis	>180	*or*	>120

From Whelton PK, Carey RM, Aronow WS, Casey DE Jr, Collins KJ, et al.: 2017 ACC/AHA/AAPA/ABC/ACPM/AGS/APhA/ASH/ASPC/NMA/PCNA guideline for the prevention, detection, evaluation, and management of high blood pressure in adults: A report of the American College of Cardiology/American Heart Association Task Force on Clinical Practice Guidelines. *J Am Coll Cardiol*, 71:e127–248, 2018.

TECHNIQUES / **FINDINGS**

Pain Assessment

Explain how to use the pain assessment tool. See the following figures. Ask the patient to indicate the pain level at each body site and then to describe the pain characteristics. Observe for pain behaviors.

EXPECTED: The patient does not have pain, or the painful condition is well managed.

UNEXPECTED: Pain level greater than 3 or pain level that interferes with usual activities. Pain characteristics, such as stabbing, sharp, dull, burning, throbbing, or aching. Behaviors indicating pain such as guarding, facial grimace or other expression of pain, groaning, or rubbing or holding painful site.

Pain Assessment Tools

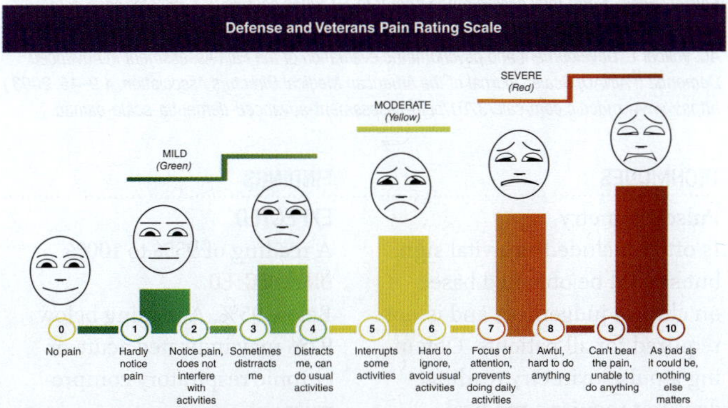

Defense and Veterans Pain Rating Scale.
(From https://www.dvcipm.org/clinical-resources/defense-veterans-pain-rating-scale-dvprs/.)

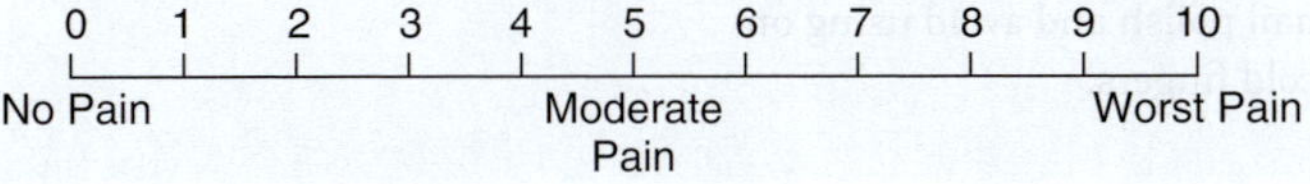

Numeric Pain Intensity Scale.

No Pain — Worst Pain

Visual analog scale.

TECHNIQUES | **FINDINGS**

For nonverbal older adults, use the Pain Assessment in Advanced Dementia (PAINAD) Scale to assess pain behaviors (Paulson et al., 2014).

	0	1	2	Score
Breathing Independent of vocalization	Normal	Occasional labored breathing. Short period of hyperventilation.	Noisy labored breathing. Long period of hyperventilation. Cheyne-Stokes respirations.	
Negative vocalization	None	Occasional moan or groan. Low-level speech with a negative or disapproving quality.	Repeated troubled calling out. Loud moaning or groaning. Crying.	
Facial expression	Smiling, or inexpressive	Sad. Frightened. Frown.	Facial grimacing.	
Body language	Relaxed	Tense. Distressed pacing. Fidgeting.	Rigid. Fists clenched. Knees pulled up. Pulling or pushing away. Striking out.	
Consolability	No need to console	Distracted or reassured by voice or touch.	Unable to console, distract, or reassure.	
			TOTAL	

PAINAD Scale. Note: Total scores range from 0 to 10, when scoring 0, 1, or 2 for each item. A score of 0 = no observable pain and 10 = highest observable pain. (From Warden V, Hurley AC, Volicer L: Development and psychometric evaluation of the Pain Assessment in Advanced Dementia (PAINAD) Scale, Journal of the American Medical Directors Association, 4:9–15, 2003.) https://www.mdcalc.com/calc/3701/pain-assessment-advanced-dementia-scale-painad.

TECHNIQUES

Pulse Oximetry

Is often included as a vital sign, but should be obtained based on clinical judgement and is not required for all patients. Obtaining a pulse oximetry reading does not require a medical order (Joint Commission, 2022). Place on right hand's middle finger for best results. Remove nail polish and avoid using on cold fingers.

FINDINGS

EXPECTED

A reading of 95% to 100%

UNEXPECTED

Below 95%. A reading below 92% may indicated acute or chronic respiratory compromise.

PEDIATRIC VARIATIONS

EXAMINATION

TECHNIQUES	FINDINGS

Pulse rate

Palpate the pulse or use a stethoscope to auscultate the apical pulse.

EXPECTED:

Age (year)	*Beats/min*
Newborn	120–130
1	116–119
2–3	106–108
4–5	94–97
6–11	77–88
12–19	72–80

Respiratory rate

Observe abdominal rise to count the respiratory rate in infants and toddlers, and chest rise in older children.

EXPECTED:

Age (years)	*Breaths/min*
Newborn	24–50
1	20–40
3	20–30
6	16–22
10	16–20
17	12–20

UNEXPECTED: Sustained rate higher or lower than expected range.

Measure the blood pressure

Select the appropriate size cuff to measure the infant's or child's blood pressure.

- The cuff width should cover approximately 70% of the distance between the shoulder and the elbow.

EXPECTED: For children aged 1 to 13 years, <90th percentile for age, gender, and height percentile. Refer to expected blood pressure values for children at https://nhlbi.nih.gov/files/docs/guidelines/child_tbl.pdf.

TECHNIQUES	FINDINGS
	Use adult blood pressure ranges for adolescents older than 13 years (Flynn, Kaelber, et al., 2017).
• The bladder length should be 80% to 100% of the upper arm circumference, and the bladder width should be at least 40% of the arm circumference at the midpoint of the acromion-olecranon distance.	**UNEXPECTED:** ≥90th percentile for age, gender, and height percentile is an elevated blood pressure. Stage 1 hypertension is ≥95th percentile. Stage 2 hypertension is 95th percentile + 12 mm Hg. Use adult ranges for elevated blood pressure and Stage 1 and Stage 2 hypertension for adolescents older than 13 years (Flynn, Kaelber, et al., 2017).

Pain Assessment

Select a self-report pain scale when the child understands higher lower and more-less concepts, such as the Wong–Baker Faces Pain Rating Scale. See the following figure.	**EXPECTED:** Reported pain is less than 3. **UNEXPECTED:** Pain score >3 and pain behaviors.

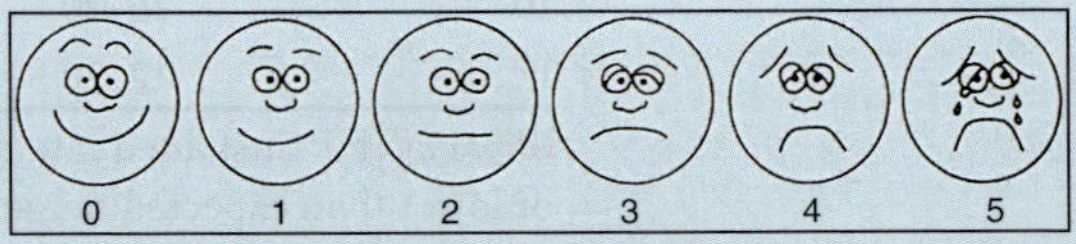

Wong–Baker FACES pain rating scale. (From Hockenberry MJ, Wilson D, Rodgers CC: Wong's essentials of pediatric nursing, ed 11, St. Louis, 2022, Elsevier.)

TECHNIQUES	FINDINGS
For nonverbal children, observe for pain behaviors using a tool, such as the Face, Legs, Activity, Cry, and Consolability (FLACC) Behavioral Pain Assessment Scale, when the child is unable to use a self-report pain assessment tool. See the following FLACC figure.	**UNEXPECTED:** The child has pain behaviors such as crying, posturing, restlessness, or facial grimace and is difficult to comfort.

CATEGORIES	SCORING 0	SCORING 1	SCORING 2
Face	No particular expression or smile	Occasional grimace or frown; withdrawn, disinterested	Frequent to constant frown, clenched jaw, quivering chin
Legs	Normal position or relaxed	Uneasy, restless, tense	Kicking or legs drawn up
Activity	Lying quietly, normal position, moves easily	Squirming, shifting back and forth, tense	Arched, rigid, or jerking
Cry	No cry (awake or asleep)	Moans or whimpers, occasional complaint	Crying steadily, screams or sobs; frequent complaints
Consolability	Content, relaxed	Reassured by occasional touching, hugging, or being talked to; distractable	Difficult to console or comfort

Guidelines for Scoring the FLACC

Face

Score 0 if the patient has a relaxed face, makes eye contact, shows interest in surroundings.

Score 1 if the patient has a worried facial expression, with eyebrows lowered, eyes partially closed, cheeks raised, mouth pursed.

Score 2 if the patient has deep furrows in the forehead, closed eyes, an open mouth, deep lines around nose and lips.

Legs

Score 0 if the muscle tone and motion in the limbs are normal.

Score 1 if patient has increased tone, rigidity, or tension; if there is intermittent flexion or extension of the limbs.

Score 2 if patient has hypertonicity, the legs are pulled tight, there is exaggerated flexion or extension of the limbs, tremors.

Activity

Score 0 if the patient moves easily and freely, normal activity or restrictions.

Score 1 if the patient shifts positions, appears hesitant to move, demonstrates guarding, a tense torso, pressure on a body part.

Score 2 if the patient is in a fixed position, rocking; demonstrates side-to-side head movement or rubbing of a body part.

Cry

Score 0 if the patient has no cry or moan, awake or asleep.

Score 1 if the patient has occasional moans, cries, whimpers, sighs.

Score 2 if the patient has frequent or continuous moans, cries, grunts.

Consolability

Score 0 if the patient is calm and does not require consoling.

Score 1 if the patient responds to comfort by touching or talking in 30 seconds to 1 minute.

Score 2 if the patient requires constant comforting or is inconsolable.

Interpreting the Behavioral Score

Each category is scored on the 0–2 scale, which results in a total score of 0–10.

0 = Relaxed and comfortable

1–3 = Mild discomfort

4–6 = Moderate pain

7–10 = Severe discomfort or pain or both

FLACC Behavioral Pain Assessment Scale for nonverbal children. (From Merkel SI, et al.: The FLACC: A behavioral scale for scoring postoperative pain in young children, Pediatr Nurs, 23(2):293–297, 1997. https://www.dshs.wa.gov/sites/default/files/ALTSA/stakeholders/documents/duals/toolkit/forms/Pain%20Scale%20FLACC.pdf)

CHAPTER

4 Mental Status

Equipment

- Familiar objects (coins, glasses, and watches)
- Paper and pencil

EXAMINATION

Perform the mental status examination throughout the patient interaction. Focus on the patient's alertness, orientation, mood, and cognition or complex mental processes (learning, perceiving, decision-making, and memory). Use a mental status screening examination for health visits when no cognitive, emotional, or behavioral problems are apparent. Information is generally observed during the history in the following areas:

APPEARANCE AND BEHAVIOR	EMOTIONAL STABILITY
Grooming	Mood and feelings
Emotional status	Thought process and content
Body language	

COGNITIVE ABILITIES	SPEECH AND LANGUAGE
State of consciousness	Voice quality
Memory	Articulation
Attention span	Comprehension
Judgment	Coherence
	Aphasia

Note any reliance on another adult to answer questions. When concerned about any of the patient's responses or behaviors, ask a family member or close friend if the patient has had any challenges with memory or cognitive function, such as forgetting important appointments or events, paying bills, or taking medications. Additionally, determine if the patient shops independently for food or clothing, gets lost while walking or driving, and makes decisions about daily life.

TECHNIQUE	FINDINGS

Mental Status and Speech Patterns

Observe Physical Appearance and Behavior

• *Grooming*	**UNEXPECTED:** Poor hygiene; lack of concern with appearance; or inappropriate dress for season or occasion in previously well-groomed patient.
• *Emotional status*	**EXPECTED:** Cooperative; friendly; expresses concern appropriate for emotional content of topics discussed. **UNEXPECTED:** Behavior conveys carelessness, apathy, loss of sympathetic responses, unusual docility, rage reactions, agitation, or excessive irritability.
• *Body language*	**EXPECTED:** Erect posture and eye contact (if culturally appropriate). **UNEXPECTED:** Slumped posture, lack of facial expression, excessively energetic movements, or constantly watchful eyes.
• *State of consciousness*	**EXPECTED:** Oriented to person, place, and time; appropriate responses to questions and environmental stimuli. **UNEXPECTED:** Disoriented to person, place, or time. Verbal response is confused, incoherent, or inappropriate, or there is no verbal response. Lethargic or difficult to arouse.

Investigate Cognitive Abilities

Assess cognitive function during history and physical examination.	**EXPECTED:** Responses indicate good memory, ability to follow one- and two-step instructions, and appropriate decision-making. **UNEXPECTED:** Confusion, difficulty following directions, risky behavior, validation of concerns by family member or friend.

TECHNIQUE	FINDINGS
• *Mini-Cog* Ask patient to remember and immediately repeat three unrelated words (e.g., *red, plate,* and *milk*). Ask patient to draw a clock face with numbers, then draw the clock hands pointing to the time you specify. Allow 3 minutes. Ask the patient to repeat the three words. Score 1 point for each word recalled. Score 2 points when all numbers of the clock face are near the rim, in correct sequence, and hands point to the specified time. Total of 5 points (Yang et al., 2016).	**EXPECTED:** All three words are remembered, and the clock face has all numbers in proper position and hands pointing to the specified time. **UNEXPECTED:** A score of ≤2 may indicate dementia. 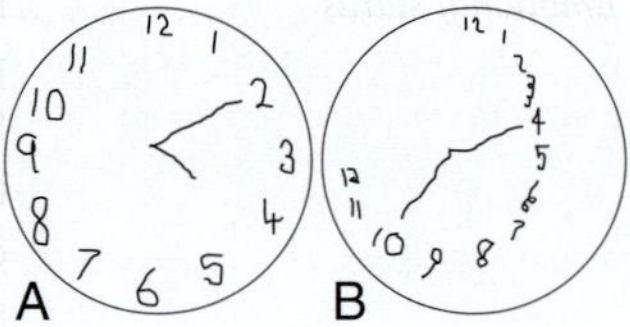
• *Montreal Cognitive Assessment low literacy (MoCA-Basic)* This more extensive test of memory recall and executive functioning takes 10 to 20 minutes to administer. It can be used for all literacy levels and helps identify mild cognitive impairment (Julayanont et al., 2015). See www.mocatest.org to access the screening tool.	**EXPECTED:** Score of ≥24 for MoCA-Basic out of 30 points; scores do not vary significantly by literacy level. **UNEXPECTED:** Score ≤23 points indicates multiple-domain mild cognitive impairment associated with a higher risk for dementia.
• *Analogies* Ask patient to describe analogies: first simple, then more complex.	**EXPECTED:** Correct responses when patient has average intelligence. **UNEXPECTED:** Unable to describe similarities or differences.

TECHNIQUE	FINDINGS
• What is similar about peaches and lemons, oceans and lakes, trumpet and flute? • An engine is to an airplane as an oar is to a ________? • What is different about a magazine and a cookbook, or a bush and a tree?	
• *Abstract reasoning* Ask patient to explain meaning of fable, proverb, or metaphor. • A stitch in time saves nine. • A bird in the hand is worth two in the bush. • A rolling stone gathers no moss.	**EXPECTED:** Adequate interpretation when patient has average intelligence. **UNEXPECTED:** Unable to give adequate explanation.
• *Arithmetic calculations* Ask patient to perform simple calculations without paper and pencil. • 50 – 7, –7, –7, etc., until answer is 8. • 50 + 8, +8, +8, etc., until answer is 98.	**EXPECTED:** Able to complete with few errors within a minute. **UNEXPECTED:** Unable to perform calculations.
• *Writing ability* Ask patient to write name and address or a phrase you recite. If low literacy, ask the patient to draw figures (e.g., triangle, circle, square, flower, house, clockface).	**UNEXPECTED:** Omission or addition of letters, syllables, or words; mirror writing. Uncoordinated writing or figure drawings unrelated to a neurologic condition.
• *Execution of motor skills* Ask patient to do a motor task, such as zipping up a jacket or typing on a computer.	**UNEXPECTED:** Inability to complete a task that is not related to paralysis.

TECHNIQUE	FINDINGS
• *Memory* *Immediate recall or new learning:* Ask patient to listen to, then repeat, a sentence or series of numbers. *Recent memory:* Ask the patient to remember the four or five objects shown, or give a visually impaired patient four unrelated words with distinct sounds to remember (e.g., carpet, iris, bench, fortune). In 10 minutes, ask patient to list objects. *Remote memory:* Ask patient about verifiable past events (e.g., mother's maiden name, name of high school, subject of common knowledge).	**EXPECTED:** *Immediate recall:* Able to repeat sentence or numbers (e.g., five to eight numbers forward, four to six numbers backward). *Recent memory:* Able to remember test objects. *Remote memory:* Able to recall verifiable past events. **UNEXPECTED:** Impaired memory. Loss of immediate and recent memory with retention of remote memory.
• *Attention span* Ask patient to follow a series of short commands (e.g., stand up from chair, put on patient gown, sit on examining table), or spell *world* forward and backward. Arithmetic calculation is another test of attention span.	**EXPECTED:** Responds to directions appropriately. **UNEXPECTED:** Easy distraction or confusion, negativism.
• *Judgment* Explore: • How patient meets social and family obligations, patient's future plans.	**EXPECTED:** Able to evaluate situation and provide appropriate response; managing family and finances appropriately. **UNEXPECTED:** Response indicating risky behavior or inappropriate action.

TECHNIQUE	FINDINGS
• Patient's solutions to hypothetical situations (e.g., found stamped envelope or was stopped by police for driving through a red light).	
Observe Speech and Language	
• *Voice quality*	**EXPECTED:** Uses inflections, speaks clearly and strongly, is able to increase voice volume and pitch. **UNEXPECTED:** Difficulty or discomfort making laryngeal speech sounds or varying volume; harsh, nasal, or monotone speech quality.
• *Articulation*	**EXPECTED:** Proper pronunciation of consonants; fluent and rhythmic speech; easily expresses thoughts. **UNEXPECTED:** Imperfect or slurring pronunciation, difficulty articulating single speech sound, or speech with hesitancy, stuttering, or repetitions.
• *Comprehension*	**EXPECTED:** Able to follow simple one- and two-step instructions.
• *Coherence*	**EXPECTED:** Able to clearly convey intentions or perceptions. **UNEXPECTED:** Word substitutions, perseveration, disordered or disconnected words or sentences, gibberish, made-up words, clang association, repetition of another's words, or unusual sounds may be associated with a psychiatric disorder. Hesitations, omissions, inappropriate word substitutions, made-up words, and disturbance of rhythm or words in sequence may be signs of aphasia.

TECHNIQUE	FINDINGS
Evaluate Emotional Stability	
• *Mood and feelings* Ask patient how they feel, whether feelings interfere with daily life, and whether they have particularly difficult times or experiences.	**EXPECTED:** Expresses appropriate feelings for the situation. **UNEXPECTED:** Unresponsiveness, hopelessness, agitation, irritability, hostility, hypervigilance, euphoria, or mood swings.
• *Depression screening questions* using the Patient Health Questionnaire 2 (PHQ-2) • Over the past 2 weeks, have you felt down, depressed, or hopeless? • Over the past 2 weeks, have you felt little interest or pleasure in doing things?	**EXPECTED:** Negative response to one or both questions. **UNEXPECTED:** Positive response to both questions indicates a need to ask more questions about depression symptoms of fatigue, restlessness, and poor concentration. The Patient Health Questionnaire 9 (PHQ-9) may be used for further assessment. See www.phqscreeners.com for access to the tool.
• *Suicide screening questions* using the Columbia-Suicide Severity Risk Screener • Have you wished you were dead or wished you could go to sleep and not wake up? • Have you actually had any thoughts of killing yourself? If a positive response to second question, ask about preparations made to end their life.	**UNEXPECTED:** A positive response to either question indicates higher risk. A more thorough suicide risk assessment is needed (Posner et al., 2016). See https://cssrs.columbia.edu/wp-content/uploads/C-SSRS_Pediatric-SLC_11.14.16.pdf. A positive response to the second question with any recent preparations requires implementation of a patient safety monitoring plan.

Ask the patient to choose the best answer for how he or she felt over the previous week.

1. Are you basically satisfied with your life?	YES / NO
2. Have you dropped many of your activities and interests?	YES / NO
3. Do you feel that your life is empty?	YES / NO
4. Do you often get bored?	YES / NO
5. Are you in good spirits most of the time?	YES / NO
6. Are you afraid that something bad is going to happen to you?	YES / NO
7. Do you feel happy most of the time?	YES / NO
8. Do you feel helpless?	YES / NO
9. Do you prefer to stay at home, rather than going out and doing new things?	YES / NO
10. Do you feel you have more problems with memory than most?	YES / NO
11. Do you think it is wonderful to be alive now?	YES / NO
12. Do you feel pretty worthless the way you are now?	YES / NO
13. Do you feel full of energy?	YES / NO
14. Do you feel that your situation is hopeless?	YES / NO
15. Do you think most people are better off than you are?	YES / NO

Correct responses are the following:
Yes for questions 2, 3, 4, 6, 8, 9, 10, 12, 14, and 15.
No for questions 1, 5, 7, 11, and 13.
Give one point for each correct answer. A score greater than five suggests depression.

Geriatric Depression Scale. (From Sheikh JI, Yesavage JA: Geriatric depression scale: recent evidence and development of a shorter version, Clin Gerontol 5:165-172, 1986.)

TECHNIQUE	FINDINGS
• *Thought process and content* • Ask patient about obsessive thoughts related to fears, guilt, or making decisions. • Ask patient about the need to compulsively repeat actions, check, and recheck (or observe the patient's actions).	**EXPECTED:** Patient's thought processes can be followed, and ideas expressed are logical and goal-oriented. **UNEXPECTED:** Illogical or unrealistic thought processes; blocking or disturbance in stream of thinking. Obsessive thought content, compulsive behavior, phobias, anxieties that interfere with daily life or are disabling; delusions.

TECHNIQUE	FINDINGS
• Observe sequence, logic, coherence, and relevance of topics discussed. • Does patient have delusions (of grandeur, of being controlled by external force)? Does the patient feel watched, followed, persecuted, or paranoid?	
• *Perceptual distortions and hallucinations* • Ask patient about any sensations you believe are not caused by external stimuli. • Find out when these experiences occur.	**UNEXPECTED:** Sensory hallucinations—hears voices, sees vivid images or shadowy figures, smells offensive odors, feels worms crawling on skin.

AIDS TO DIFFERENTIAL DIAGNOSIS

SUBJECTIVE DATA	OBJECTIVE DATA
Dementia	
Forgets significant events; gets lost in familiar areas; unable to manage shopping, food preparation, medications; mood changes (depression, uncharacteristic anger, anxiety, or agitation); apathy; behavior changes (e.g., impulsiveness, socially inappropriate dress).	Impaired memory, social and occupational functioning, and activities of daily living; impaired use of language; impaired executive functioning; progressive deterioration in cognitive function.
Delirium	
Sudden impairment of memory and attentiveness, mood swings, increased, or decreased activity.	Altered consciousness; fearful, suspicious; rambling and irrelevant conversation, illogical flow of ideas. Misperceptions, illusions, hallucinations, and delusions; symptoms increase and decrease during the day.

SUBJECTIVE DATA	OBJECTIVE DATA
Depression	
Feels sad, hopeless, worthless; guilt, loss of pleasure or interest; loss of energy, insomnia or excessive sleeping; increased or decreased appetite. May have experienced a loss, change in health status, or stressful life event.	Altered mood and affect with extreme sadness, anxiety, irritability; impaired concentration, reduced attention span, indecisiveness, slower thought processes.
Mania	
Persistently elevated and expansive mood, hyperactivity, overconfidence, exaggerated view of own abilities, hyperactivity, racing thoughts.	Increased talkativeness or pressure to keep talking with excessive rhyming, puns, or flight of ideas; impaired attention, judgment, social, occupational, and interpersonal functioning; grandiose or persecutory delusions; hypersexual behavior.
Anxiety Disorder	
Anxiety or fear that interferes with personal, social, or occupational functioning. Panic attacks (palpitations, sweating, shaking, dizziness, nausea, chest pain, abdominal distress); nightmares; flashbacks; poor concentration; chronic worry; sleeps poorly.	Tachycardia, diaphoresis, tremors, impaired attention, ritualized acts performed compulsively; impulsive behavior, hyperarousal, detachment from others.

PEDIATRIC VARIATIONS

EXAMINATION

TECHNIQUE	FINDINGS
Mental Status	
Use parent's impression of infant's responsiveness to guide your assessment. Questionnaires completed by parents (e.g., Ages and Stages Questionnaire or Parent's Evaluation of Developmental Status) are effective developmental screening tools.	EXPECTED: Infant responds appropriately to parent's voice, is attentive, comforts easily. Social smile can be elicited; babbling or cooing or language appropriate for age. Child follows simple directions. UNEXPECTED: Nonresponsive, inconsolable, combative, lethargic.

AIDS TO DIFFERENTIAL DIAGNOSIS

SUBJECTIVE DATA	OBJECTIVE DATA
Intellectual Disability	
Delayed motor, speech, and language development.	Delayed developmental milestones, impaired cognitive functioning and short-term memory; poor academic performance; lack of motivation.
Autism	
Does not make eye contact or point to share experiences with others; resists being held or touched; odd and repetitive behaviors, ritualized play, preoccupation with objects; motor development appropriate for age.	Impaired social interactions and language, odd intonation to speech, pronoun reversal, nonsensical rhyming; lacks awareness of others.
Attention-Deficit/Hyperactivity Disorder	
Short attention span, easily distracted, fidgets and squirms, often moving, disruptive behavior, talks excessively, temper outbursts; has problems in more than one setting.	Increased motor activity, difficulty organizing tasks, difficulty maintaining attention, poor school performance, and low self-esteem.

CHAPTER

Growth and Nutrition 5

Equipment

- Standing platform scale with height attachment
- Measuring tape with millimeter markings
- Infant scale
- Recumbent measuring device (for infants)
- Stature measuring device (for children)
- Calculator

EXAMINATION

TECHNIQUE	FINDINGS
Anthropometrics	
Measure Height and Weight	
• For weight, ask the patient to remove excess clothing and shoes. Have the patient stand in the middle of the scale platform and note the digital reading.	**EXPECTED:** *Women:* 100 lb for first 5 ft, plus 5 lb for each inch thereafter. *Men:* 106 lb for first 5 ft, plus 6 lb for each inch thereafter.
• For height, have the patient stand erect with their back to the stature-measuring device. Pull up the height attachment and position the headpiece on the top of the head. Make the reading at the nearest centimeter or half inch.	
• Calculate percent weight change: $\left(\frac{\text{Usual weight} - \text{Current weight}}{\text{Usual weight}}\right) \times 100$	**UNEXPECTED:** Weight loss that equals or exceeds 1% to 2% in 1 week, 5% in 1 month, 7.5% in 3 months, 10% in 6 months.

TECHNIQUE	FINDINGS
• Calculate body mass index (BMI) kg/m^2 or calculate using pounds by: $$\frac{(\text{Weight in pounds} \times 703)}{(\text{Height in inches} \times \text{Height in inches})}$$	**EXPECTED:** BMI (children age 2 and above) of 18.5–24.9 is classified as healthy weight. **UNEXPECTED:** BMI <18.5 is classified as underweight. BMI 25–29.9 is overweight. BMI ≥30 is obesity.
Measure Waist Circumference Indicator of visceral fat. Using a tape measure with millimeter markings, measure waist at high point of iliac crest when patient is standing and at minimal respiration.	**EXPECTED:** Waist circumference <40 in for men and <35 in for women. **UNEXPECTED:** Measurements >40 in in men and >35 in in women are associated with increased risk for type 2 diabetes, dyslipidemia, hypertension, and cardiovascular disease.
Calculate Waist-Height Ratio	**EXPECTED:** Ratio <0.5. **UNEXPECTED:** Ratios >0.5 in is associated with increased risk for type 2 diabetes and cardiovascular disease in adults.

TECHNIQUE	FINDINGS

Determine Diet Adequacy

24-hour Diet Recall and Food Diary

Ask patient to complete 24-hour food and beverage recall or a 3- or 4-day food diary that includes 1 weekend day. Ask specific questions about methods of food preparation, portion sizes, amount of sugar-sweetened beverages, and the use of salt or other additives. The US Department of Agriculture (USDA) MyPlate website and mobile device application are useful tools for tracking daily food and beverage intake by food groups (grains, vegetables, fruits, dairy, and protein foods) based on the 2020–2025 *Dietary Guidelines for Americans.*

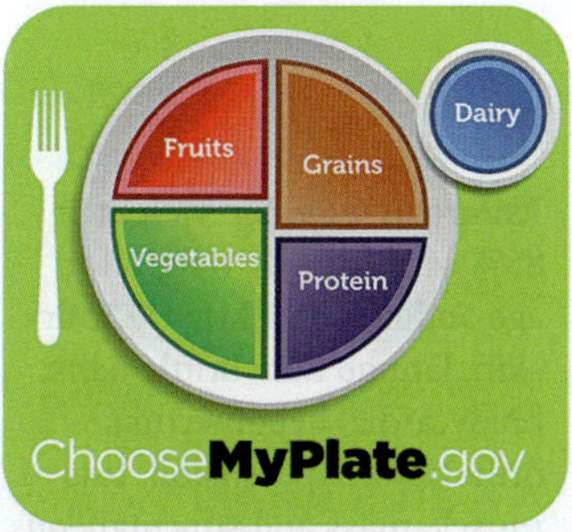

(From U.S. Department of Agriculture, 2020, https://www.dietaryguidelines.gov/sites/default/files/2020-12/Dietary_Guidelines_for_Americans_2020-2025.pdf.)

EXPECTED: Plate of food should have half fruits and vegetables with a focus on whole fruits and a variety of vegetables. Half of the plate should have grains and protein. Dairy milk or yogurt should be low fat or fat free. Recommended daily amounts of fruits, vegetables, grains, and protein are based on the individual's age, gender, weight, height, and level of physical activity. The 2020–2025 *Dietary Guidelines for Americans* emphasize the following key recommendations:

- Follow a healthy diet at every life stage.
- Customize nutrient-dense food and beverages based on personal preferences, culture, and budget.
- Consume nutrient-dense foods and beverages (rich in vitamins and minerals with little to no added sugars, saturated fat, or sodium) and stay within calorie limits.
- Limit foods and beverages high in added sugars, saturated fat, and sodium; limit alcoholic beverages.

Calorie Needs and Nutritional Adequacy

An interactive Dietary Reference Intake (DRI) calculator can be found on the USDA Food and Nutrition Information Center website (https://www.nal.usda.gov/fnic/dri-calculator/).

AIDS TO DIFFERENTIAL DIAGNOSIS

SUBJECTIVE DATA	OBJECTIVE DATA
Obesity	
Excessive caloric intake and high-fat foods, weight gain, decrease in physical activity, recent life change or stressors, medications. Obesity-related symptoms or conditions include snoring and sleep apnea, shortness of breath, headaches, musculoskeletal symptoms, depression, irregular menses, polyuria, and polydipsia. Obesity may contribute to an increased risk of developing cardiovascular and metabolic diseases later in life.	Body mass index (BMI)—for adults, overweight: 25–29.9, obesity: ≥30; excess fat located in breasts, buttocks, thighs; may have pale striae or acanthosis nigricans.
Anorexia Nervosa	
Preoccupation with weight, excessive exercise, and unusual eating habits, including voluntary starvation, purging, vomiting, and weight control measures, such as diet pills, use of laxatives, and diuretics. Symptoms may include fatigue, dizziness, low energy, amenorrhea, weight loss or gain, constipation, bloating, abdominal discomfort, heartburn, intolerance to cold, palpitations, depression or irritability, decreased libido, and interrupted sleep.	Failure to maintain weight at 85% of ideal body weight for age and height, BMI ≤ 17.5; dry skin, lanugo hair, brittle nails, bradycardia, hypothermia, orthostatic hypotension, loss of muscle mass and subcutaneous fat; may have hypoglycemia, elevated liver enzymes, and thyroid hormone abnormalities.

SUBJECTIVE DATA	OBJECTIVE DATA
Bulimia	
Binge-eating episodes on average of two times per week, usually high-calorie or high-carbohydrate foods, followed by purging behaviors (e.g., vomiting, laxatives, diuretics); bloating, fullness, abdominal pain, heartburn.	Body weight may be normal, underweight, or overweight; knuckle calluses, dental enamel erosion, salivary gland enlargement; may have metabolic alkalosis, hypokalemia, or elevated salivary amylase.

PEDIATRIC VARIATIONS

EXAMINATION

TECHNIQUE	FINDINGS
Anthropometrics	
Growth Assessment	
Measure the length of infants and children until age 24 months of age in a supine position on a measuring device. For children 2 years and older, obtain a standing height using a stature-measuring device (stadiometer). Weigh infants and children on a scale that measures grams and kilograms. Calculate body mass index (BMI) starting at 2 years of age. Use growth charts for pediatric patients (available at www.cdc.gov/growthcharts).	**EXPECTED:** Child is following a growth curve pattern for length or height and weight. Length or height and weight are approximately same percentiles. BMI is following a growth pattern expected for age and gender. **UNEXPECTED (2–18 years):** • Underweight—BMI < 5th percentile • Overweight—BMI > 85th percentile to <95th percentile • Obese—BMI > 95th percentile

TECHNIQUE	FINDINGS
Measure Head Circumference	
Wrap tape measure snugly around the head at the occipital protuberance and supraorbital prominence for infants and children younger than 2 years. Plot the measurement on the appropriate growth curve and identify the child's percentile in comparison with the population standard. Compare measurements over time.	UNEXPECTED: Head circumference <3rd percentile or increasing in size at a rate faster than expected for age.

CHAPTER 6

Skin, Hair, and Nails

Equipment

- Centimeter ruler (flexible, clear)
- Flashlight with transilluminator
- Handheld magnifying lens or dermatoscope (optional)
- Wood's lamp (to view fluorescing lesions)

EXAMINATION

TECHNIQUE	FINDINGS
Skin	
Perform overall inspection of whole body	
In particular, check areas not usually exposed and intertriginous surfaces.	**EXPECTED:** Skin color differences among body areas and between sun-exposed and non-sun-exposed areas. **UNEXPECTED:** Lesions.
Inspect skin of each body area and mucous membranes	
• *Color/uniformity* Inspect sclerae, conjunctivae, buccal mucosa, tongue, lips, nail beds, and palms.	**EXPECTED:** General uniformity—dark brown to light tan, with pink, or yellow overtones. Sun-darkened areas. Darker skin around knees and elbows. Calloused areas yellow. Knuckles darker and palms/soles lighter in dark-skinned patients. Vascular flush areas pink or red, especially with anxiety or excitement. Pigmented nevi. Nonpigmented striae. Freckles. Birthmarks.

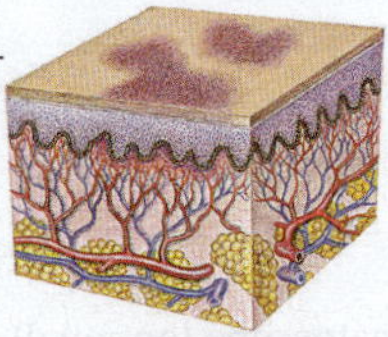

Purpura—red-purple nonblanchable discoloration greater than 0.5 cm diameter
Cause: Intravascular defects, infection

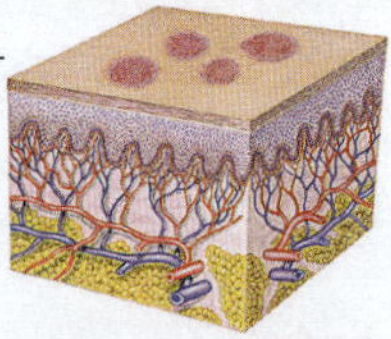

Petechiae—red-purple nonblanchable discoloration less than 0.5 cm diameter
Cause: Intravascular defects, infection

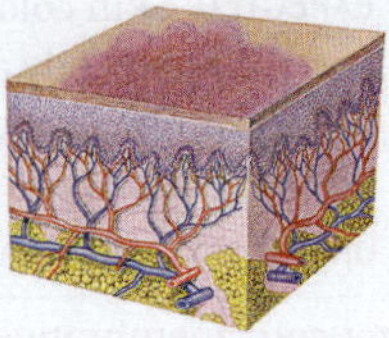

Ecchymoses—red-purple nonblanchable discoloration of variable size
Cause: Vascular wall destruction, trauma, vasculitis

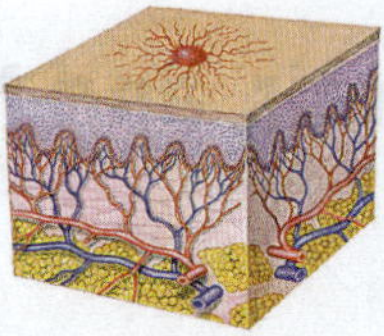

Spider angioma—red central body with radiating spiderlike legs that blanch with pressure to the central body
Cause: Liver disease, vitamin B deficiency, idiopathic

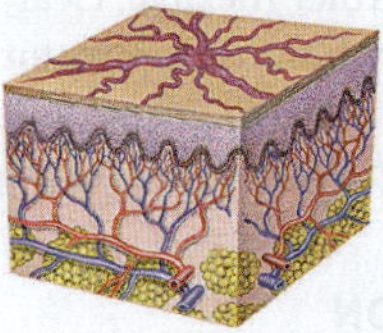

Venous star—bluish spider, linear or irregularly shaped; does not blanch with pressure
Cause: Increased pressure in superficial veins

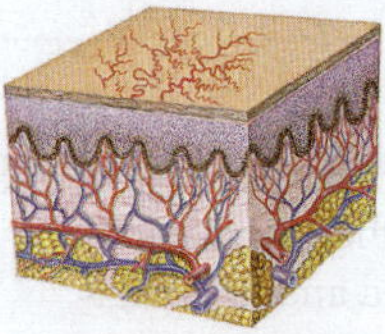

Telangiectasia—fine, irregular red line
Cause: Dilation of capillaries

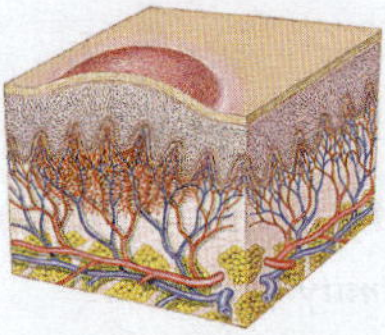

Capillary hemangioma (nevus flammeus)—red irregular macular patches
Cause: Dilation of dermal capillaries

Cutaneous Color Changes

COLOR	CAUSE	DISTRIBUTION	SELECT CONDITIONS
Brown	Darkening of melanin pigment	Generalized	Pituitary, adrenal, liver disease Nevi, neurofibromatosis
White	Absence of pigmentation	Generalized Localized	Albinism Vitiligo
Red (erythema)	Increased cutaneous blood flow	Localized Generalized	Inflammation Fever, viral exanthems, urticaria
	Increased intravascular red blood cells	Generalized	Polycythemia

Cutaneous Color Changes—cont'd

COLOR	CAUSE	DISTRIBUTION	SELECT CONDITIONS
Yellow	Increased bile pigmentation (jaundice)	Generalized	Liver disease
	Increased carotene pigmentation	Generalized (except sclera)	Hypothyroidism, increased intake of vegetables containing carotene
	Decreased visibility of oxyhemoglobin	Generalized	Anemia, chronic renal disease
Blue	Increased unsaturated hemoglobin secondary to hypoxia	Lips, mouth, and nail beds	Cardiovascular and pulmonary disease

TECHNIQUE	FINDINGS
	UNEXPECTED: Dysplastic, precancerous, or cancerous nevi. Chloasma. Unpigmented skin. Generalized or localized color changes. Vascular skin lesions. Vascular changes.
• *Thickness*	**EXPECTED:** Thickness variations, with eyelids thinnest, areas of rubbing thickest. Calluses on hands and feet. **UNEXPECTED:** Atrophy. Hyperkeratosis. Corns.
• *Symmetry*	**EXPECTED:** Bilateral symmetry.
• *Hygiene*	**EXPECTED:** Clean.
Palpate skin	
• *Moisture*	**EXPECTED:** Minimal perspiration or oiliness. Increased perspiration (associated with activity, environment, obesity, anxiety, excitement) noticeable on palms, scalp, forehead, axillae. **UNEXPECTED:** Damp intertriginous areas.
• *Temperature* Palpate with dorsal surface of hand or fingers.	**EXPECTED:** Cool to warm. Bilateral symmetry.

TECHNIQUE	FINDINGS
• *Texture*	**EXPECTED:** Smooth, soft, and even. Roughness resulting from heavy clothing, cold weather, or soap. **UNEXPECTED:** Extensive or widespread roughness.
• *Turgor and mobility* Gently pinch skin on forearm or in sternal area, and release.	**EXPECTED:** Resilience. **UNEXPECTED:** Failure of skin to return to place quickly.

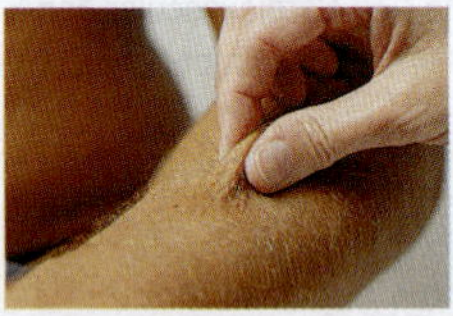

Inspect and palpate lesions

TECHNIQUE	FINDINGS
• *Size* Measure all dimensions. • *Shape* • *Color* Use Wood's lamp to distinguish fluorescing lesions. • *Blanching* • *Texture* Transilluminate to determine presence of fluid. • *Elevation/depression* • *Pedunculation* • *Exudate* Note color, odor, amount, and consistency of lesion. • *Configuration* Check lesion for annular, grouped, linear, arciform, or diffuse arrangement. • *Location/distribution* Check lesion for generalized/localized, body region, patterns, or discrete/confluent.	**UNEXPECTED:** See table on pp. 48–51.

Primary Skin Lesions

DESCRIPTION	EXAMPLES

Macule

Flat, circumscribed area that is a change in skin color; <1 cm in diameter

Examples: Freckles, flat moles (nevi), petechiae, measles, scarlet fever

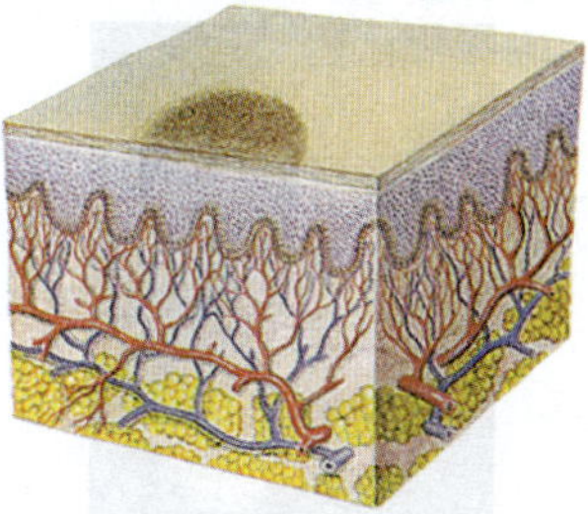

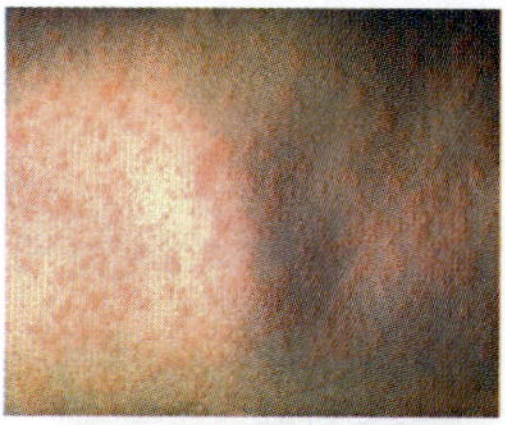

Measles.

Papule

Elevated, firm, circumscribed area <1 cm in diameter

Examples: Wart (verruca), elevated moles, lichen planus

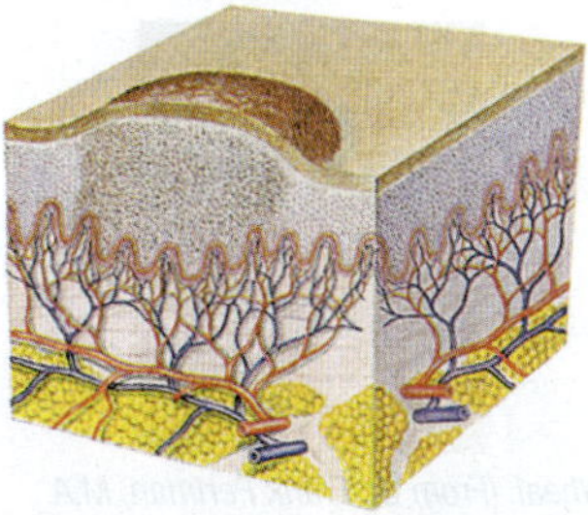

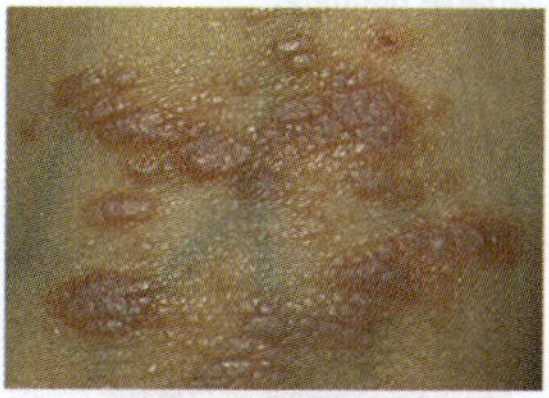

Lichen planus.

Patch

Flat, nonpalpable, irregular-shaped macule >1 cm in diameter

Examples: Vitiligo, port-wine stains, Mongolian spots, café-au-lait spots

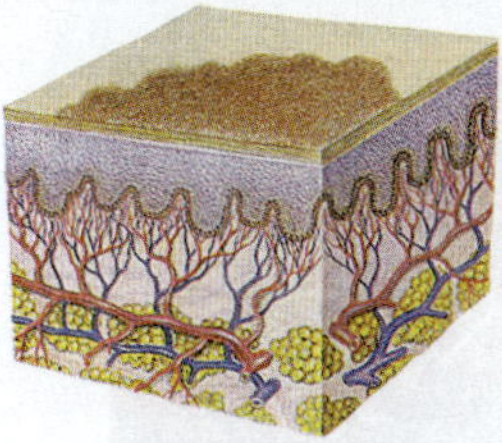

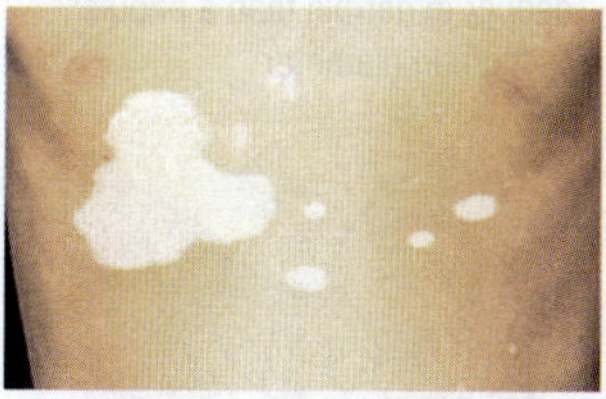

Vitiligo.

Continued

Primary Skin Lesions—cont'd

DESCRIPTION	EXAMPLES
Plaque Elevated, firm, and rough lesion with flat-top surface >1 cm in diameter	Psoriasis, seborrheic and actinic keratosis

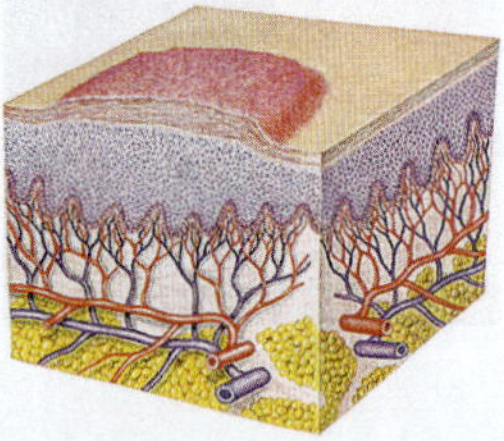

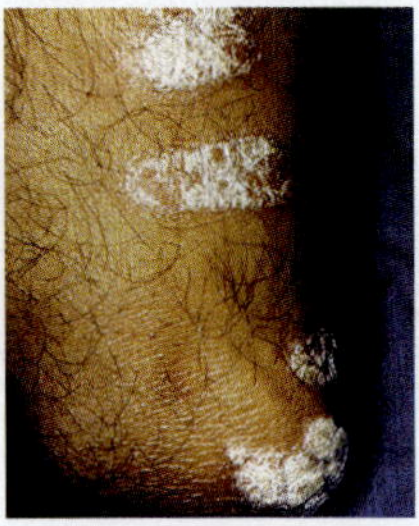

Psoriasis.

DESCRIPTION	EXAMPLES
Wheal Elevated irregular-shaped area of cutaneous edema; solid, transient; variable diameter	Insect bites, urticaria, allergic reaction

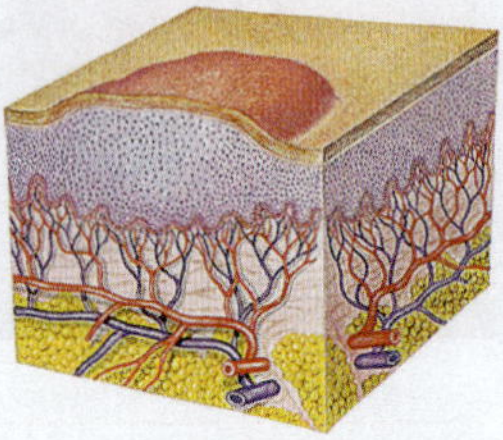

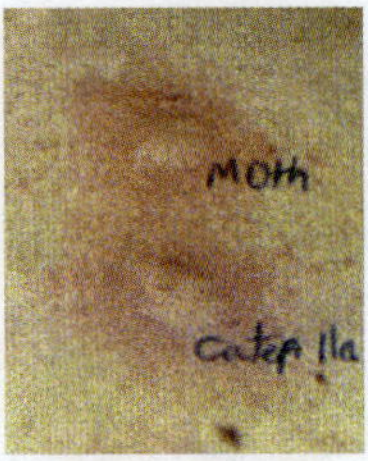

Wheal. (From Dr. Frank Perlman, M.A. Parsons; PHIL, CDC.)

DESCRIPTION	EXAMPLES
Nodule Elevated, firm, circumscribed lesion; deeper in dermis than a papule; 1–2 cm in diameter	Erythema nodosum, lipomas

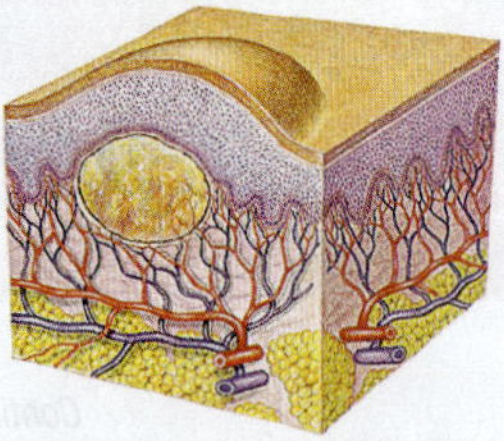

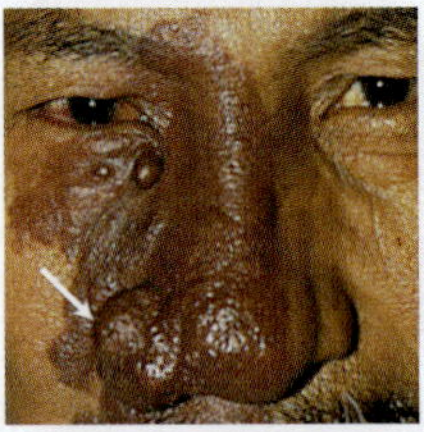

Hypertrophic nodule.

Primary Skin Lesions—cont'd

DESCRIPTION	EXAMPLES
Tumor Elevated and solid lesion; may or may not be clearly demarcated; deeper in dermis; >2 cm in diameter 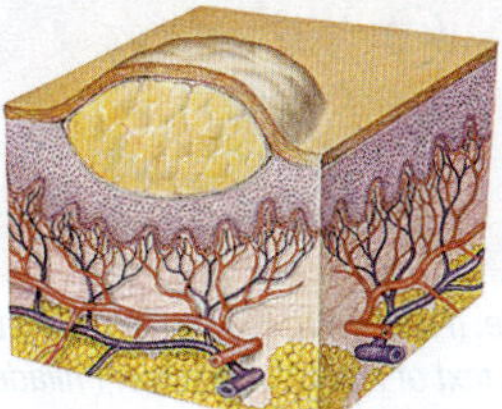	Neoplasms, benign tumor, lipoma, hemangioma 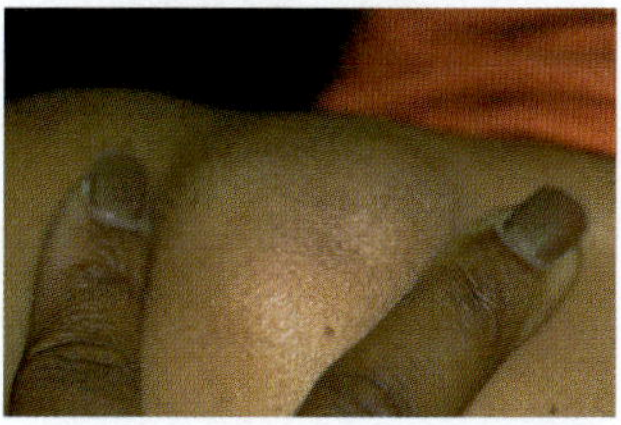 *Lipoma.*
Vesicle Elevated, circumscribed, superficial, not into dermis; filled with serous fluid; <1 cm in diameter 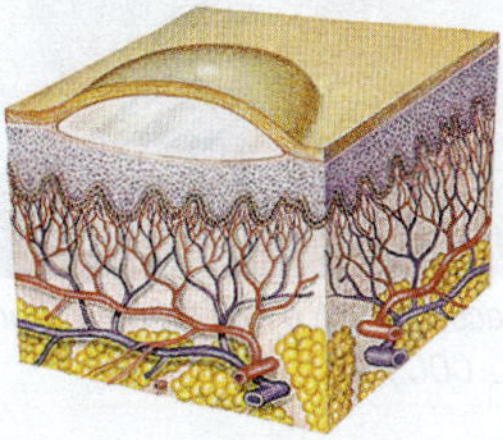	Varicella (chickenpox), herpes zoster (shingles) 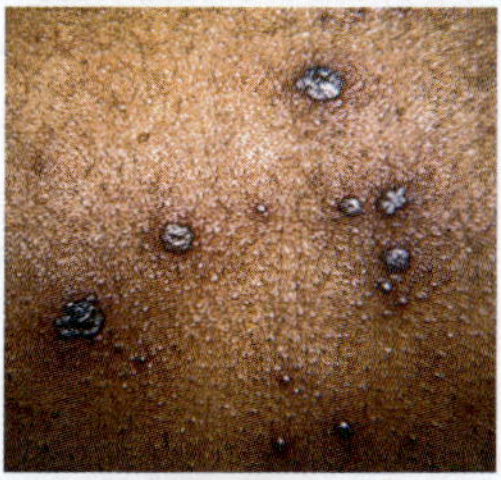 *Vesicles caused by varicella. (From Dr. John Noble, Jr.; PHIL, CDC.)*
Bulla Vesicle >1 cm in diameter 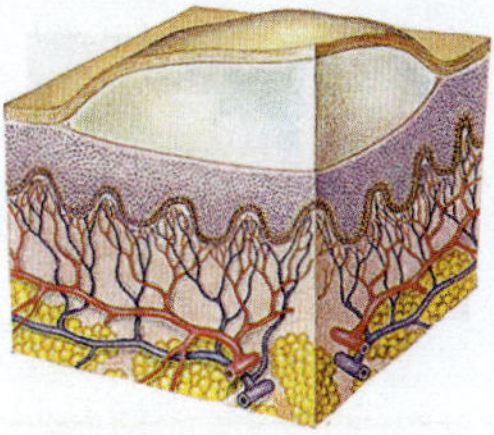	Blister, pemphigus vulgaris 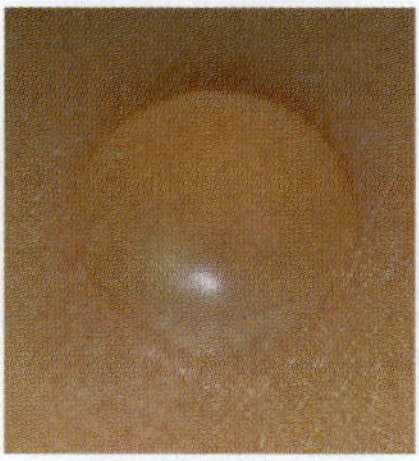 *Blister.*

Continued

Primary Skin Lesions—cont'd

DESCRIPTION	EXAMPLES
Pustule Elevated, superficial lesion; similar to a vesicle but filled with purulent fluid 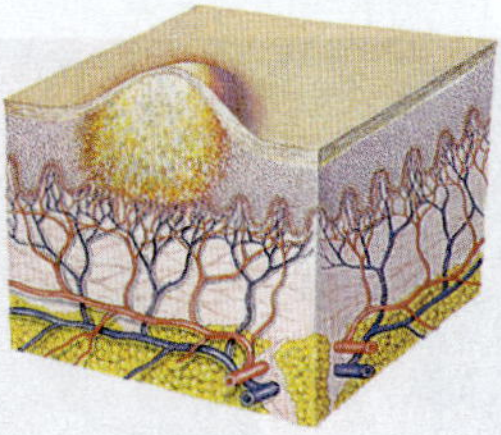	Impetigo, acne 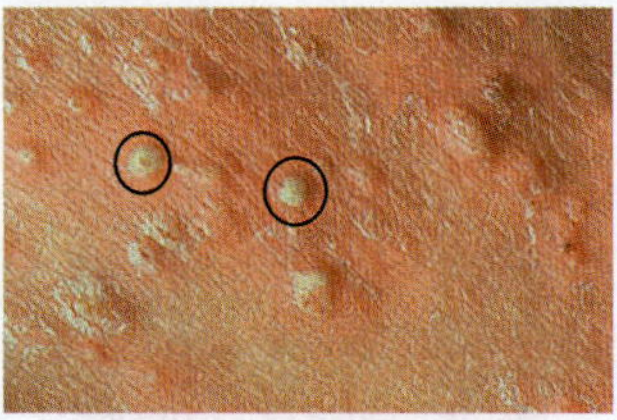 *Acne. (From Ferri, FF: Ferri's color atlas and text of clinical medicine, Philadelphia, 2009, Saunders.)*
Cyst Elevated, circumscribed, encapsulated lesion; in dermis or subcutaneous layer; filled with liquid or semisolid material 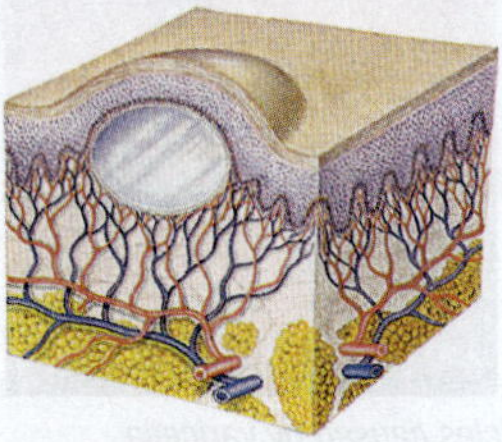	Sebaceous cyst, cystic acne 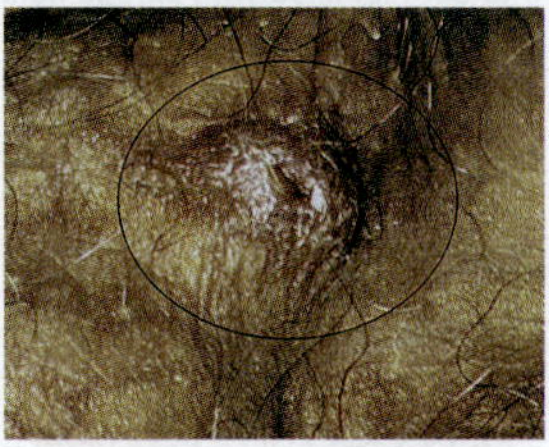 *Sebaceous cyst. (From Dr. Gavin Hart; PHIL, CDC.)*
Telangiectasia Fine, irregular red lines produced by capillary dilation 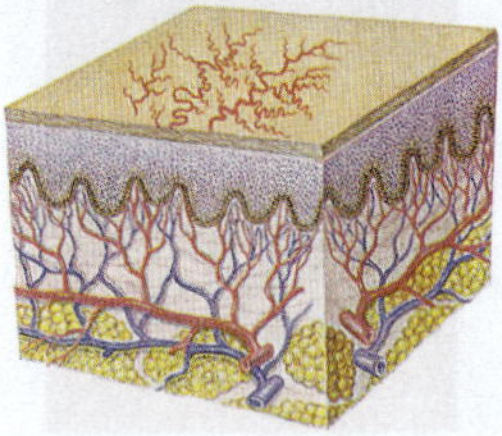	Hereditary hemorrhagic telangiectasia  *Telangiectasia.*

TECHNIQUE	FINDINGS
Hair	
Inspect hair over entire body	
• *Color*	**EXPECTED:** Light blond to black and gray, with alterations caused by rinses, dyes, and permanents.
• *Distribution/quantity*	**EXPECTED:** Hair present on scalp, lower face, neck, nares, ears, chest, axillae, back, shoulders, arms, legs, pubic area, and around nipples. Scalp hair loss in adult men, adrenal androgenic female-pattern alopecia in adult women.
	UNEXPECTED: Localized or generalized hair loss, inflammation, or scarring. Broken/absent hair shafts. Hirsutism in women.
Palpate for texture	**EXPECTED:** Coarse or fine, curly or straight, shiny, smooth, and resilient. Fine vellus covering body; coarse terminal hair on scalp, on pubis, on axillary areas, and in male beard.
	UNEXPECTED: Dryness and brittleness.
Nails	
Inspect nails	
• *Color*	**EXPECTED:** Variations of pink with varying opacity. Pigment deposits in persons with dark skin. White spots.
	UNEXPECTED: Yellow or green–black discoloration. Diffuse darkening. Pigment deposits in persons with light skin. Longitudinal red, brown, or white streaks or white bands. White, yellow, or green tinge. Blue nail beds. Blue–black discoloration.

TECHNIQUE	FINDINGS
• *Length/configuration/ symmetry*	**EXPECTED:** Varying shape, smooth and flat/slightly convex, with edges smooth and rounded. **UNEXPECTED:** Jagged, broken, or bitten edges or cuticles. Peeling. Absence of nail.
• *Cleanliness*	**EXPECTED:** Clean and neat. **UNEXPECTED:** Unkempt.
• *Ridging and beading*	**EXPECTED:** Longitudinal ridging and beading. **UNEXPECTED:** Longitudinal ridging and grooving with lichen planus. Transverse grooving, rippling, and depressions. Pitting.
Palpate nail plate	
• *Texture/firmness/ thickness/uniformity*	**EXPECTED:** Hard and smooth with uniform thickness. **UNEXPECTED:** Thickening or thinning.
• *Adherence to nail bed*	**EXPECTED:** Firmness.
Gently squeeze between thumb and finger.	**UNEXPECTED:** Separation. Boggy nail base.
Measure nail base angle	
Inspect fingers when patient places dorsal surfaces of fingertips together.	**EXPECTED:** 160-degree angle. **UNEXPECTED:** Clubbing.

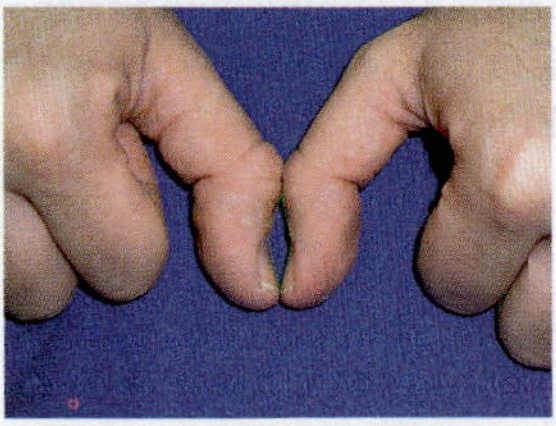
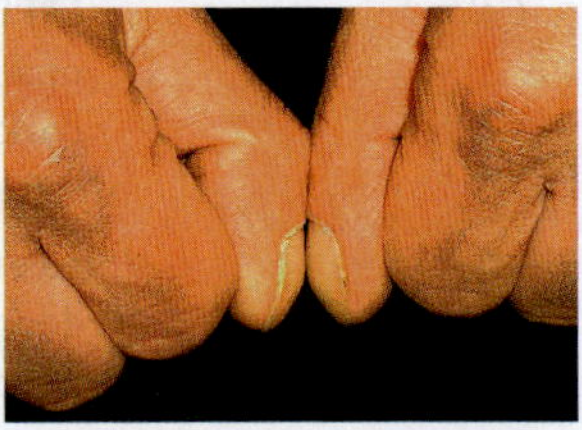

Clubbing deformity. The finger on the right is clubbed compared with the normal-shaped finger on the left.

Inspect and palpate proximal and lateral nail folds	
	UNEXPECTED: Redness, swelling, pus, warts, cysts, tumors, and pain.

AIDS TO DIFFERENTIAL DIAGNOSIS

SUBJECTIVE DATA	OBJECTIVE DATA
Eczematous Dermatitis	
Itching may or may not be present; those with atopic dermatitis often report allergy history (allergic rhinitis and asthma).	Acute: erythematous, pruritic, weeping vesicles; subacute: erythema and scaling; chronic: thick, lichenified, pruritic plaques. Atopic dermatitis: during childhood, lesions involve flexures, the nape, and the dorsal aspects of the limbs. In adolescence and adulthood, lichenified plaques affect the flexures, head, and neck.
Folliculitis	
Acute onset of papules and pustules associated with pruritus or mild discomfort; may have pain with deep folliculitis.	Primary lesion is a small pustule 1–2 cm in diameter located over a pilosebaceous orifice and may be perforated by a hair. Pustule may be surrounded by inflammation or nodular lesions. A crust forms after the pustule ruptures.
Tinea (Dermatophytosis)	
Pruritus.	Papular, pustular, vesicular, erythematous, or scaling lesions. Possible secondary bacterial infection. Hyphae on microscopic examination of skin scraping with KOH solution.
Rosacea	
Common triggers: sun, cold weather, sudden emotion, hot beverages, spicy foods, and alcohol.	Telangiectasia, erythema, papules, and pustules, particularly in the central area of the face; rhinophyma may occur.

SUBJECTIVE DATA	OBJECTIVE DATA
Herpes Zoster (Shingles)	
Pain, itching, or burning usually precedes eruption by 4–5 days.	Red, swollen plaques or vesicles along a single dermatome.
Basal Cell Carcinoma	
Persistent sore or lesions that have not healed; crusting; itching.	Shiny nodule that is pearly or translucent; may be pink, red, white, tan, black, or brown growth with a slightly elevated rolled border and a crusted indentation in the center.
Squamous Cell Carcinoma	
Persistent sore or lesion that has not healed or that has grown in size; crusting and/or bleeding.	Elevated growth with a central depression, wartlike growth; scaly red patch with irregular borders; open sore.
Malignant Melanoma	
New or preexisting mole that has changed or is changing; history of melanoma, dysplastic or atypical nevi; family history of melanoma.	Characteristic asymmetry, irregular borders, variegated colors, and is growing or >6 mm (see ABCDs of Melanoma on pp. 57–58).
Hirsutism	
Growth of terminal hair in women in the male distribution pattern on the face, body, and pubic areas.	Presence of thick, dark terminal hairs in androgen-sensitive sites: face, chest, areola, external genitalia, upper and lower back, buttock, inner thigh, and linea.
Paronychia	
Acute: history of nail trauma or manipulation; acute onset. Chronic: history of repeated exposure to moisture (e.g., through hand-washing). Initially evolves slowly with tenderness and mild swelling.	Redness, swelling, tenderness at lateral and proximal nail folds. Possible purulent drainage under cuticle. Acute or chronic (with nail rippling).

SUBJECTIVE DATA	OBJECTIVE DATA
Onychomycosis	
Yellow, crumbling nail.	Distal nail plate turns yellow or white as hyperkeratotic debris accumulates, causing the nail to separate from the nail bed. Redness and swelling where nail pierces the lateral nail fold and grows into the dermis.

PEDIATRIC VARIATIONS

EXAMINATION

TECHNIQUE	FINDINGS
Skin	
Inspect hands and feet of newborns for skin creases	
	EXPECTED: Number of creases is indication of maturity of newborn; the older the gestational age, the more creases.
	UNEXPECTED: Single transverse crease across palm often seen in infants with Down syndrome.

AIDS TO DIFFERENTIAL DIAGNOSIS

SUBJECTIVE DATA	OBJECTIVE DATA
Seborrheic Dermatitis	
Thick, greasy scalp scales, or body rash.	Thick, yellow, adherent, crusted scalp, ear, or neck lesions.
Impetigo	
Lesion, typically on the face, that itches and burns.	Crusted or ruptured honey-colored vesicles.
Miliaria (Prickly Heat)	
Parent reports rash noted while undressing infant.	Irregular, red, macular rash on covered areas.

SUBJECTIVE DATA	OBJECTIVE DATA
Chickenpox (varicella)	
Fever, headache, sore throat, malaise.	Pruritic maculopapular skin eruption that becomes vesicular in a matter of hours.
German Measles (Rubella)	
Fever, coryza, sore throat, cough.	Koplik spots on buccal mucosa; generalized light pink to red maculopapular rash.

The ABCDs of Melanoma

Characteristics that should alert you to the possibility of malignant melanoma:

- **AAA** Asymmetry of lesion: Half of a mole or birthmark does not match the other half.
- **ABA** Borders: Edges are irregular, ragged, notched, or blurred. Pigment may be streaming from the border.
- **ACA** Color: The color is not the same all over and may show differing shades of brown or black, sometimes with patches of red, white, or blue.
- **ADA** Diameter: The diameter is larger than 6 mm (about the size of a pencil eraser) or is growing larger.
- **AEA** Evolution: Changes seen in existing pigmented lesions, particularly in a nonuniform, asymmetric manner.

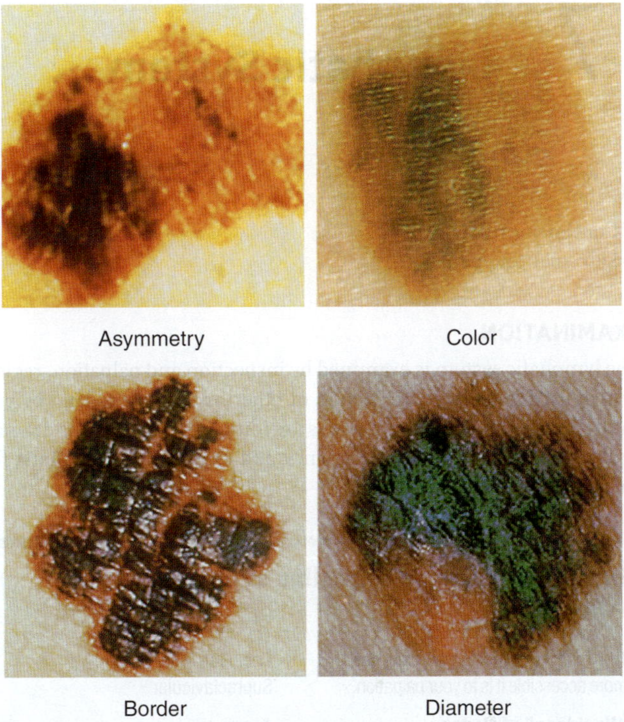

Melanoma. (Reproduced with permission from the American Academy of Dermatology, 2010. All rights reserved.)

CHAPTER

7 Lymphatic System

Equipment

- Centimeter ruler
- Skin-marking pencil

EXAMINATION

The lymphatic system is examined by inspection and palpation, region by region, during the examination of other body systems, and by palpating the spleen. If enlarged nodes are found, inspect regions drained by nodes for infection or malignancy and examine other regions for enlargement.

Lymph Nodes Most Accessible to Inspection and Palpation

The more superficial the node, the more accessible it is to your palpation.

"Necklace" of Nodes
Parotid and retropharyngeal (tonsillar)
Submandibular
Submental
Sublingual (facial)
Superficial anterior cervical
Superficial posterior cervical
Preauricular and postauricular
Occipital
Supraclavicular

Arms
Axillary
Epitrochlear (cubital)

Legs
Superficial superior inguinal
Superficial inferior inguinal
Occasionally, popliteal

TECHNIQUE	FINDINGS
Head and Neck	
Inspect for visible nodes	
Ask if patient is aware of any lumps.	**UNEXPECTED:** Edema, erythema, red streaks, or lesions.

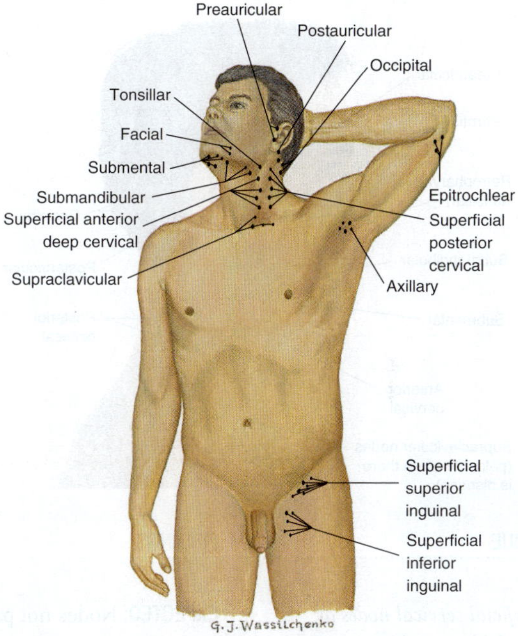

TECHNIQUE	FINDINGS

Palpate superficial nodes; note size, consistency, mobility, tenderness, warmth

Bend patient's head slightly forward or to side. Palpate gently with pads of second, third, and fourth fingers.

- *Occipital nodes at base of skull*
- *Postauricular nodes over mastoid process*
- *Preauricular nodes in front of ears*
- *Parotid and retropharyngeal nodes at angle of mandible*
- *Submandibular nodes between angle and tip of mandible*
- *Submental nodes behind tip of mandible*

EXPECTED: Nodes not palpable. **UNEXPECTED:** Enlarged, tender, red or discolored, fixed, matted, inflamed, or warm nodes; increased vascularity.

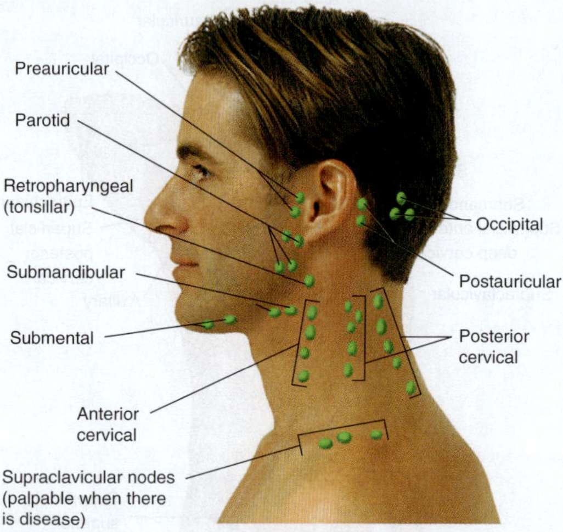

TECHNIQUE	FINDINGS

Neck

- *Superficial cervical nodes at sternocleidomastoid*
- *Posterior cervical nodes along anterior border of trapezius*
- *Deep cervical nodes along anterior border of trapezius*

EXPECTED: Nodes not palpable.

UNEXPECTED: Enlarged, tender, red or discolored, fixed, matted, inflamed, or warm nodes; increased vascularity.

- *Supraclavicular areas*
  Hook fingers over clavicle and rotate over supraclavicular fossa while patient turns head toward same side and raises shoulder.

UNEXPECTED: Detection of Virchow nodes.

NOTE: A palpable supraclavicular node should always make you suspect the probability of a malignancy.

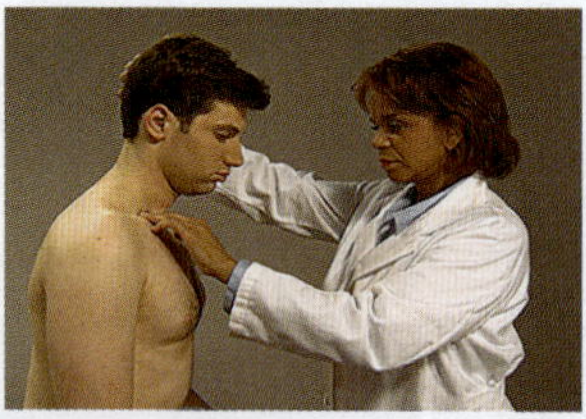

TECHNIQUE	FINDINGS
Axillae	
Inspect for visible nodes	
Ask if patient is aware of any lumps.	UNEXPECTED: Edema, erythema, red streaks, or lesions.
Palpate superficial nodes for size, consistency, mobility, tenderness, and warmth	
Using firm, deliberate, gentle touch, rotate fingertips and palm. Attempt to glide fingers beneath nodes.	
Axillary Nodes	
Support patient's forearm and bring palm of examining hand flat into axilla. With palmar surface of fingers, reach deep into hollow, pushing firmly upward, then bring fingers down, rotating your fingers and gently rolling soft tissue against chest wall and axilla. Explore apex, medial, lateral aspects along rib cage; lateral aspects along upper surface of arm; anterior and posterior walls of axilla. Repeat mirror image of this maneuver for the other axilla.	EXPECTED: Nodes not palpable. UNEXPECTED: Enlarged, tender, red or discolored, fixed, matted, inflamed, or warm nodes; increased vascularity.

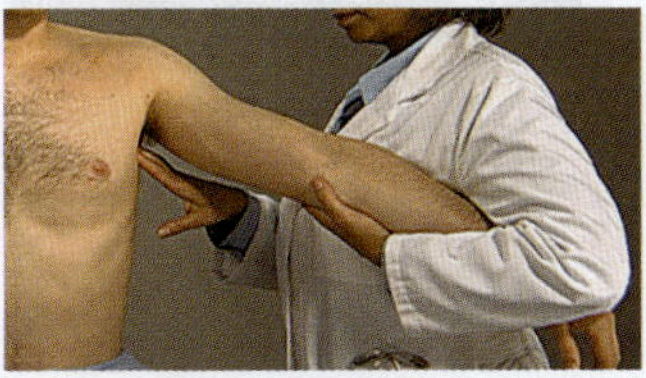

TECHNIQUE	FINDINGS
Other Lymph Nodes	
Inspect visible nodes	
Ask if patient is aware of any lumps.	UNEXPECTED: Edema, erythema, red streaks, or lesions.

TECHNIQUE	FINDINGS

Palpate superficial nodes for size, consistency, mobility, tenderness, and warmth

Systematically palpate other areas, moving hand in circular fashion, probing without pressing hard.

EXPECTED: Nodes not palpable.

UNEXPECTED: Enlarged, tender, red or discolored, fixed, matted, inflamed, or warm nodes; increased vascularity.

- *Epitrochlear nodes*
  Support elbow in one hand while exploring with other. Palpate the groove between the triceps and biceps muscle with your fingers using a circular motion.

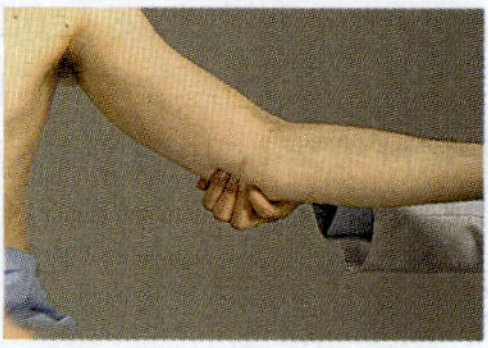

- *Inguinal area*
  Have patient lie supine with knee slightly flexed. The superior superficial inguinal (femoral) nodes are close to the surface over the inguinal canals. The inferior superficial inguinal nodes lie deeper in the groin.

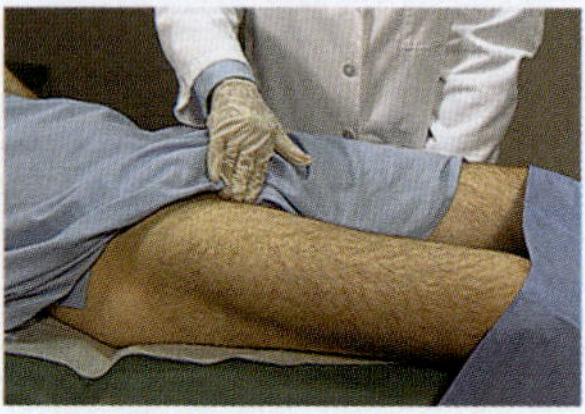

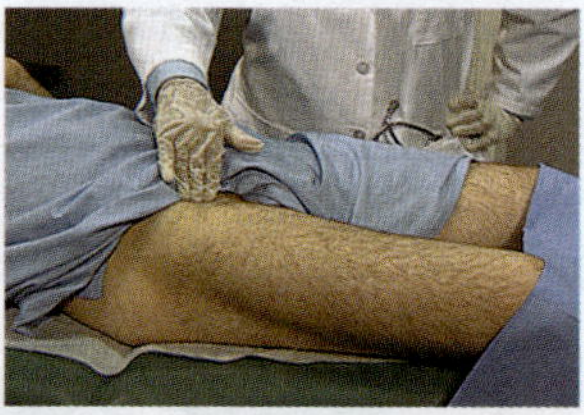

- *Popliteal nodes*
  Relax the posterior popliteal fossa by flexing the knee. Wrap your hand around the knee and palpate the fossa with your fingers.

AIDS TO DIFFERENTIAL DIAGNOSIS

SUBJECTIVE DATA	OBJECTIVE DATA
Acute Lymphangitis	
Pain, malaise, illness, possible fever.	Red streak (tracing of fine lines) may follow course of lymphatic collecting duct. Inflamed area was indurated and tender to gentle touch. Related infection possible distally, particularly interdigitally.
Non-Hodgkin Lymphoma	
Painless enlarged lymph node(s); fever, weight loss, night sweats, abdominal pain or fullness.	Nodes may be localized in the posterior cervical triangle or may become matted, crossing into the anterior triangle nodes; usually well-defined and solid.
Hodgkin Lymphoma	
Painless progressive enlargement of cervical lymph nodes. Generally asymmetric.	Nodes sometimes matted and generally very firm, almost rubbery.
Epstein-Barr Virus; Mononucleosis	
Pharyngitis, fever, fatigue, malaise.	Commonly splenomegaly and/or rash. Palpable nodes are generalized but more commonly in anterior and posterior cervical chains. Nodes vary in firmness, are generally discrete, and are occasionally tender.
Roseola Infantum (Human Herpesvirus 6)	
Fever: usually high grade and persistent over 3 to 4 days; sometimes associated with a mild respiratory illness.	Discrete and nontender nodes in the occipital and postauricular chains.

SUBJECTIVE DATA	OBJECTIVE DATA
Herpes Simplex	
Burning, itching lesions; enlarged lymph nodes.	Discrete labial and gingival ulcers, high fever, and enlargement of anterior cervical and submandibular nodes. Nodes tend to be firm, discrete, movable, and tender.
Human Immunodeficiency Virus/Acquired Immunodeficiency Syndrome (HIV/AIDS)	
Severe fatigue, malaise, weakness, persistent diarrhea; arthralgias.	Lymphadenopathy, fever, and unexplained weight loss.

Terms

Conditions

Lymphadenopathy (adenopathy)—enlarged lymph node(s)
Lymphadenitis—inflamed and enlarged lymph node(s)
Lymphangitis—inflammation of the lymphatics that drain an area of infection; tender erythematous streaks extend proximally from the infected area; regional nodes may also be tender
Lymphedema—edematous swelling caused by excess accumulation of lymph fluid in tissues caused by inadequate lymph drainage
Lymphangioma—congenital malformation of dilated lymphatics

Nodes

Shotty—small nontender nodes that feel like BBs (small round pellets) under the skin
Fluctuant—wavelike motion that is felt when the node is palpated
Matted—group of nodes that feel connected and seem to move as a unit

Some Conditions That Simulate Lymph Node Enlargement

Lymphangioma
Hemangioma (tends to feel spongy; appears reddish blue, depending on size and extent of angiomatous involvement)
Branchial cleft cyst (sometimes accompanied by tiny orifice in neck on line extending to ear)
Thyroglossal duct cyst
Laryngocele
Esophageal diverticulum
Thyroid goiter
Graves disease
Hashimoto thyroiditis
Parotid swelling (e.g., from mumps or tumor)

Differential Diagnosis: Lymphedema or Edema?

- Both can be either pitting or nonpitting.
- Except in early stages, lymphedema does not resolve with elevation of the affected area.
- Edema secondary to increased capillary filtration (e.g., chronic venous insufficiency) usually improves.
- Diuretics do not help lymphedema. They may help edema from other causes.
- Be aware that some patients may have both edema and lymphedema.

PEDIATRIC VARIATIONS

EXAMINATION

TECHNIQUE	FINDINGS
Head and Neck	
Palpate superficial nodes	
• *Occipital nodes at base of skull* • *Postauricular nodes over mastoid process*	**EXPECTED:** In children: small, firm, discrete, nontender, nonmovable nodes in occipital, postauricular chains.
Other Lymph Nodes	
Palpate superficial nodes	
• *Inguinal and popliteal areas*	**EXPECTED:** In children: small, firm, discrete nodes; nontender, movable in inguinal chain.

CHAPTER

8

Head and Neck

Equipment

- Tape measure
- Cup of water
- Stethoscope
- Transilluminator

EXAMINATION

Ask patient to sit.

TECHNIQUE	FINDINGS
Head and Face	
Observe head position	**EXPECTED:** Upright, midline, still. **UNEXPECTED:** Tilted, horizontal jerking or bobbing, tics, nodding.
Inspect facial features	
• *Shape* Observe eyelids, eyebrows, palpebral fissures, nasolabial folds, mouth at rest, during movement, with expression.	**EXPECTED:** Variations according to race, sex, age, body build. **UNEXPECTED:** Change in shape. Unusual features: edema, puffiness, coarsened features, prominent eyes, hirsutism, lack of expression, excessive perspiration, pallor, or pigmentation variations.
• *Symmetry* Note if asymmetry affects all features of one side or a portion of the face.	**EXPECTED:** Slight asymmetry. **UNEXPECTED:** Facial nerve weakness or paralysis, or problem with peripheral trigeminal nerve.

HEAD AND NECK

TECHNIQUE	FINDINGS
Inspect skull and scalp	
• *Size/shape/symmetry*	**EXPECTED:** Symmetric.
• *Scalp condition* • *Systematically part hair from frontal to occipital region.*	**UNEXPECTED:** Lesions, scabs, tenderness, parasites, nits, scaliness.
• *Hair pattern* Pay special attention to areas behind ears, at hairline, at crown.	**EXPECTED:** Bitemporal recession or balding over crown in men. **UNEXPECTED:** Random areas of alopecia or alopecia totalis.
Palpate head and scalp	
• *Symmetry* Palpate in gentle rotary motion from front to back.	**EXPECTED:** Symmetric and smooth with bones indistinguishable. Ridge of sagittal fissure occasionally palpable. **UNEXPECTED:** Indentations or depressions.
Palpate hair	
• *Texture/color distribution*	**EXPECTED:** Smooth, symmetrically distributed. **UNEXPECTED:** Splitting or cracked ends. Coarse, dry, or brittle. Fine and silky.
Palpate temporal arteries	
Note course of arteries.	**UNEXPECTED:** Thickening, hardness, or tenderness.
Auscultate temporal arteries and over skull and eyes	
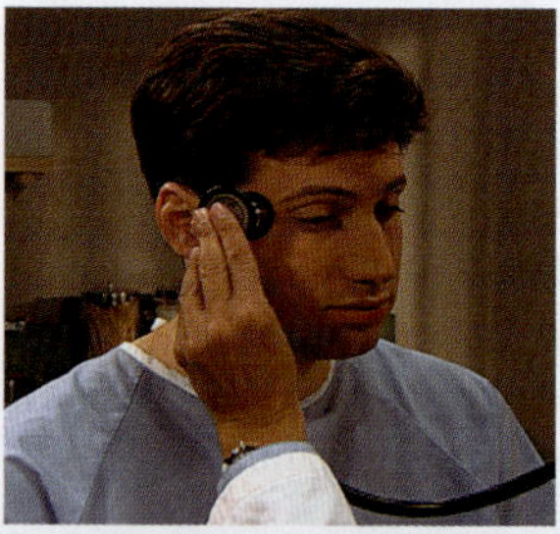	**EXPECTED:** No bruits.

TECHNIQUE	FINDINGS
Inspect salivary glands	
• *Symmetry/size* Palpate if asymmetry noted. Have patient open mouth, then press on salivary duct in attempt to express material.	**UNEXPECTED:** Asymmetry or enlargement. Tenderness. Discrete nodule.

Neck

TECHNIQUE	FINDINGS
Inspect neck	
• *Symmetry* Inspect in usual position, in slight hyperextension, and during swallowing. Look for landmarks of anterior and posterior triangles.	**EXPECTED:** Bilateral symmetry of sternocleidomastoid and trapezius muscles. **UNEXPECTED:** Asymmetry, torticollis, webbing, excessive posterior skinfolds, unusually short neck, distention of jugular vein; prominence of carotid arteries or edema.
• *Trachea* Inspect in usual position, in slight hyperextension, and while patient swallows.	**EXPECTED:** Midline placement. **UNEXPECTED:** Masses, deviation.
Evaluate range of motion	
Have patient flex, extend, rotate, laterally turn head, and neck.	**EXPECTED:** Smooth. **UNEXPECTED:** Pain, dizziness, or limitation of motion.
Palpate neck	
• *Trachea* Place thumb on each side of trachea in lower portion of neck, and compare space between trachea and sternocleidomastoid on each side.	**EXPECTED:** Midline position. **UNEXPECTED:** Deviation to right or left.

TECHNIQUE	FINDINGS
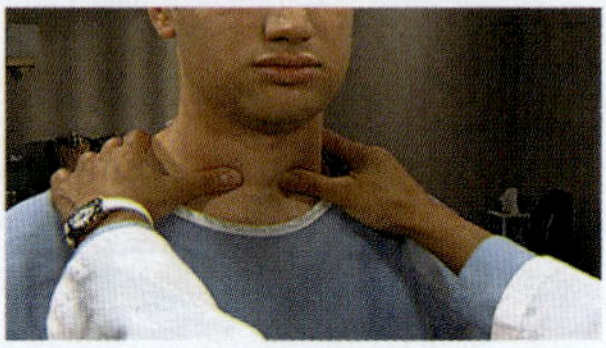	
• *Hyoid bone/thyroid and cricoid cartilages* Have patient swallow.	**EXPECTED:** Smooth. Moves during swallowing. **UNEXPECTED:** Tender
• *Cartilaginous rings of trachea* Have patient swallow.	**EXPECTED:** Distinct. **UNEXPECTED:** Tender.
• *Tracheal tug* With neck extended, palpate for movement with index finger and thumb on each side of trachea below thyroid isthmus.	**UNEXPECTED:** Tug synchronous with pulse.
Palpate lymph nodes	
• *Size/consistency, mobility/condition*	**UNEXPECTED:** Enlarged, matted, tender, fixed, warm.
Palpate thyroid gland	
• *Symmetry* Observe from frontal and lateral positions while patient hyperextends neck. Then observe as patient sips water while neck is hyperextended.	**UNEXPECTED:** Asymmetry. Enlarged and visible thyroid gland.

TECHNIQUE	FINDINGS
• *Size/shape/configuration/consistency* Stand either facing or behind patient. Have patient hold head slightly forward and tipped toward side being examined. Lightly palpate isthmus and lateral lobes. Give water to patient to facilitate swallowing. From the front, examine the left lobe by sitting on the left side of the patient and pressing the trachea to the left with the left thumb. Place the first three fingers in the thyroid bed just medial to the sternocleidomastoid. Keep your fingers still while the patient again swallows, thereby moving the gland beneath your fingers. Repeat on the right side. If gland is enlarged, auscultate for vascular sounds with stethoscope bell.	**EXPECTED:** Lobes small and smooth. Gland rises freely with swallowing. Right lobe as much as 25% larger than left. Tissue firm and pliable. **UNEXPECTED:** Enlarged, tender nodules (smooth or irregular, soft or hard); coarse tissue; gritty sensation. **UNEXPECTED:** Bruit.

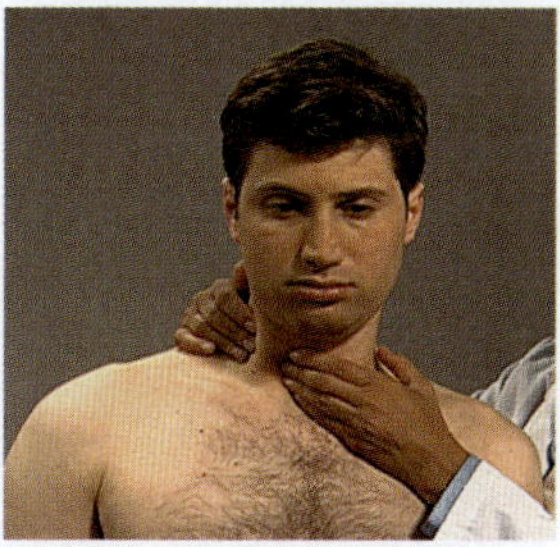

AIDS TO DIFFERENTIAL DIAGNOSIS

SUBJECTIVE DATA	OBJECTIVE DATA
Myxedema	
Cognitive impairment, slowed mentation, poor concentration, decreased short-term memory, social withdrawal, psychomotor retardation, depressed mood, and apathy.	Dull, puffy, yellow skin. Coarse, sparse hair. Temporal loss of eyebrows. Periorbital edema. Prominent tongue. Hypothyroidism (see table on p. 9).
Graves Disease	
Symptoms of hyperthyroidism, palpitations, heat intolerance, weight loss, fatigue, increased appetite, tachycardia.	Diffuse thyroid enlargement, hyperthyroidism. Various pathologic conditions—ophthalmologic (prominent eyes, lid retraction, staring or startled expression), dermatologic (fine and moist skin, fine hair), musculoskeletal (muscle weakness), cardiac (tachycardia) (see table on p. 76).

Headaches

Headaches are one of the most common concerns and probably one of the most self-medicated. They are not always benign. A history of insistent headache that is severe and recurrent must be given attention. Sometimes the underlying cause is life-threatening, such as a brain tumor. Sometimes it affects daily activities. The patient's history is fully as important as the physical examination in getting at the root of a headache. Various kinds of headaches can be compared as follows:

CHARACTERISTIC	CLASSIC MIGRAINE	MEDICATION REBOUND	CLUSTER	HYPERTENSIVE	MUSCULAR TENSION	TEMPORAL ARTERITIS	SPACE-OCCUPYING LESION
Age at onset	Childhood		Adulthood	Adulthood	Adulthood	Older adulthood	Any
Location	Unilateral or generalized	Holocranial or diffuse	Unilateral	Bilateral or occipital	Unilateral or bilateral	Unilateral or bilateral	Localized
Duration	Hours to days	Hours	0.5 to 2 hours	Hours	Hours to days	Hours to days	Rapidly increasing frequency
Time of onset	Morning or night	Predictably begins within hours to days of the last medication dose	Night	Morning	Anytime, commonly in afternoon or evening	Anytime	Awakening from sleep
Quality of pain	Pulsating or throbbing	Dull or throbbing	Intense burning, boring, searing, knifelike	Throbbing	Bandlike, constricting	Throbbing	

Continued

Headaches—cont'd

CHARACTERISTIC	CLASSIC MIGRAINE	MEDICATION REBOUND	CLUSTER	HYPERTENSIVE	MUSCULAR TENSION	TEMPORAL ARTERITIS	SPACE-OCCUPYING LESION
Prodromal event	Vague neurologic changes, personality changes, fluid retention, appetite loss Well-defined neurologic event, scotoma, aphasia, hemianopsia, aura	Daily analgesic use	Personality changes, sleep disturbances	None	None	None	Aggravated by coughing or bending forward
Precipitating event	Menstrual period, missing meals, birth control pills, letdown after stress	Abrupt discontinuation of analgesics	Alcohol consumption	None	Stress, anger, bruxism	None	Develops in temporal relation to the neoplasm
Frequency	Twice a week	Gradual increase to daily headache frequency	Several times nightly for several nights, then none	Daily	Daily	Daily	Progressive
Sex predilection	Females	Females	Males	Equal	Equal	Equal	Equal
Other symptoms	Nausea, vomiting	Alternate or preventive medications fail to control the headache	Increased lacrimation, nasal discharge	Generally remits as day progresses	None	None	Vomiting, confusion, abnormal neurologic findings, gait abnormality, papilledema, nystagmus

Hyperthyroidism Versus Hypothyroidism

SYSTEM OR STRUCTURE AFFECTED	HYPERTHYROIDISM	HYPOTHYROIDISM
Constitutional		
Temperature preference	Cool climate	Warm climate
Weight	Loss	Gain
Emotional state	Nervous, easily irritated, highly energetic	Lethargic, complacent, uninterested
Hair	Fine, with hair loss; failure to hold permanent wave	Coarse, with tendency to break
Skin	Warm, fine, hyperpigmentation at pressure points	Coarse, scaling, dry
Fingernails	Thin, with tendency to break; may show onycholysis	Thick
Eyes	Bilateral or unilateral proptosis, lid retraction, double vision	Puffiness in periorbital region
Neck	Goiter, change in shirt neck size, pain over thyroid	No goiter
Cardiac	Tachycardia, dysrhythmia, palpitations	No change noted
Gastrointestinal	Increased frequency of bowel movements; diarrhea rare	Constipation
Menstrual	Scant flow, amenorrhea	Menorrhagia
Neuromuscular	Increasing weakness, especially of proximal muscles	Lethargic but good muscular strength

PEDIATRIC VARIATIONS

EXAMINATION

TECHNIQUE	FINDINGS
Head and Face	
Palpate head and scalp	
• *Symmetry*	**EXPECTED:** An infant's head circumference is 2 cm greater than chest circumference up to the age of 2 years. **UNEXPECTED:** Head circumference much larger or smaller than 2 cm more than the chest circumference.
• *Skull condition*	**EXPECTED:** In infants, posterior fontanel closed at 2 months; anterior fontanel closed at 12–15 months. **UNEXPECTED:** Tenderness or depressions; sunken areas; swelling, bulging, or depressed fontanels.
• *Scalp*	**EXPECTED:** Free movement. **UNEXPECTED:** Fixation of scalp, bulging either on one side or crossing midline of scalp.
Auscultate Temporal Arteries and Over Skull and Eyes	**EXPECTED:** Bruits are common in children up to age 5 years.
Neck	
Palpate Thyroid Gland	
• *Symmetry*	**EXPECTED:** In children, thyroid gland may be palpable. **UNEXPECTED:** Tenderness.

CHAPTER 9

Eyes

Equipment

- Snellen chart or Lea cards, Landolt C, or HOTV chart
- Eye cover, gauze, or opaque card
- Rosenbaum or Jaeger near-vision card
- Penlight
- Cotton wisp
- Ophthalmoscope

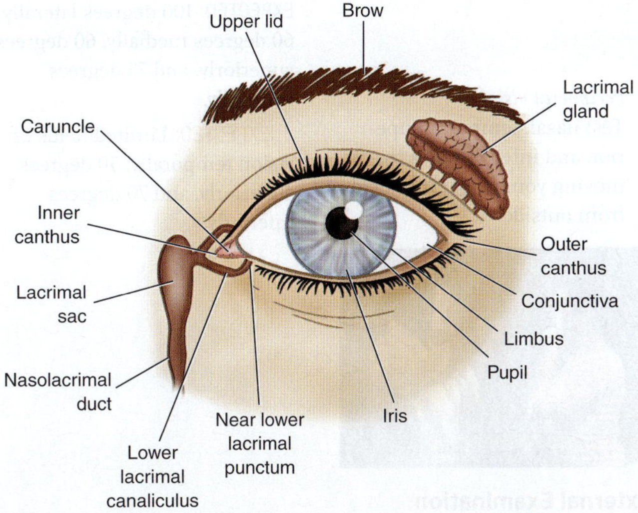

(From Thompson JM, et al.: Mosby's clinical nursing*, ed 5, St. Louis, 2002, Mosby.)*

EXAMINATION

Ask patient to sit or stand.

TECHNIQUE	FINDINGS

Visual Testing

Measure visual acuity in each eye separately

TECHNIQUE	FINDINGS
• *Distance vision* Use Snellen chart, Landolt C, or HOTV chart. If testing with and without corrective lenses, test without lenses first and record readings separately.	**EXPECTED:** Vision 20/20 with or without lenses with near and far vision in both eyes. **UNEXPECTED:** Myopia, amblyopia, or presbyopia.
• *Near vision* Use near-vision card.	**EXPECTED:** Vision 20/20. **UNEXPECTED:** Myopia, amblyopia, or presbyopia.
• *Peripheral vision* Test nasal, temporal, superior, and inferior fields by moving your finger into field from outside.	**EXPECTED:** 100 degrees laterally, 60 degrees medially, 60 degrees superiorly, and 75 degrees inferiorly. **UNEXPECTED:** Limited fields of vision temporally, 50 degrees superiorly, and 70 degrees inferiorly.

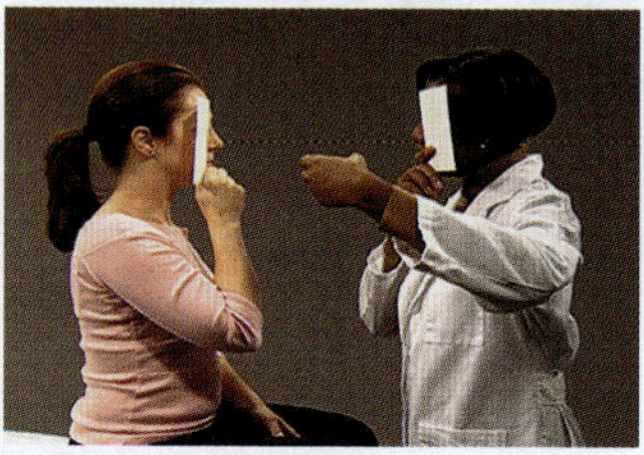

External Examination

Inspect eyebrows

TECHNIQUE	FINDINGS
• *Size/extension*	**EXPECTED:** Unusually thin if plucked. **UNEXPECTED:** Ending short of temporal canthus.
• *Hair texture*	**UNEXPECTED:** Coarse.

TECHNIQUE	FINDINGS
Inspect orbital area	UNEXPECTED: Edema, puffiness not related to aging, or sagging tissue below orbit. Xanthelasma.
Inspect eyelids	
• *Eyelid position*	UNEXPECTED: Ectropion or entropion.
• *Ability to open wide and close completely* Examine with eyes lightly closed, closed tightly, and open wide.	EXPECTED: Superior eyelid covering a portion of iris when open. UNEXPECTED: Fasciculations when lightly closed. Ptosis. Lagophthalmos.
• *Eyelid margin*	UNEXPECTED: Flakiness, redness, or swelling. Hordeola.
• *Eyelashes*	EXPECTED: Present on both lids. Turned outward.
Palpate eyelids	UNEXPECTED: Nodules.
Palpate eye	EXPECTED: Can be gently pushed into orbit without discomfort. UNEXPECTED: Firm and resists palpation.
Pull down lower lids and inspect conjunctivae and sclerae	
• *Color* Inspect upper tarsal conjunctivae only if the presence of a foreign body is suspected.	EXPECTED: Conjunctivae clear and inapparent. Sclerae white and visible above irides only when eyelids are wide open. UNEXPECTED: Conjunctivae with erythema or hemorrhage. Sclerae yellow or green. Sclerae with dark, rust-colored pigment anterior to insertion of medial rectus muscle.

TECHNIQUE	FINDINGS
• *Appearance*	**UNEXPECTED:** Exudate. Pterygium. Corneal arcus senilis or opacities.
Inspect lacrimal gland region	
• *Lacrimal gland puncta* Palpate lower orbital rim near inner canthus. If temporal aspect of upper lid feels full, evert lid and inspect gland.	**EXPECTED:** Slight elevations with central depression on both upper and lower lid margins. **UNEXPECTED:** Enlarged glands. Dry eyes.
Test corneal sensitivity	
Touch wisp of cotton to cornea.	**EXPECTED:** Bilateral blink reflex.
Inspect external eyes	
• *Corneal clarity* Shine light tangentially on cornea.	**EXPECTED:** clear, transparent **UNEXPECTED:** Blood vessels present. Abrasions, swelling (hydrops).
• *Irides*	**EXPECTED:** Clearly visible pattern. Similar color. **UNEXPECTED:** different colors, Brushfield spots.
• *Pupillary size/shape*	**EXPECTED:** Round, regular, and equal in size. **UNEXPECTED:** Miosis, mydriasis, anisocoria, or coloboma.
• *Pupillary response to light*	**EXPECTED:** Constricting with consensual response of opposite pupil.
• *Pupillary accommodation*	**EXPECTED:** Constricting when pupils focus on near object or dilating when focus changes from near to distant object.
• *Afferent pupillary testing*	**EXPECTED:** The pupil toward which the light is moving dilates and then constricts as light shines onto it. **UNEXPECTED:** The pupil continues to dilate when light shines onto it.

TECHNIQUE | **FINDINGS**

Extraocular Eye Muscles

Evaluate muscle balance and movement of eyes

- *Six cardinal fields of gaze*
  Hold patient's chin and ask patient to watch finger or penlight.

EXPECTED: A few horizontal nystagmic beats. Smooth, full, coordinated movement of eyes.

UNEXPECTED: Sustained or jerking nystagmus. Exposure of sclera from lid lag. Inability of eye to move in all directions.

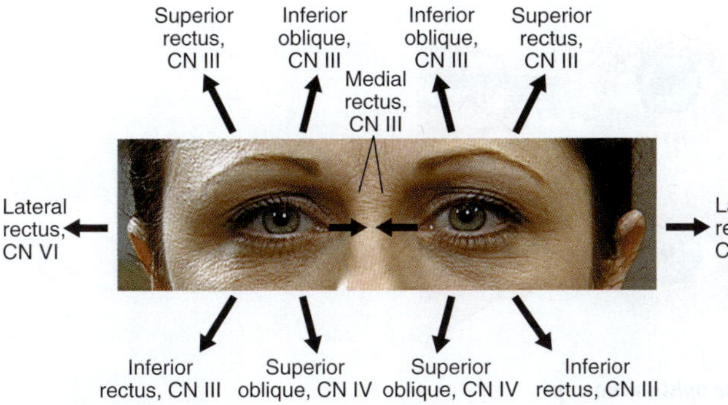

- *Corneal light reflex*
  Direct light at nasal bridge from 30 cm (12 in). Have patient look at nearby object.

EXPECTED: Light reflected symmetrically from both eyes.

- *Cover–uncover test*
  Perform if imbalance found with corneal light reflex test. Have patient stare ahead at near, fixed object. Cover one eye and observe the other; remove cover and observe uncovered eye. Repeat with other eye.

UNEXPECTED: strabismus, movement of covered or uncovered eye.

TECHNIQUE	FINDINGS

Ophthalmoscopic Examination

Inspect internal eye

- *Lens clarity*

UNEXPECTED: Cloudiness or opacity. Shallow chamber. If observed, avoid mydriatics.

- *Anterior chamber*
  Shine focused light tangentially at limbus. Note illumination of iris nasally.

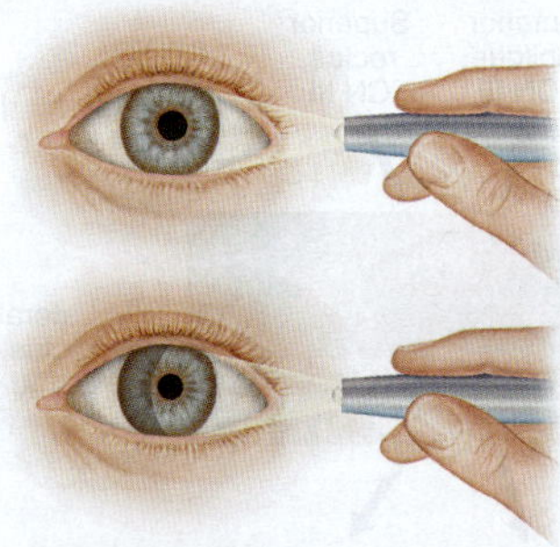

- *Use ophthalmoscope*
  With patient looking at distant object, direct light at pupil from about 30 cm (12 in). Move toward patient, observing:
- *Red reflex*

UNEXPECTED: Opacities.

- *Fundus*

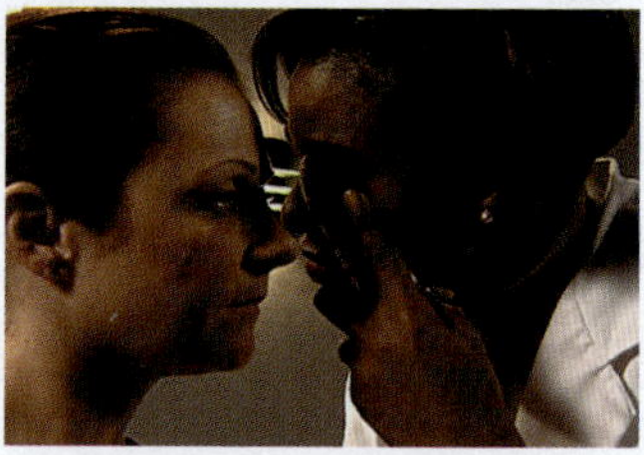

EXPECTED: Yellow or pink background, depending on race. Possible crescents or dots of pigment at disc margin, usually temporally.

UNEXPECTED: Discrete areas of pigmentation away from disc. Lesions. Drusen bodies. Hemorrhages.

TECHNIQUE	FINDINGS
• *Blood vessel characteristics* Follow blood vessels distally in each quadrant, noting crossings of arterioles and venules.	**EXPECTED:** Possible venous pulsations (should be documented). Arteriole/venule ratio 3:5 or 2:3. **UNEXPECTED:** Nicking, tortuosity.

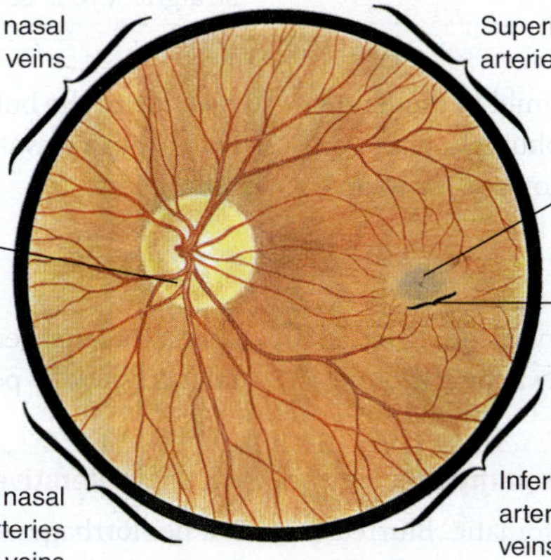

TECHNIQUE	FINDINGS
• *Disc characteristics*	**EXPECTED:** Yellow to creamy pink, varying by race. Sharp, well-defined margin, especially in temporal region; 1.5-mm diameter. **UNEXPECTED:** Myelinated nerve fibers. Papilledema. Glaucomatous cupping.
• *Macula densa characteristics* Ask patient to look directly at light.	**EXPECTED:** Yellow dot surrounded by deep pink.

AIDS TO DIFFERENTIAL DIAGNOSIS

SUBJECTIVE DATA	OBJECTIVE DATA
Strabismus (Paralytic and Nonparalytic)	
Eyes cannot focus simultaneously. Can focus separately in nonparalytic type.	Eye movement on the cover–uncover test; strabismic eye will fixate on the object after the "straight" eye is covered.
Episcleritis	
Acute onset of mild to moderate discomfort or photophobia. Painless injection and/or watery discharge.	Injection of the bulbar conjunctiva purplish elevation of a few millimeters.
Cataracts	
Cloudy or blurry vision, faded colors; halo may appear around lights.	Opacity of lens, generally central, occasionally peripheral.
Diabetic Retinopathy (Background or Nonproliferative)	
Initially asymptomatic. Blurred vision, distortion, or visual acuity loss in more advanced stages.	Dot hemorrhages, microaneurysms, and hard exudates.
Diabetic Retinopathy (Proliferative)	
Generally asymptomatic, floaters, blurred vision, or progressive visual acuity loss in advanced stages.	New vessel formation; extension out of the retina, hemorrhage.

PEDIATRIC VARIATIONS

EXAMINATION

TECHNIQUE	FINDINGS
Visual Testing	
Measure visual acuity	
• *Distance vision* When child is cooperative, visual acuity is tested with Lea cards, Landolt C, or HOTV chart, usually at about 3 years of age.	**EXPECTED:** Infants should be able to focus on and track a face or light through 60 degrees. Age 3 to 5 years: 20/50 or better. Age 6 years: 20/30 or better.

Extraocular Eye Muscles

Evaluate muscle balance and movement of eyes

Evaluation of six cardinal fields of gaze is performed as with adults. You may, however, need to hold child's head still.

CHAPTER

10 Ears, Nose, and Throat

Equipment

- Otoscope with pneumatic attachment
- Nasal speculum
- Tongue blades
- Tuning fork (512 and 1024 Hz approximate vocal frequencies)
- Gauze
- Gloves
- Penlight or light from otoscope

EXAMINATION

Ask patient to sit.

TECHNIQUE | **FINDINGS**

Ears

Inspect auricles and mastoid area

Examine lateral and medial surfaces and surrounding tissue.

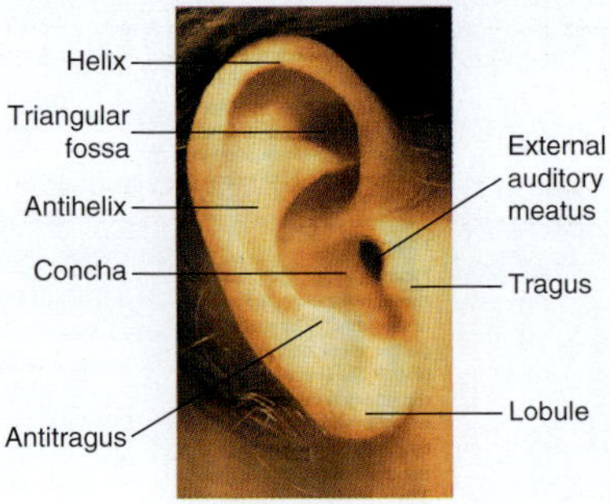

Auricle landmarks.

- *Size/shape/symmetry*

EXPECTED: Familial variations. Auricles of equal size and similar appearance. Darwin tubercle (congenital thickening along upper ridge of helix).

TECHNIQUE	FINDINGS
	UNEXPECTED: Unequal size or configuration. Cauliflower ear and other deformities.
• *Lesions*	**UNEXPECTED:** Moles, cysts, or other lesions, nodules, or tophi (small whitish uric acid crystal deposition along peripheral margins of the auricles).
• *Color*	**EXPECTED:** Same color as facial skin. **UNEXPECTED:** Blueness, pallor, or excessive redness.
• *Position* Draw imaginary line between inner canthus of the eye and most prominent protuberance of occiput. Draw imaginary line perpendicular to first line and anterior to auricle.	**EXPECTED:** Top of auricle above or touching horizontal line. Auricle is in vertical position. **UNEXPECTED:** Auricle positioned below line (low-set); unequal alignment. Lateral posterior angle >10 degrees.
• *Preauricular area*	**EXPECTED:** Smooth skin. **UNEXPECTED:** Skin tags or preauricular pits with or without discharge.
• *External auditory canal*	**EXPECTED:** No discharge, no odor; canal walls pink. **UNEXPECTED:** Serous, bloody, or purulent discharge; foul smell.

Palpate auricles and mastoid area

TECHNIQUE	FINDINGS
	EXPECTED: Firm and mobile, readily recoils from folded position; no tenderness in postauricular or mastoid area. **UNEXPECTED:** Tenderness, swelling, nodules. Pain when pulling on lobule.

TECHNIQUE	FINDINGS
Inspect auditory canal with otoscope	
Using largest speculum that fits comfortably in the ear, slowly insert the otoscope speculum to a depth of 1 to 1.5 cm (0.5 in) inspecting the auditory canal from the meatus to the tympanic membrane.	**EXPECTED:** Minimal cerumen in varying color and texture. Uniformly pink canal. Hairs in outer third of canal. **UNEXPECTED:** Cerumen obscures tympanic membrane, odor, lesions, discharge, scaling, excessive redness, swelling, and foreign body.
Inspect tympanic membrane	
Tilt the patient's head toward the opposite shoulder, and as the speculum is inserted, pull the patient's auricle upward and back to straighten the auditory canal for the best view. • *Landmarks* Vary light direction to observe entire membrane and annulus.	**EXPECTED:** Visible landmarks (umbo, handle of malleus, light reflex). **UNEXPECTED:** Perforations, landmarks not visible.
• *Color*	**EXPECTED:** Translucent, pearly gray. **UNEXPECTED:** Amber, yellow, blue, deep red, chalky white, dull, white flecks, or dense white plaques; air bubbles or fluid level.

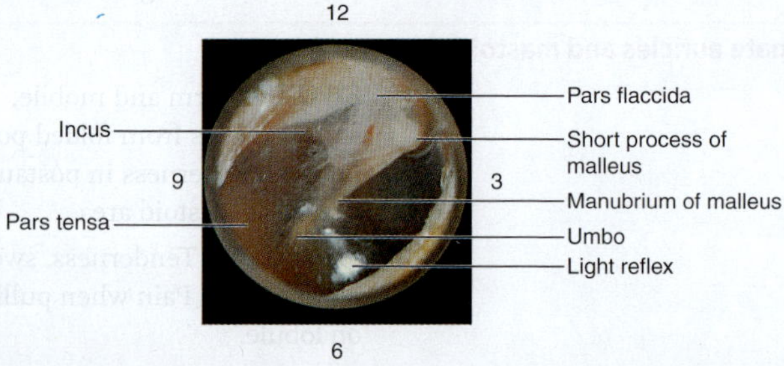

Tympanic membrane. (From Barkauskas VH, et al.: Health and physical assessment, ed 3, St. Louis, 2002, Mosby.)

TECHNIQUE	FINDINGS
• *Contour*	**EXPECTED:** Slightly conical with concavity at umbo. **UNEXPECTED:** Bulging (more conical, usually with loss of bony landmarks and distorted light reflex) or retracted (more concave, usually with accentuated bony landmarks and distorted light reflex).
• *Mobility* Seal canal with speculum, and gently apply positive (squeeze bulb) and negative (release bulb) pressure with pneumatic attachment.	**EXPECTED:** Tympanic membrane moves in and out. **UNEXPECTED:** Minimal to no movement of tympanic membrane.

Assess hearing

TECHNIQUE	FINDINGS
• *Questions asked during history*	**EXPECTED:** Responds to questions appropriately. **UNEXPECTED:** Excessive requests for repetition. Speech with monotonous tone and erratic volume.
• *Whispered voice* Have patient mask hearing in one ear by having patient gently occlude the nontested ear. Stand behind and to the side of patient at arm's length from the nontested ear and softly whisper combinations of three letters and numbers (e.g., 3, T, 9 or 5, M, 2). Ask patient to repeat what was heard. Use a different letter-number combination in other ear.	**EXPECTED:** Patient repeats numbers and letters correctly more than 50% of time. **UNEXPECTED:** Patient unable to repeat whispered words.

TECHNIQUE	FINDINGS
• *Weber test* Place base of vibrating tuning fork on midline vertex of head. To test patient's reliability, repeat with one ear occluded.	**EXPECTED:** Sound heard equally in both ears when ears are not occluded. Sound heard better in occluded ear. **UNEXPECTED:** See table on p. 92.

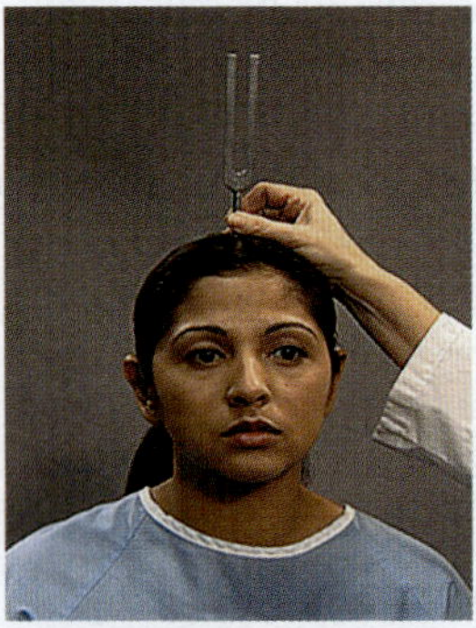

Weber test.

TECHNIQUE	FINDINGS
• *Rinne test* Place base of vibrating tuning fork against mastoid bone, note seconds until sound is no longer heard; then quickly move fork 1 to 2 cm (0.5 to 1 in) from auditory canal and note seconds until sound is no longer heard. Repeat with other ear.	**EXPECTED:** Measurement of air-conducted sound twice as long as measurement of bone-conducted sound. **UNEXPECTED:** See table on p. 92.

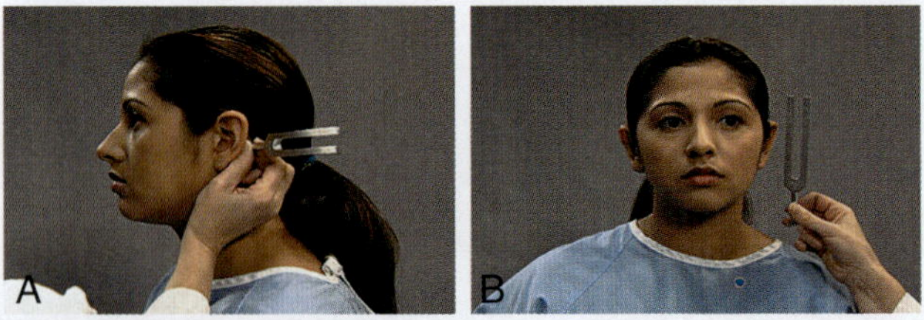

Rinne test. ***A,*** *Tuning fork against mastoid bone.* ***B,*** *Tuning fork near ear.*

Interpretation of Tuning Fork Tests

	WEBER TEST	RINNE TEST
Expected findings	No lateralization, but will lateralize to ear occluded by patient	Air conduction heard longer than bone conduction by 2:1 ratio (Rinne positive)
Conductive hearing loss	Lateralization to affected ear unless sensorineural loss	Bone conduction heard longer than air conduction in affected ear (Rinne negative)
Sensorineural hearing loss	Lateralization to better hearing ear unless conductive loss	Air conduction heard longer than bone conduction in affected ear, but <2:1 ratio

TECHNIQUE | **FINDINGS**

Nose and Sinuses

Inspect external nose

- *Shape/size*

EXPECTED: Smooth. Columella directly midline, width is not greater than diameter of a naris.

UNEXPECTED: Swelling or depression of nasal bridge. Transverse crease at junction of nose cartilage and bone.

- *Color*

EXPECTED: Conforms to face color.

- *Nares*

EXPECTED: Oval. Symmetrically positioned.

UNEXPECTED: Asymmetry, narrowing, discharge, and nasal flaring on inspiration.

Palpate ridge and soft tissues of nose

Place one finger on each side of nasal arch and gently palpate from nasal bridge to tip.

EXPECTED: Firm and stable structures.

UNEXPECTED: Displacement of bone and cartilage, tenderness, crepitus (crackling sensation), or masses.

TECHNIQUE	FINDINGS
Evaluate patency of nares	
Occlude one naris with finger on side of nose and ask patient to breathe through nose. Repeat with other naris.	**EXPECTED:** Noiseless, easy breathing. **UNEXPECTED:** Noisy breathing; occlusion.
Inspect nasal mucosa and nasal septum	
With the thumb of your nondominant hand, tip the nose upward. With your dominant hand, using a large speculum tip, slowly and cautiously insert without touching nasal septum.	
• *Color*	**EXPECTED:** Mucosa and turbinates deep pink and glistening. **UNEXPECTED:** Increased redness of mucosa or localized redness and swelling in vestibule. Turbinates bluish gray or pale pink.
• *Shape*	**EXPECTED:** Septum close to midline and fairly straight, thicker anteriorly than posteriorly. Inferior and middle turbinates visible. **UNEXPECTED:** Asymmetry of posterior nasal cavities, septal deviation.
• *Condition*	**EXPECTED:** Possibly film of clear discharge on septum. Possibly hairs in vestibule. Turbinates firm consistency. **UNEXPECTED:** Discharge, bleeding, crusting, masses, or lesions. Swollen, boggy turbinates. Perforated septum. Polyps.
Sense of smell	
See Chapter 20.	

TECHNIQUE	FINDINGS

Inspect frontal and maxillary sinus area

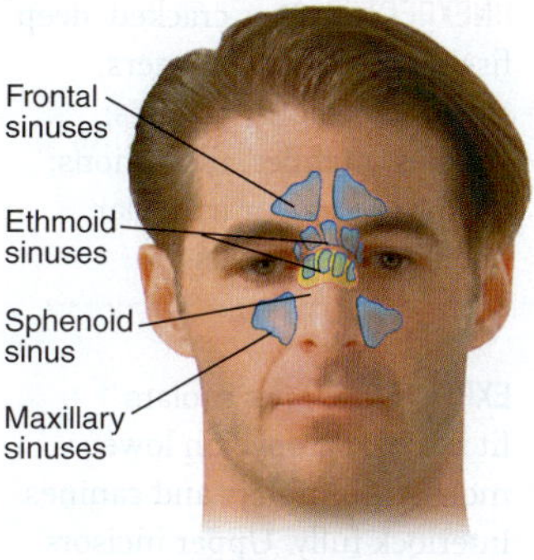

Sinuses.

UNEXPECTED: Swelling on face over sinus areas.

Palpate frontal and maxillary sinuses

Press thumbs up under bony brow on each side of nose. Palpate with thumbs or index and middle fingers just below the cheekbones.

EXPECTED: Nontender on palpation.

UNEXPECTED: Tenderness or pain, swelling.

Mouth

Inspect and palpate lips with mouth closed

- *Symmetry*

EXPECTED: Symmetric vertically and horizontally at rest and while moving.

UNEXPECTED: Asymmetric.

- *Color*

EXPECTED: Pink in persons with lighter skin, more bluish in persons with darker skin, distinct border between lips and facial skin.

UNEXPECTED: Pallor, circumoral pallor, bluish purple, or cherry red.

TECHNIQUE	FINDINGS
• *Condition*	**EXPECTED:** Smooth. **UNEXPECTED:** Dry, cracked; deep fissures in mouth corners, swelling; lesions; plaques; vesicles; nodules, ulcerations; or round, oval, or irregular bluish-gray macules.

Inspect teeth

TECHNIQUE	FINDINGS
• *Occlusion* Have patient clench teeth and smile with lips spread.	**EXPECTED:** Upper molars fit into the groove on lower molars. Premolars and canines interlock fully. Upper incisors slightly override lower incisors. **UNEXPECTED:** Malocclusion. Protrusion of upper incisors (overbite). Protrusion of lower incisors. Problems with bite.

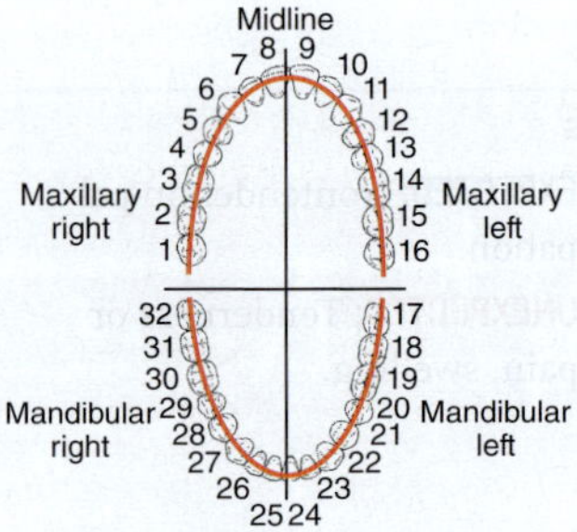

Teeth occlusion line and individual tooth numbers. (From Miyasaki-Ching, 1997.)

TECHNIQUE	FINDINGS
• *Color*	**EXPECTED:** Ivory, stained yellow, or brown. **UNEXPECTED:** Discolorations on crown may indicate caries.
• *Condition*	**EXPECTED:** 32 teeth, firmly anchored. **UNEXPECTED:** Caries and loose or missing teeth.

Inspect buccal mucosa

Have patient remove any dental appliances and then partially open mouth. Use tongue blade and bright light to assess.

TECHNIQUE	FINDINGS
• *Color*	**EXPECTED:** Pinkish red, patchy pigmented mucosa in individuals with dark skin. **UNEXPECTED:** Deeply pigmented. Whitish or pinkish scars.
• *Condition*	**EXPECTED:** Smooth and moist. Whitish yellow or whitish pink Stensen duct. Fordyce spots (yellow-white raised lesions). **UNEXPECTED:** Adherent thickened white patch; white, round, or oval ulcerative lesions; red spot at opening of Stensen duct; stones or exudate from Stensen duct.
Inspect and palpate gingiva Use Gloves to Palpate.	
• *Color*	**EXPECTED:** Slightly stippled and pink, may be more hyperpigmented in individuals with dark skin.
• *Condition*	**EXPECTED:** Clearly defined, tight margin at each tooth. Gingival enlargement with pregnancy, puberty, and certain medications. **UNEXPECTED:** Inflammation, swelling, bleeding, or lesions under dentures or on gingiva; induration, thickening, masses, or tenderness. Enlarged crevices between teeth and gum margins. Pockets containing debris at tooth margins.
Inspect tongue	
• *Size/symmetry* Ask patient to extend tongue.	**EXPECTED:** Midline, no fasciculations. **UNEXPECTED:** Atrophied, deviation to one side.
• *Color*	**EXPECTED:** Dull red.

TECHNIQUE	FINDINGS
• *Dorsum surface* Have patient extend tongue and hold extended.	**EXPECTED:** Moist and glistening. Anterior: smooth yet roughened surface with papillae and small fissures. Posterior: smooth, slightly uneven, or rugated surface with thinner mucosa than anterior. Possibly geographic. **UNEXPECTED:** Smooth, red, slick; hairy; swollen; coated; ulcerated; fasciculations; or limitation of movement.
• *Ventral surface and floor of mouth* Have patient touch tip of tongue to palate behind upper incisors.	**EXPECTED:** Ventral surface pink and smooth with large veins between frenulum and fimbriated folds. Wharton ducts apparent on each side of frenulum. **UNEXPECTED:** Difficulty touching hard palate. Swelling, varicosities, and ranula (mucocele).
• *Lateral borders* Wrap tongue with gauze and pull to each side. With tongue blade, scrape white or red margins to remove food particles.	**UNEXPECTED:** Leukoplakia or any other fixed lesion, ulceration.

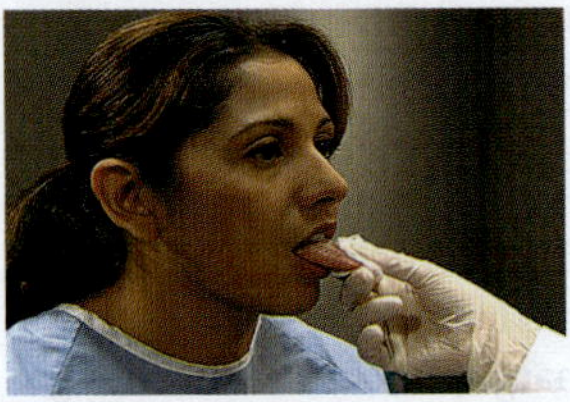

Inspecting lateral border of tongue.

Palpate tongue and floor of mouth

EXPECTED: Smooth and even texture.

UNEXPECTED: Lumps, nodules, induration, ulcerations, or thickened white patches.

TECHNIQUE	FINDINGS
Inspect palate and uvula	
Have Patient Tilt Head Back.	
• *Color and landmarks*	**EXPECTED:** Hard palate (whitish and dome-shaped with transverse rugae) contiguous with pinker soft palate. Uvula at midline. Bony protuberance of hard palate at midline (torus palatinus). **UNEXPECTED:** Nodule or other lesions on palate, not at midline.
• *Movement* Ask patient to say "ah" while observing soft palate. Depress tongue if necessary.	**EXPECTED:** Soft palate rises symmetrically, with uvula remaining in midline. **UNEXPECTED:** Failure of soft palate to rise bilaterally. Uvula deviation. Bifid uvula.
Inspect oropharynx	
Depress tongue with tongue blade.	
• *Tonsils* Inspect the tonsillar pillars and size of tonsils.	**EXPECTED:** Tonsils, if present, blend into pink color of pharynx. Possible crypts in tonsils where cellular debris and food particles collect. **UNEXPECTED:** Tonsils projecting beyond limits of tonsillar pillars. Tonsils red, enlarged, and covered with exudate.
• *Posterior wall of pharynx*	**EXPECTED:** Smooth, glistening, pink mucosa with some small, irregular spots of lymphatic tissue and small blood vessels. **UNEXPECTED:** Red bulge adjacent to tonsil extending beyond midline. Yellowish mucoid film in pharynx.

TECHNIQUE	FINDINGS
Elicit gag reflex	
Prepare patient and touch posterior wall of pharynx on each side.	**EXPECTED:** Bilateral response. **UNEXPECTED:** Unequal response or no response.

AIDS TO DIFFERENTIAL DIAGNOSIS

Differentiating Between Otitis Externa, Acute Otitis Media, and Middle-Ear Effusion

SIGNS AND SYMPTOMS	OTITIS EXTERNA	ACUTE OTITIS MEDIA	OTITIS MEDIA WITH EFFUSION
Initial symptoms	Itching in ear canal	Abrupt onset, fever, irritability, feeling of blockage; preceding or concurrent upper respiratory symptoms	Sticking or cracking sound on yawning or swallowing; no signs of acute infection
Pain	Intense with movement of pinna or chewing	Deep-seated earache that interferes with activity or sleep, pulling at ear	Discomfort; feeling of fullness
Discharge	Watery, then purulent and thick; musty, foul smelling	Only if tympanic membrane ruptures or through tympanostomy tube; foul smelling	Uncommon
Hearing	Conductive loss caused by exudate and swelling of ear canal	Conductive loss as middle ear fills with purulent material	Conductive loss as middle ear fills with fluid
Inspection	Canal is red, edematous; tympanic membrane is obscured	Tympanic membrane with distinct erythema, thickened or clouding, bulging; limited movement to positive and negative pressure, air–fluid level, and/or bubbles; vesicles or bullae may be seen	Tympanic membrane is retracted or full, yellowish; impaired mobility; air-fluid level and/or bubbles

SUBJECTIVE DATA	OBJECTIVE DATA
Otitis Externa	
Swimming underwater, water retained in ear canal.	See differential diagnosis table on p. 99.
Otitis Media With Effusion	
Upper respiratory infection, ear feels full, reduced hearing.	See differential diagnosis table on p. 99.
Acute Otitis Media	
Recent upper respiratory infection, fever, ear pain or pressure, reduced hearing.	See differential diagnosis table on p. 99.
Sinusitis	
Upper respiratory infection worsens or persists after 7 to 10 days, headache, facial pain or pressure, tooth pain, nasal discharge or congestion, persistent cough (worse at night).	Fever, tenderness of sinuses, swelling over orbit or sinus; purulent nasal discharge; may also have no physical findings.
Acute Bacterial Pharyngitis	
Sore throat, referred pain to ears, dysphagia, fever, fetid breath, malaise, abdominal pain, rash.	Tonsils are red and swollen; crypts filled with purulent exudate; enlarged anterior cervical lymph nodes; palatal petechiae.
Peritonsillar Abscess	
Difficulty and painful swallowing, severe sore throat with pain radiating to ear, fever, and malaise.	Drooling, unilateral red and swollen tonsil and adjacent soft palate; tonsil may appear pushed forward or backward, possibly displacing uvula; muffled voice, fetid breath, trismus, enlarged cervical lymph nodes.
Retropharyngeal Abscess	
Recent upper respiratory infection, pain in neck and jaw referred to ear, anxious, limited neck movement, drooling, and poor appetite.	Fever, restlessness, pain with lateral neck movement, lateral pharyngeal wall is distorted medially, trismus, respiratory distress, muffled voice.

SUBJECTIVE DATA	OBJECTIVE DATA
Oral Cancer	
Painless sore in mouth that does not heal; often discovered by clinician or dentist; major risk factors including tobacco and excessive alcohol use.	Ulcerative lesion (red or white) on lateral border of tongue, floor of mouth, or other mucosa. Firm non-mobile mass, tooth mobility when no periodontal disease present; cervical lymphadenopathy.
Periodontal Disease	
Red, swollen gums that easily bleed, tender gums, loose teeth, teeth sensitive to temperature.	Plaque and tartar buildup on teeth, deep pockets between teeth and gum margins, loose or missing teeth, halitosis.

PEDIATRIC VARIATIONS

EXAMINATION

Ear and Oral Assessments Are Typically Performed at the End of the Physical Examination. Place Infant in Supine or Prone Position So Head Can Be Turned Side to Side. Position Young Child on Caregiver's Lap

TECHNIQUE	FINDINGS
Ears	
Inspect tympanic membrane	
In infants, pull auricle downward and back to straighten canal.	**EXPECTED:** Tympanic membrane may be mildly red from crying. **UNEXPECTED:** Bulging, limited or absent mobility, drainage in canal.
Assess hearing	
To conduct an informal assessment, use a bell, whisper, or rub your fingers together to create a sound stimulus.	**EXPECTED:** For infants, see table on p. 102. Young children should turn toward sound consistently. When asked, children should repeat words whispered.

Sequences of Expected Hearing and Speech Response in Infants

AGE	RESPONSE
Birth to 3 months	Turns or looks toward voices; quiets or smiles when hearing caregiver voice; makes different sounds if happy or upset; coos, makes sounds "oh," "ah," or "mm"
4–6 months	Reacts to toys that make sounds; giggles and laughs; vocalizes during play using vowel sounds sometimes with a consonant like "da" or "um"
7–9 months	Looks at person calling name; stops in response to "no"; recognizes names of some people and objects; babbles long strings of sounds like "mamama"
10–12 months	Points, waves, and shows or gives objects; imitates or initiates gestures in play like peek-a-boo; tries to copy sounds; responds to words and phrase like "go bye-bye"; says one or two words like "mama" or "dada"

Modified from American Speech-Language-Hearing Association: *Communication Milestones: Birth to 1 Year (asha.org)*. 2024. https://www.asha.org/public/developmental-milestones/communication-milestones-birth-to-1-year/.

TECHNIQUE	FINDINGS

Nose and Sinuses

Evaluate patency of nares

TECHNIQUE	FINDINGS
With infant's mouth closed or with infant sucking on bottle or pacifier, occlude one naris and then the other. Observe respiratory pattern.	**EXPECTED:** Breathes easily; obligatory nose breathing until 2 to 3 months of age. **UNEXPECTED:** Noisy breathing.

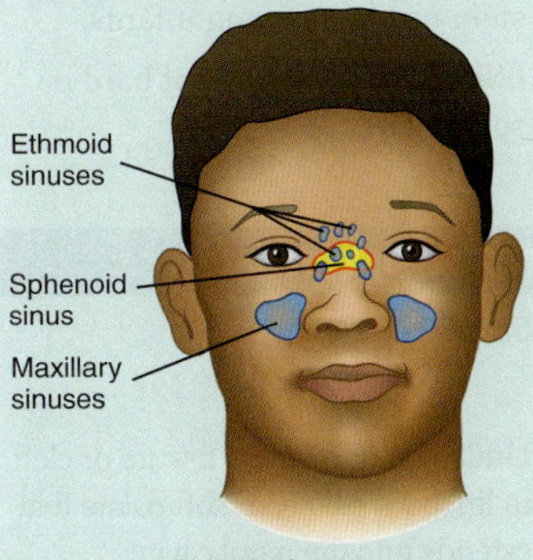

Pediatric sinuses.

TECHNIQUE	FINDINGS
Mouth	
Inspect and palpate lips with mouth closed	
	EXPECTED: Drooling in infants age 6 weeks to 6 months, sucking calluses in newborns.
	UNEXPECTED: Drooling persistent after age 6 months not associated with teething, or drooling beyond 2 years of age.
Inspect teeth	
Ask child to let you see his or her teeth.	**EXPECTED:** Zero to 20 teeth until age 6 years. Permanent teeth start erupting around age 6 years.
	UNEXPECTED: Natal teeth.
Inspect buccal mucosa	
	EXPECTED: In infants, nonadherent white patches (milk).
	UNEXPECTED: In infants, adherent white patches (thrush).
Inspect and palpate gingiva	
	EXPECTED: In infants up to 2 months, pearl-like retention cysts.
Inspect and palpate hard palate	
	EXPECTED: Strong suck and Epstein pearls in young infants.
	UNEXPECTED: No cleft of hard or soft palate.

AIDS TO DIFFERENTIAL DIAGNOSIS

SUBJECTIVE DATA	OBJECTIVE DATA
Cleft Lip and Palate	
Difficulty sucking, formula comes out of nose, failure to gain weight.	Unilateral or bilateral fissure or cleft in lip, hard palate, or soft palate that extends into the nasal cavity.

CHAPTER

11

Chest and Lungs

Equipment

- Drape
- Skin-marking pencil
- Ruler and tape measure
- Stethoscope with bell and diaphragm

EXAMINATION

Have patient sit, disrobed to waist.

TECHNIQUE	FINDINGS
Chest and Lungs	
Inspect Front and Back of Chest	
See thoracic landmarks.	
• *Size/shape/symmetry*	
• *Landmarks*	**EXPECTED:** Supernumerary nipples possible (can be clue to other congenital abnormalities, particularly in white individuals).
• *Compare anteroposterior diameter with transverse diameter*	**EXPECTED:** Ribs prominent, clavicles prominent superiorly, sternum usually flat and free of abundance of overlying tissue. Chest somewhat asymmetric. Anteroposterior diameter often half of transverse diameter.
	UNEXPECTED: Barrel chest, posterior or lateral deviation, pigeon chest, or funnel chest.
• *Assess nails, lips, nares*	**UNEXPECTED:** Clubbed fingernails (usually symmetric and painless; may indicate disease, may be hereditary), pursed lips, flared alae nasi.

TECHNIQUE	FINDINGS
• *Color* Assess skin, lips, and nails.	**UNEXPECTED:** Superficial venous patterns. Cyanosis or pallor of lips or nails.
• *Breath*	**UNEXPECTED:** Malodorous.

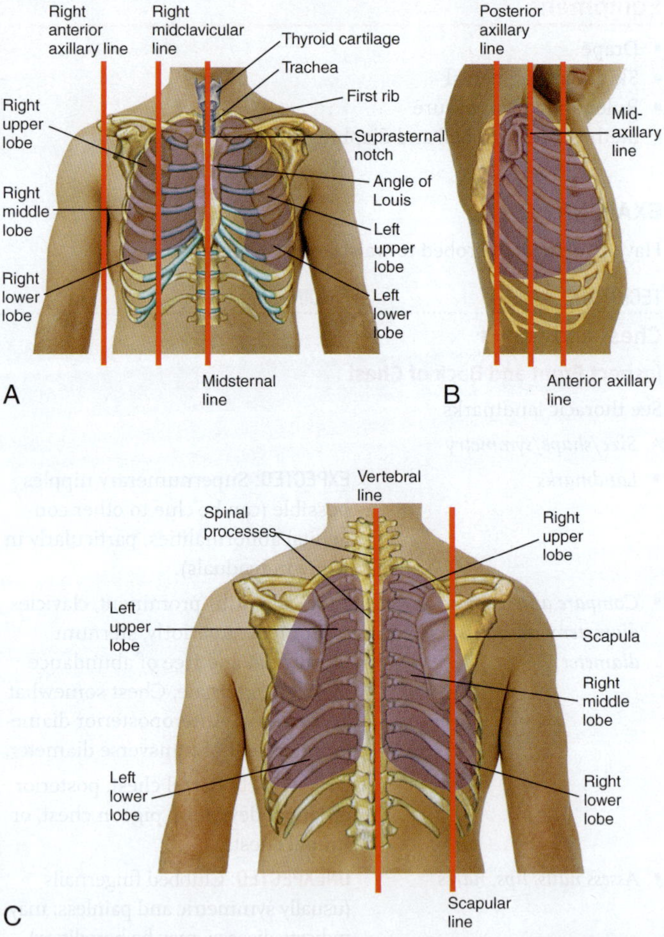

*Thoracic landmarks. (**A**) Anterior thorax. (**B**) Right lateral thorax. (**C**) Posterior thorax.*

TECHNIQUE	FINDINGS

Evaluate respirations

- *Rhythm or pattern and rate*
  See patterns of respiration in the following figure.

EXPECTED: Breathing easy, regular, without distress. Pattern even. Rate 12–16 respirations/min. Ratio of respirations to heartbeats about 1:4.
UNEXPECTED: Dyspnea, orthopnea, paroxysmal nocturnal dyspnea, platypnea, tachypnea, hypopnea. Use of accessory muscles, retractions.

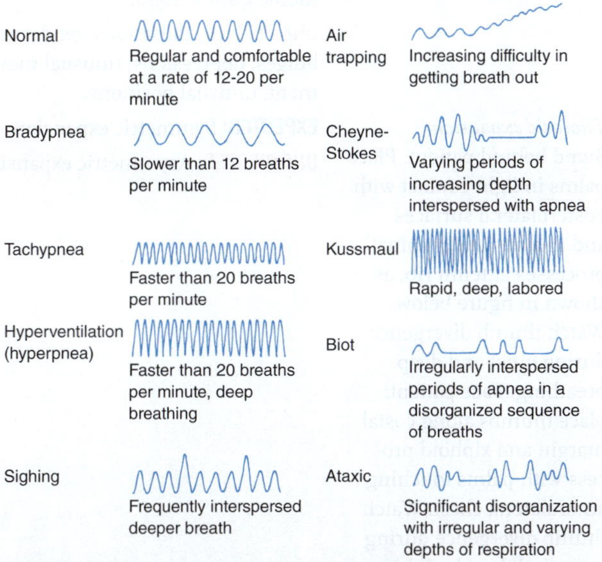

Patterns of respiration. The horizontal axis indicates the relative rates of these patterns. The vertical swings of the lines indicate the relative depth of respiration.

- *Inspiration/expiration ratio*

UNEXPECTED: Air trapping, prolonged expiration.

Inspect chest movement with breathing

- *Symmetry*

EXPECTED: Chest expansion bilaterally symmetric.
UNEXPECTED: Asymmetry. Unilateral or bilateral bulging. Bulging on expiration.

TECHNIQUE	FINDINGS
Listen to respiration sounds audible without stethoscope	
	EXPECTED: Generally bronchovesicular. **UNEXPECTED:** Crepitus, stridor, wheezes.
Palpate thoracic muscles and skeleton	
• *Symmetry/condition*	**EXPECTED:** Bilateral symmetry. Some elasticity of rib cage, but sternum and xiphoid relatively inflexible and thoracic spine rigid. **UNEXPECTED:** Pulsations, tenderness, bulges, depressions, unusual movement, unusual positions.
• *Thoracic expansion* Stand behind patient. Place palms in light contact with posterolateral surfaces and thumbs along spinal processes at tenth rib, as shown in figure below. Watch thumb divergence during quiet and deep breathing. Face patient; place thumbs along costal margin and xiphoid process with palms touching anterolateral chest. Watch thumb divergence during quiet and deep breathing.	**EXPECTED:** Symmetric expansion. **UNEXPECTED:** Asymmetric expansion.

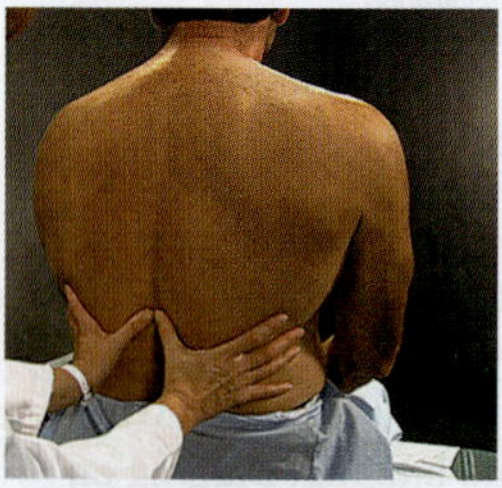

Palpating thoracic expansion. The thumbs are at the level of the tenth rib.

TECHNIQUE	FINDINGS
• *Sensations*	**EXPECTED:** Nontender sensations. **UNEXPECTED:** Crepitus or grating vibration.
• *Tactile fremitus* Ask patient to recite numbers or words while systematically palpating chest with palmar surfaces of fingers or ulnar aspect of clenched fist using firm, light touch. Assess each area, front to back, side to side, lung apices. Compare sides.	**EXPECTED:** Great variability; generally, fremitus is more intense in males (lower pitched voice). **UNEXPECTED:** Decreased or absent fremitus, increased fremitus (coarser, rougher), or gentle, more tremulous fremitus. Variation between similar positions on right and left thorax.

Note position of trachea

Using index finger or thumbs, palpate gently from suprasternal notch along upper edges of each clavicle and in spaces above, to inner borders of sternocleidomastoid muscles.	**EXPECTED:** Spaces equal side to side. Trachea midline directly above suprasternal notch. Possible slight deviation to right. **UNEXPECTED:** Significant deviation or tug. Pulsations.

Perform percussion on chest

Percuss as shown in the following figure. Compare all areas bilater—ally, following a sequence, such as that shown in figures on p. 109. See table on p. 109 for common tones, intensity, pitch, duration, and quality.

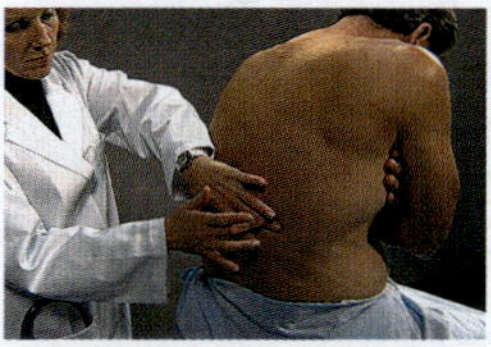

Method for percussion.

TECHNIQUE FINDINGS

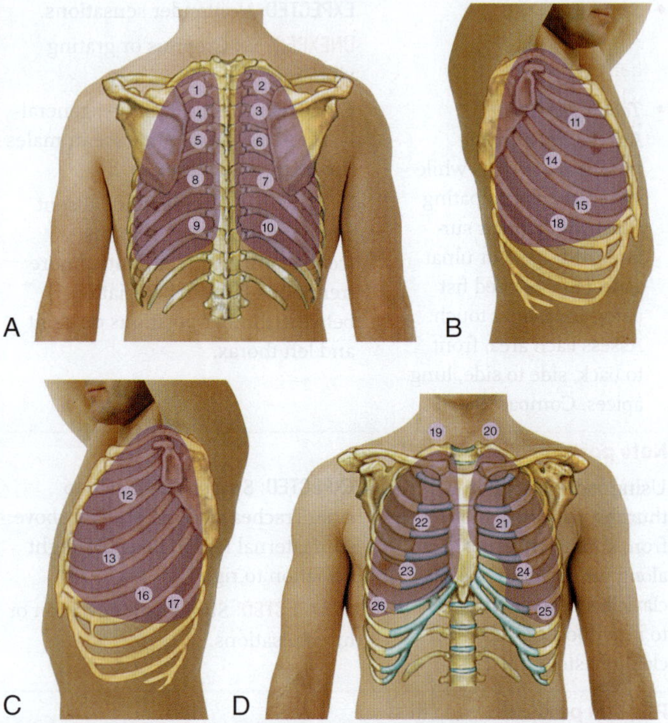

*Suggested sequence for systematic percussion and auscultation of the thorax. (**A**) Posterior thorax. (**B**) Right lateral thorax. (**C**) Left lateral thorax. (**D**) Anterior thorax. The pleximeter finger or the stethoscope is moved in the numeric sequence suggested; however, other sequences are possible.*

Percussion Tones Heard Over the Chest

TYPE OF TONE	INTENSITY	PITCH	DURATION	QUALITY
Resonant	Loud	Low	Long	Hollow
Flat	Soft	High	Short	Extremely dull
Dull	Medium	Medium-high	Medium	Thudlike
Tympanic	Loud	High	Medium	Drumlike
Hyperresonant*	Very loud	Very low	Longer	Booming

*Hyperresonance is unexpected in adults. It represents air trapping, which occurs in obstructive lung diseases.

TECHNIQUE	FINDINGS
• *Thorax* Have patient sit with head bent and arms folded in front while percussing posterior thorax, then with arms raised overhead while percussing lateral and anterior chest. Percuss at 4- to 5-cm intervals over intercostal spaces, moving superior to inferior, medial to lateral. The female breast may obscure findings. You or patient may need to shift the breast but pay careful attention to modesty.	EXPECTED: Resonance over all areas of lungs, dull over heart and liver, spleen, and areas of thorax. UNEXPECTED: Hyperresonance, dullness, or flatness.
• *Diaphragmatic excursion* Ask patient to breathe deeply and hold breath. Percuss along scapular line on one side until tone changes from resonant to dull. Mark skin. Allow patient to breathe normally, then repeat on other side. Have patient take **several** breaths, then exhale as much as possible and hold. On each side, percuss up from mark to change from dull to resonant. Tell patient to resume breathing comfortably. Measure excursion distance.	EXPECTED: 3 to 5 cm (higher on right than left). UNEXPECTED: Limited descent. 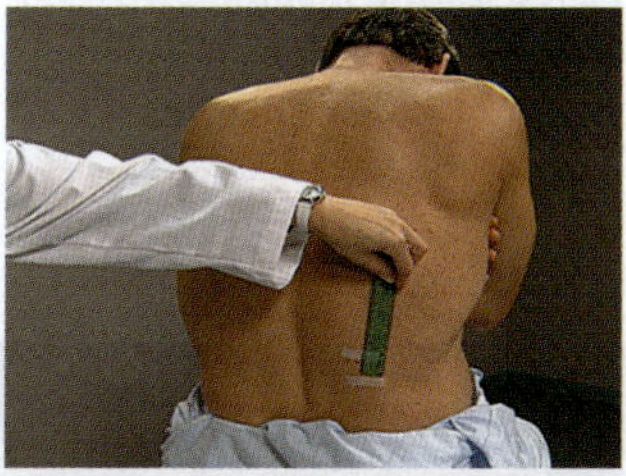 *Measuring diaphragmatic excursion. Excursion distance is usually 3 to 5 cm.*

TECHNIQUE	FINDINGS
Auscultate chest with stethoscope diaphragm, apex to base	
• *Intensity, pitch, duration, and quality of breath sounds* Have patient breathe slowly and deeply through mouth. Follow set auscultation sequence, holding stethoscope as shown in the following figure. • Ask patient to sit upright: 1. with head bent and arms folded in front while auscultating posterior thorax. 2. with arms raised overhead while auscultating lateral chest. 3. with arms down and shoulders back while auscultating anterior chest. Listen during inspiration and expiration. Auscultate downward from apex to base at intervals of several centimeters, making side-to-side comparisons.	**EXPECTED:** See expected breath sounds in table on p. 112. **UNEXPECTED:** Amphoric or cavernous breathing. Sounds difficult to hear or absent. Crackles, rhonchi, wheezes, or pleural friction rub, as described in box on pp. 112–113.

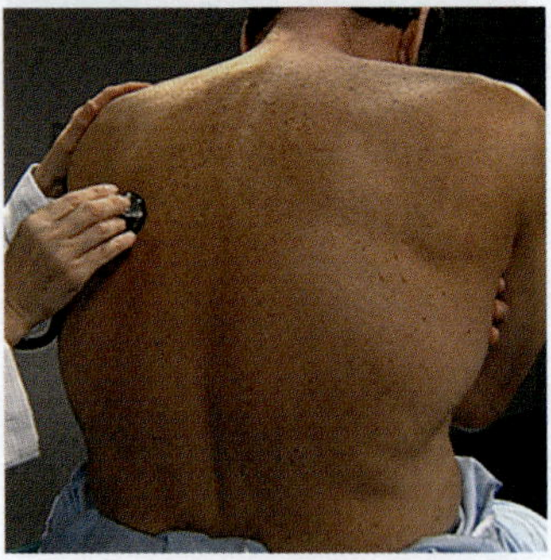

Auscultation with a stethoscope.

TECHNIQUE	FINDINGS
• *Vocal resonance* Ask patient to recite numbers or words.	**EXPECTED:** Muffled and indistinct sounds. **UNEXPECTED:** Bronchophony, whispered pectoriloquy, or egophony.

Characteristics of Expected Breath Sounds

SOUND	CHARACTERISTICS	FINDINGS
Vesicular	Heard over most of lung fields; low pitch; soft and short expirations; will be accentuated in a thin person or a child but diminished in an overweight or very muscular patient.	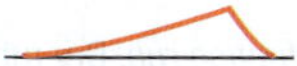
Bronchovesicular	Heard over main bronchus area and over upper right posterior lung field; medium pitch; expiration equals inspiration.	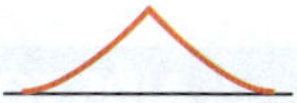
Bronchotracheal (tubular)	Heard only over trachea; high pitch; loud and long expirations, often somewhat longer than inspiration.	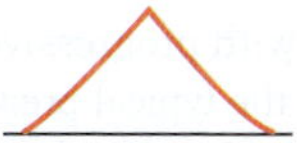

Adventitious Breath Sounds

Fine crackles: High-pitched, discrete, discontinuous crackling sounds heard during end of inspiration; not cleared by cough.

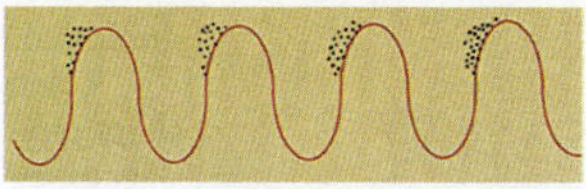

Medium crackles: Lower, more moist sound heard during midstage of inspiration; not cleared by cough.

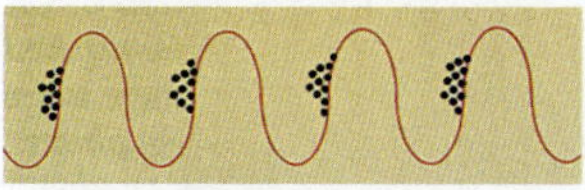

Coarse crackles: Loud, bubbly noise heard during inspiration; not cleared by cough.

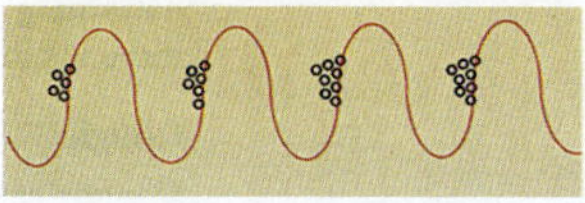

Continued

Rhonchi (sonorous wheeze): Loud, low, coarse sounds, like a snore, most often heard continuously during inspiration or expiration; coughing may clear sound (usually means mucus accumulation in trachea or large bronchi).

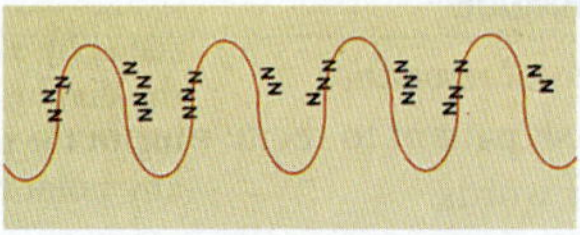

Wheeze (sibilant wheeze): Musical noise sounding like a squeak; most often heard continuously during inspiration or expiration; usually louder during expiration.

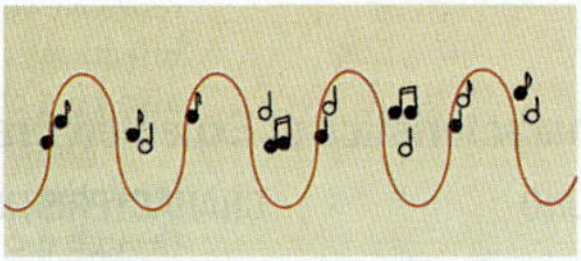

Pleural friction rub: Dry rubbing or grating sound, usually caused by inflammation of pleural surfaces; heard during inspiration or expiration; loudest over lower lateral anterior surface.

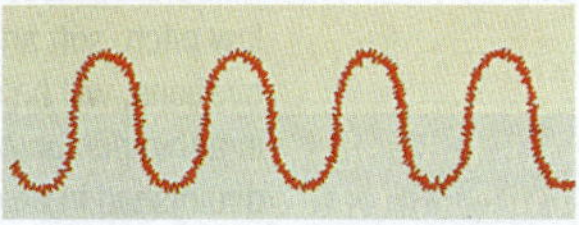

AIDS TO DIFFERENTIAL DIAGNOSIS

SUBJECTIVE DATA	OBJECTIVE DATA
Pleural Effusion	
Cough with progressive dyspnea is the typical presenting concern. Pleuritic chest pain occurs with an inflammatory effusion.	Findings on auscultation and percussion vary in the amount of fluid present and in the position of the patient. These include dullness to percussion and tactile fremitus, which are the most useful findings for pleural effusion. When the fluid is mobile, it will gravitate to the most dependent position. In the affected areas, the breath sounds are muted, and the percussion note is often hyperresonant in the area above the perfusion.

SUBJECTIVE DATA	OBJECTIVE DATA
Lung Cancer	
Cough, wheezing, a variety of patterns of emphysema and atelectasis, pneumonitis, and hemoptysis. Peripheral tumors without airway obstruction may be asymptomatic.	Findings are based on the extent of the tumor and the patterns of its invasion and metastasis. With airway obstruction, a postobstructive pneumonia can develop with consolidation. A malignant pleural effusion may develop with corresponding findings.
Pneumonia	
Rapid onset (hours to days) of cough, pleuritic chest pain, and dyspnea. Sputum production is common with bacterial infection (see table on p. 115). Chills, fever, rigors, and nonspecific abdominal symptoms of nausea and vomiting may be present. Involvement of the right lower lobe can stimulate the 10th and 11th thoracic nerves to cause right lower quadrant pain and simulate an abdominal process.	Febrile, tachypneic, and tachycardic. Crackles and rhonchi are common with diminished breath sounds. Egophony, bronchophony, and whispered pectoriloquy. Dullness to percussion occurs over the area of consolidation.
Asthma	
Episodes of paroxysmal dyspnea and cough. Chest pain is common and includes a feeling of tightness. Episodes may last for minutes, hours, or days. May be asymptomatic between episodes.	Tachypnea with wheezing on expiration and inspiration. Expiration becomes more prolonged with labored breathing, fatigue, and anxious expression as airway resistance increases. Hypoxemia by pulse oximetry.

SUBJECTIVE DATA	OBJECTIVE DATA
Chronic Bronchitis	
Dyspnea may be present, although not severe. Cough and sputum production are impressive.	Wheezing and crackles. Hyperinflation with decreased breath sounds and a flattened diaphragm. Severe chronic bronchitis may result in right ventricular failure with dependent edema.
Emphysema	
Dyspnea is common even at rest. Cough is infrequent without much production of sputum.	Chest may be barrel shaped, and scattered crackles or wheezes may be heard. Overinflated lungs are hyperresonant on percussion. Inspiration is limited with a prolonged expiratory effort (i.e., >4 or 5 seconds) to expel air.

Assessing Sputum

CAUSE	POSSIBLE SPUTUM CHARACTERISTICS
Bacterial infection	Yellow, green, rust colored (blood mixed with yellow sputum), clear, or transparent; purulent; blood streaked; mucoid, viscid
Viral infection	Mucoid, viscid; blood streaked (not common)
Chronic infectious disease	All of the above; particularly abundant in early morning; slight, intermittent blood streaking; occasionally large amounts of blood
Carcinoma	Slight, persistent blood streaking
Infarction	Blood clotted; large amounts of blood
Tuberculous cavity	Large amounts of blood

PEDIATRIC VARIATIONS

EXAMINATION

TECHNIQUE	FINDINGS
Chest and Lungs	
Inspect Front and Back of Chest	
• *Compare anteroposterior diameter with transverse diameter*	**EXPECTED:** Infant's chest is expected to measure 2 to 3 cm less than head circumference.
Evaluate respirations	
• *Rhythm or pattern and rate*	**EXPECTED:**
Perform direct or indirect percussion on chest	
• *Thorax*	**EXPECTED:** Hyperresonance may be heard in children.
Auscultate chest with stethoscope diaphragm, apex to base	
• *Intensity, pitch, duration, and quality of breath sounds*	**EXPECTED:** In infants and children, expect transmitted breath sounds throughout chest. Vesicular sound is accentuated in a child, making absent or diminished breath sounds harder to detect.

Respirations expected (Evaluate respirations):

Age (years)	*Respirations/Min*
Newborn	30 to 80
1	20 to 40
3	20 to 30
6	16 to 22
10	16 to 20
17	12 to 16

CHAPTER

12 Heart

Equipment

- Tangential light source
- Skin-marking pencil
- Stethoscope with bell and diaphragm
- Centimeter ruler

EXAMINATION

TECHNIQUE	FINDINGS
Heart	
Inspect precordium	
Have patient supine and keep light source tangential. • *Apical impulse*	**EXPECTED:** Visible about midclavicular line in fifth left intercostal space. Sometimes visible only with patient sitting. **UNEXPECTED:** Visible in more than one intercostal space; exaggerated lifts or heaves.
Palpate precordium	
• *Apical impulse* Have patient supine. With warm hands, gently feel precordium using proximal halves of fingers held together or whole hand, as shown in figure. Methodically move from apex to left sternal border, base, right sternal border, epigastrium, axillae.	**EXPECTED:** Gentle, brief impulse, palpable within radius of ≤1 cm, although often not felt. **UNEXPECTED:** Heave or lift, loss of thrust, displacement to right or left and/or inferiorly; thrill.

TECHNIQUE	FINDINGS
Locate sensation in terms of its intercostal space and relationship to midsternal, midclavicular, axillary lines.	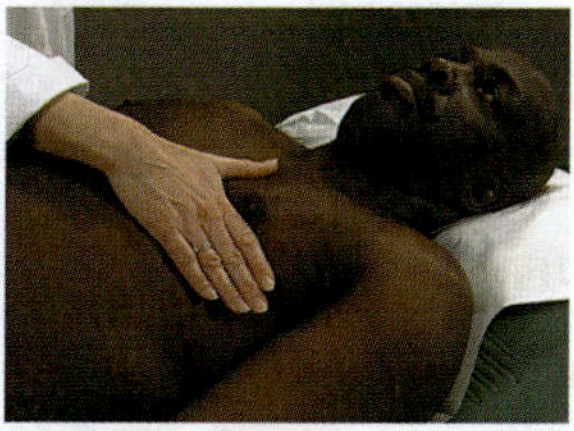

Percuss precordium (optional)

Begin by tapping at anterior axillary line, moving medially along intercostal spaces toward sternal borders until tone changes from resonance to dullness. Mark skin with marking pen.

EXPECTED: No change in tone before right sternal border; on left, loss of resonance generally close to point of maximal impulse at fifth intercostal space. Loss of resonance may outline left border of heart at second to fifth intercostal spaces.

Auscultate heart

Make certain patient is warm and relaxed. Isolate each sound and each pause in cycle, then inch along with stethoscope. Systematically approach each of the five precordial areas, base to apex or apex to base, using each position shown in figures at right and below. Use diaphragm of stethoscope first, with firm pressure, then bell, with light pressure.

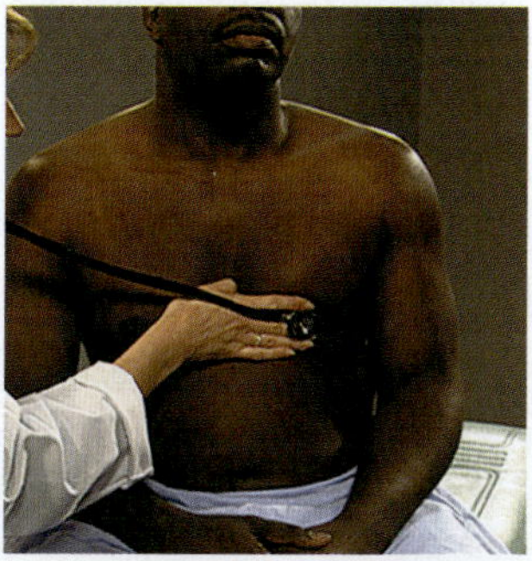

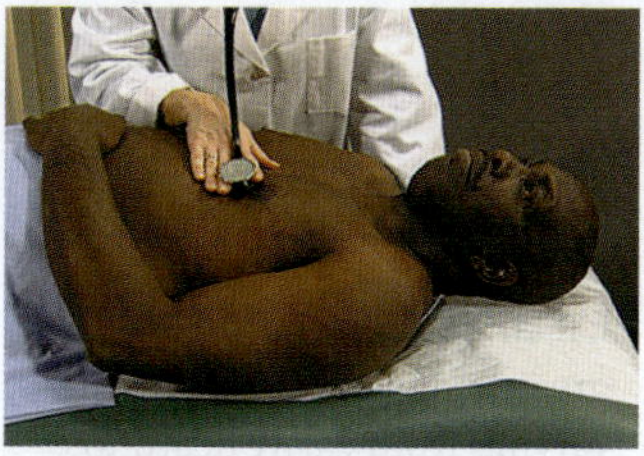

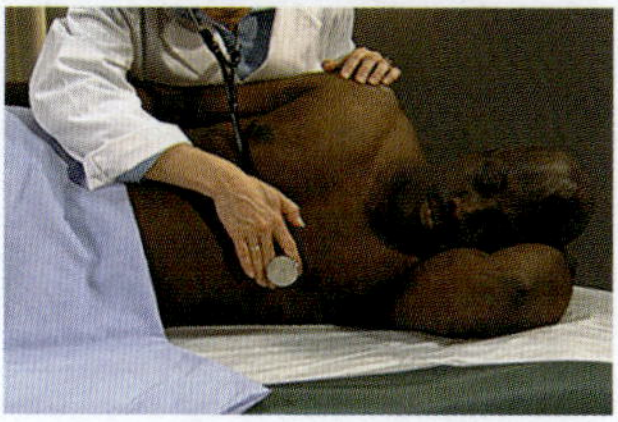

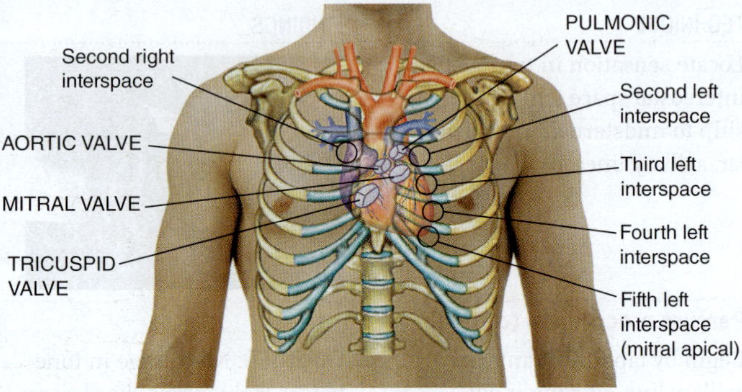

TECHNIQUE	FINDINGS
• *Rate and rhythm* Assess overall rate and rhythm.	**EXPECTED:** Rate 60 to 90 bpm, regular rhythm. **UNEXPECTED:** Bradycardia, tachycardia, dysrhythmia.
• *S1* Ask patient to breathe comfortably then hold breath in expiration. Listen for S1 (best heard toward apex) while palpating carotid pulse. Note intensity, variations, effect of respiration, splitting. Concentrate on systole, then diastole.	**EXPECTED:** S1 usually heard as one sound and coincides with rise of carotid pulse. See table on p. 119. **UNEXPECTED:** Extra sounds or murmurs.
• *S2* Ask patient to breathe comfortably as you listen for S2 (best heard in aortic and pulmonic areas) to become two components during inspiration. Ask patient to inhale and hold breath.	**EXPECTED:** S2 to become two components during inspiration. S2 to become an apparent single sound as breath is exhaled. See table on p. 119.
• *S2 splitting*	**EXPECTED:** S2 splitting—greatest at peak of inspiration—varying from easily heard to nondetectable.

TECHNIQUE	FINDINGS
• *S3 and S4* If needed, ask patient to raise a leg to increase venous return, or to grip your hand vigorously and repeatedly to increase venous return.	**EXPECTED:** Both S3 and S4 quiet and difficult to hear. S3 has rhythm of Kentucky; S4, Tennessee. **UNEXPECTED:** Increased intensity (and ease of hearing) of either.
• *Extra heart sounds*	**UNEXPECTED:** Extra heart sounds—snaps, clicks, friction rubs, murmurs. See the following table.

Assess characteristics of murmurs

Timing and duration, pitch, intensity, pattern, quality, location, radiation, respiratory phase variations.

Heart Sounds According to Auscultatory Area

	AORTIC	PULMONIC	SECOND PULMONIC	MITRAL	TRICUSPID
Pitch	S1 < S2	S1 < S2	S1 < S2	S1 > S2	S1 = S2
Loudness	S1 < S2	S1 < S2	S1 < S2*	S1 > S2†	S1 > S2
Duration	S1 < S2	S1 > S2	S1 < S2	S1 < S2	S1 = S2
S2 split	>Inhale <Exhale	>Inhale <Exhale	>Inhale <Exhale	>Inhale‡ <Exhale	>Inhale <Exhale
A2	Loudest	Loud	Decreased		
P2	Decreased	Louder	Loudest		

*S1 is relatively louder in second pulmonic area than in aortic area.
†S1 may be louder in mitral area than in tricuspid area.
‡S2 split may not be audible in mitral area if P2 is inaudible.

Extra Heart Sounds

SOUND	DETECTION	DESCRIPTION
Increased S3	Bell at apex; patient left lateral recumbent	Early diastole, low pitch
Increased S4	Bell at apex; patient supine or semilateral	Late diastole or early systole, low pitch
Gallops	Bell at apex; patient supine or left lateral recumbent	Presystole, intense, easily heard

Continued

Extra Heart Sounds—cont'd

SOUND	DETECTION	DESCRIPTION
Mitral valve opening snap	Diaphragm medial to apex, may radiate to base; any position, second left intercostal	Early diastole briefly, before S3; high pitch, sharp snap or click; not affected by respiration; easily confused with S2
Ejection clicks	Diaphragm; patient sitting or supine	
Aortic valve	Diaphragm, right second intercostal space	Early systole, intense, high pitch; radiates, not affected by respirations
Pulmonary valve	Diaphragm; left second intercostal right space	Early systole, less intense than aortic click; intensifies on expiration, decreases on inspiration
Pericardial friction rub	Diaphragm, widely heard, sound clearest toward apex	May occupy all of systole and diastole; intense, grating, machinelike; may have three components and obliterate heart sounds; if only one or two components, may sound like murmur

AIDS TO DIFFERENTIAL DIAGNOSIS

SUBJECTIVE DATA	OBJECTIVE DATA
Left Ventricular Hypertrophy	
Initially asymptomatic, may cause shortness of breath or chest pain.	Vigorous, sustained lift palpable during ventricular systole, sometimes over broader area than usual (by ≥2 cm). Displacement of apical impulse can be well lateral of midclavicular line and downward.

SUBJECTIVE DATA	OBJECTIVE DATA
Right Ventricular Hypertrophy	
Fatigue, shortness of breath, syncope may indicate more severe disease.	Lift along left sternal border in third and fourth left intercostal spaces accompanied by occasional systolic retraction at apex. Left ventricle displaced and turned posteriorly by enlarged right ventricle.
Congestive Heart Failure	
May Be Left or Right Sided: Left Sided is Either Systolic or Diastolic	
Fatigue, orthopnea, shortness of breath, edema.	Congestion in pulmonary or systemic circulation. Can develop gradually or suddenly with acute pulmonary or systemic edema.
Cor Pulmonale	
Tachypnea, fatigue, exertional dyspnea, cough hemoptysis.	Left parasternal systolic lift and loud S2 in pulmonic region, evidence of pulmonary disease.
Myocardial Infarction	
Deep substernal or visceral pain, often radiating to jaw, neck, left arm (although discomfort is sometimes mild); women may experience milder and different symptoms.	Dysrhythmias; S4 often present. Heart sounds distant, with soft, systolic, blowing murmur; pulse possibly thready; varied blood pressure (although hypertension usual in early phases).
Myocarditis	
Initially symptoms vague; fatigue, dyspnea, fever, palpitations. Symptoms may progress.	Cardiac enlargement, murmur, gallop rhythms, tachycardia, dysrhythmias, pulsus alternans.
Conduction Disturbances	
Transient weakness, syncope, stroke-like episodes, palpitations.	Labile heart rates.

SUBJECTIVE DATA	OBJECTIVE DATA
Atherosclerotic Heart Disease	
May be asymptomatic or cause angina pectoris, shortness of breath, and palpitations.	May cause myocardial insufficiency, dysrhythmias, congestive heart failure.
Angina	
Substernal pain or intense pressure radiating at times to neck, jaws, arms, particularly left arm, often accompanied by shortness of breath, fatigue, diaphoresis, faintness, syncope. Cessation of activity may relieve pain.	No pathognomonic examination findings, tachycardia, hypertension, diaphoresis, decreased S1 intensity, S4.

Chest Pain

TYPE OF CHEST PAIN	CHARACTERISTICS
Anginal	Substernal; provoked by effort, emotion, eating; relieved by rest and/or nitroglycerin
Pleural	Precipitated by breathing or coughing; usually described as sharp
Esophageal	Burning, substernal, occasional radiation to shoulder; nocturnal occurrence, usually when lying flat; relief with food, antacids, sometimes nitroglycerin
From a peptic ulcer	Almost always infradiaphragmatic and epigastric; nocturnal occurrence and daytime attacks; should not be relieved by food; unrelated to activity
Biliary	Usually under right scapula, prolonged in duration; will trigger angina more often than mimic it
From arthritis/bursitis	Usually of hours' long duration; local tenderness and/or pain with movement
Cervical	Associated with injury; provoked by activity, persists after activity; painful on palpation and/or movement
Musculoskeletal (chest)	Intensified or provoked by movement, particularly twisting or costochondral bending; long lasting; often associated with local tenderness
Psychoneurotic	Associated with or occurring after anxiety; poorly described, located in intramammary region

PEDIATRIC VARIATIONS

EXAMINATION

TECHNIQUE	FINDINGS
Assess characteristics of murmurs	
Timing and duration, intensity, pattern, quality, location, radiation, respiratory phase variations.	In children, it is necessary to distinguish innocent murmurs from murmurs caused by congenital defect or infection.

AIDS TO DIFFERENTIAL DIAGNOSIS

SUBJECTIVE DATA	OBJECTIVE DATA
Chest pain	
Unlike in adults, chest pain in children and adolescents is seldom caused by a cardiac problem. It is very often difficult to find a cause; however, trauma, exercise-induced asthma, and use of cocaine, even in a somewhat younger child, as in the adolescent and adult, should be among the considerations.	Examination is usually normal.
Congenital defects	
Tetralogy of Fallot	
Dyspnea with feeding, poor growth, exercise intolerance, tetralogy spells.	Parasternal heave and precordial prominence, cyanosis, systolic ejection murmur heard over third intercostal space, sometimes radiating to left side of neck. Single S2.

HEART

SUBJECTIVE DATA	OBJECTIVE DATA
Ventricular Septal Defect	
Tachypnea, symptoms of right-sided congestive heart failure, poor growth, recurrent respiratory infections.	Arterial pulse small; jugular venous pulse unaffected; regurgitation occurs through septal defect, resulting in holosystolic murmur that is often loud, coarse, high pitched, best heard along left sternal border in third to fifth intercostal spaces. Distinct lift often discernible along left sternal border and apical area. Does not radiate to neck.
Patent Ductus Arteriosus	
Asymptomatic if small; a larger patent ductus arteriosus cause dyspnea on exertion.	Neck vessels dilate and pulsate, and pulse pressure wide. Harsh, loud, continuous murmur with machinelike quality heard at first to third intercostal spaces and lower sternal border. Murmur usually unaltered by postural change.
Atrial Septal Defect	
Often asymptomatic, congestive heart failure in adults.	Systolic ejection murmur best heard over pulmonic area that is diamond-shaped, often loud, high in pitch, and harsh. May be accompanied by brief, rumbling, early diastolic murmur. Does not usually radiate beyond precordium. Systolic thrill may be felt over area of murmur along with palpable parasternal thrust. S2 may be split fairly widely. Particularly significant with palpable thrust and occasional radiation through to back.

CHAPTER

13

Blood Vessels

Equipment

- Tangential light source
- Stethoscope with bell and diaphragm
- Sphygmomanometer
- Centimeter ruler

EXAMINATION

TECHNIQUE / **FINDINGS**

Peripheral Arteries

Palpate arterial pulses in neck and extremities

Palpate carotid, brachial, radial, femoral, popliteal, dorsalis pedis, and posterior tibial arteries using distal pads of second and third fingers, as shown in the figures on the following page.

- *Characteristics*
  Compare characteristics bilaterally, as well as between upper and lower extremities.

EXPECTED: Femoral pulse as strong as or stronger than radial pulse.

UNEXPECTED: Femoral pulse weaker than radial pulse or absent. Alternating pulse (pulsus alternans), pulsus bisferiens, bigeminal pulse (pulsus bigeminus), bounding pulse, labile pulse, paradoxical pulse (pulsus paradoxus), pulsus differens, tachycardia, trigeminal pulse (pulsus trigeminus), or water-hammer pulse (Corrigan pulse).

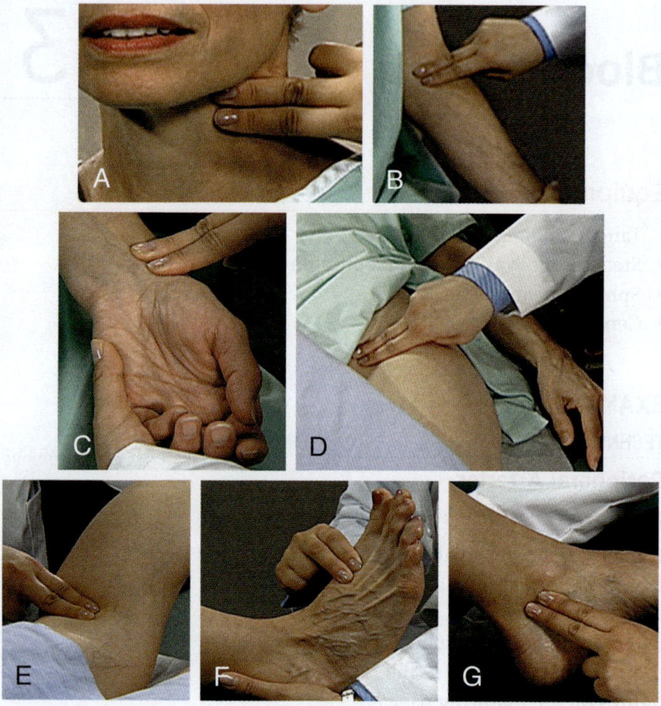

Palpation of arterial pulses: **(A)** carotid, **(B)** brachial, **(C)** radial, **(D)** femoral, **(E)** popliteal, **(F)** dorsalis pedis, and **(G)** posterior tibial.

TECHNIQUE	FINDINGS
• *Rate*	**EXPECTED:** 60–90 bpm. **UNEXPECTED:** Rate different from that observed during cardiac examination.
• *Rhythm*	**EXPECTED:** Regular. **UNEXPECTED:** Irregular, either in a pattern or patternless.
• *Contour*	**EXPECTED:** Smooth, rounded, or dome-shaped.

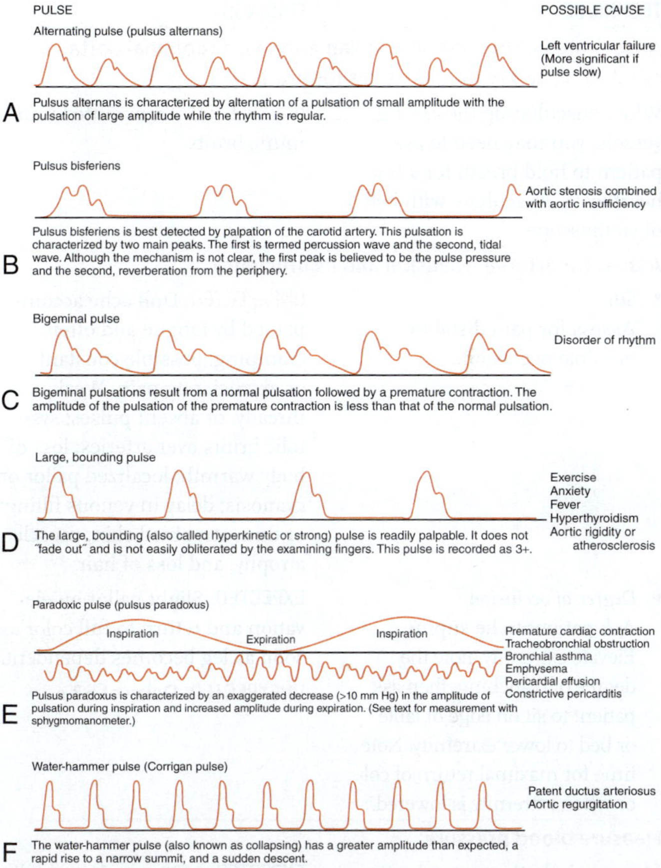

(A–F) Pulse abnormalities.

TECHNIQUE	FINDINGS
• *Amplitude*	**UNEXPECTED:** Bounding, full, diminished, or absent. Describe on a scale of 0–4: 0 = Absent, not palpable 1 = Diminished 2 = Expected 3 = Full, increased 4 = Bounding

TECHNIQUE	FINDINGS

Auscultate carotid and subclavian arteries; abdominal aorta; and renal, iliac, and femoral arteries for bruits

When auscultating the carotid vessels, you may need to ask patient to hold breath for a few heartbeats. Auscultate with bell of stethoscope.	**UNEXPECTED:** Transmitted murmurs, bruits.

Assess for arterial occlusion and insufficiency

• *Site* Assess for pain distal to possible occlusion.	**UNEXPECTED:** Dull ache accompanied by fatigue and often cramping; possible constant or excruciating pain. Weak, thready, or absent pulses; systolic bruits over arteries; loss of body warmth; localized pallor or cyanosis; delay in venous filling; or thin, atrophied skin, muscle atrophy, and loss of hair.
• *Degree of occlusion* Ask patient to lie supine. Elevate extremity, note the degree of blanching, then ask patient to sit on edge of table or bed to lower extremity. Note time for maximal return of color when extremity is lowered.	**EXPECTED:** Slight pallor on elevation and return to full color as soon as leg becomes dependent. **UNEXPECTED:** Delay of >2 s.

Measure blood pressure

Measure in both arms at least once. Patient's arm should be slightly flexed and comfortably supported on a table, pillow, or your hand.	**EXPECTED:** <120 mm Hg systolic and <80 mm Hg diastolic, with pulse pressure of 30–40 mm Hg (sometimes to 50 mm Hg). Reading between arms may vary by as much as 10 mm Hg. Prehypertension is now defined as a blood pressure between 120 and 139 mm Hg systolic or 80 and 89 mm Hg diastolic. **UNEXPECTED:** Hypertension (see Chapter 3).

TECHNIQUE	FINDINGS

Peripheral Veins

Assess jugular venous pressure

Ask patient to recline at 45-degree angle. With tangential light, observe the jugular vein. As shown in the figure, use a centimeter ruler to measure vertical distance between midaxillary line and highest level of jugular vein distention.

EXPECTED: Pressure ≤9 cm H2O, bilaterally symmetric.

UNEXPECTED: Abnormal elevation, distention, or distention on one side.

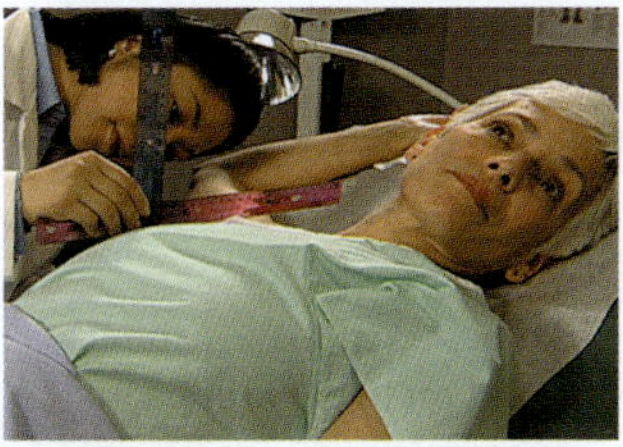

Assess for venous obstruction and insufficiency

Inspect extremities, with patient both standing and supine.

- *Affected area*

  UNEXPECTED: Constant pain with swelling and tenderness over muscles, engorgement of superficial veins, cyanosis.

- *Thrombosis*
  Examine the patient's calf for pain, swelling, erythema.

  UNEXPECTED: Redness, thickening, tenderness along superficial vein. Calf swelling.

- *Edema*
  Press index finger over bony prominence of tibia or medial malleolus for several seconds.

  UNEXPECTED: Orthostatic (pitting) edema; thickening and ulceration of skin possible.

TECHNIQUE	FINDINGS
	Grade edema from 1+ to 4+ as follows: 1+ = Slight pitting, no visible distortion, disappears rapidly 2+ = Deeper than 1+ and disappears in 10–15 s 3+ = Noticeably deep and may last >1 min, with dependent extremity full and swollen 4+ = Very deep and lasts 2–5 min, with grossly distorted dependent extremity
• *Varicose veins* If suspected, have patient stand on toes 10 times in succession.	**EXPECTED:** Pressure from toe standing disappears in seconds. **UNEXPECTED:** Veins dilated and swollen; often tortuous when extremities are dependent and pressure does not quickly disappear.
• *If varicose veins are present, assess venous incompetence with Trendelenburg test:* Ask patient to lie supine, lift leg above heart level until veins empty, then quickly lower leg.	**UNEXPECTED:** Rapid filling of veins.
• *Evaluate patency of deep veins with Perthes test:* Ask patient to lie supine. Elevate extremity and occlude subcutaneous veins with tourniquet just above knee. Then ask patient to walk.	**UNEXPECTED:** Superficial veins fail to empty.

TECHNIQUE	FINDINGS
• *Evaluate direction of blood flow and presence of compensatory circulation:* Put affected limb in dependent position, then empty or strip vein. Release pressure of one finger nearest heart to assess blood flow; if necessary, repeat and release pressure of other finger.	UNEXPECTED: Stripped vessel fills before pressure is released by distal finger, or blood refills entire vein when pressure is released by proximal finger.

AIDS TO DIFFERENTIAL DIAGNOSIS

OBJECTIVE DATA	SUBJECTIVE DATA
Arterial Aneurysm	
Generally asymptomatic until they dissect or compress an adjacent structure. With dissection, the patient may describe a severe ripping pain.	Pulsatile swelling along the course of an artery. Occurs most commonly in the aorta, although renal, femoral, and popliteal arteries are also common sites. A thrill or bruit may be evident over the aneurysm.
Venous Thrombosis	
Tenderness along the iliac vessels or the femoral canal, in the popliteal space, or over the deep calf veins. Deep vein thrombosis in the femoral and pelvic circulations may be asymptomatic. Pulmonary embolism may occur without warning.	Swelling may be distinguished only by measuring and comparing the circumference of the upper and lower legs bilaterally. There may be minimal ankle edema, low-grade fever, and tachycardia. Homan sign can be helpful but is not absolutely reliable in suggesting deep vein thrombosis.

OBJECTIVE DATA	SUBJECTIVE DATA
Raynaud Phenomenon	
Involved areas will feel cold and achy, which improves on rewarming. In secondary Raynaud phenomenon, there can be intense pain and digital ischemia with necrosis at the tips.	With primary Raynaud phenomenon, there is triphasic demarcated skin pallor (*white*), cyanosis (*blue*), and reperfusion (*red*) within the extremities. The vasospasm may last from minutes to less than an hour. In secondary Raynaud phenomenon, ulcers may appear on the tips of the digits, and eventually the skin over the digits can appear smooth, shiny, and tight from loss of subcutaneous tissue.

PEDIATRIC VARIATIONS

EXAMINATION

TECHNIQUE	FINDINGS
Palpate Arterial Pulses in Distal Extremities (see Chapter 3)	
Auscultate arteries for bruits	
	EXPECTED: In children, it is not unusual to hear a venous hum over internal jugular veins. There is usually no pathologic significance.
Measure blood pressure (see Chapter 3)	

AIDS TO DIFFERENTIAL DIAGNOSIS

SUBJECTIVE DATA	OBJECTIVE DATA
Coarctation of the aorta	
Most patients are asymptomatic unless severe hypertension or vascular insufficiency develops. In those settings, patients may experience symptoms of heart failure or vascular insufficiency of an involved upper extremity with activity.	Differences in systolic blood pressure readings when the radial and femoral pulses are palpated simultaneously.

CHAPTER

14 Breasts and Axillae

Equipment

- Ruler (if mass detected)
- Flashlight with transilluminator (if mass detected)
- Glass slide and cytologic fixative (if nipple discharge is present)
- Small pillow or folded towel

EXAMINATION

Describe any breast mass or lump that you encounter using the following characteristics:

- Location: clock positions and distance from nipple
- Size (in centimeters): length, width, thickness
- Shape: round, discoid, lobular, stellate, regular, or irregular
- Consistency: firm, soft, hard
- Tenderness
- Mobility: movable (in what directions) or fixed to overlying skin or subadjacent fascia
- Borders: discrete or poorly defined
- Retraction: presence or absence of dimpling; altered contour

All new solitary or dominant masses must be investigated with further diagnostic testing.

TECHNIQUE	FINDINGS

All Patients

With patient seated and arms hanging loosely, inspect both breasts

Inspect all quadrants and tail of Spence. If necessary, lift breasts with fingertips to expose lower and lateral aspects.

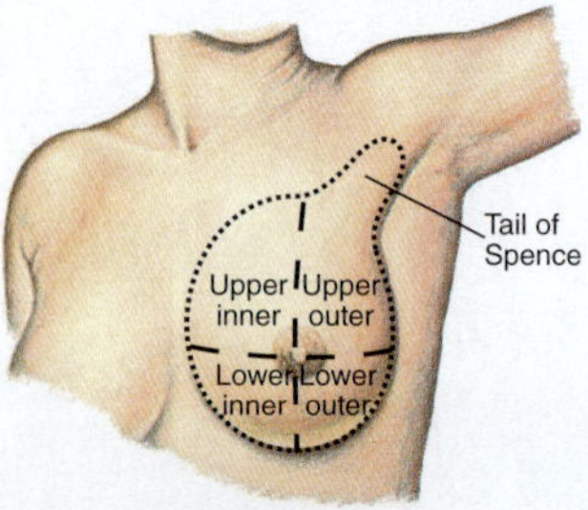

TECHNIQUE	FINDINGS
• *Size/shape/symmetry*	**EXPECTED:** Convex, pendulous, or conical. Long-standing asymmetry in size. Size and shape variations in transgender patients who have undergone gender affirming hormonal therapy or surgical modification. **UNEXPECTED:** Asymmetry in position (nipples point in different directions); new asymmetry in size. Implants that have shifted. Enlargement in cis-male patients.
• *Texture/contour*	**EXPECTED:** Smooth and uninterrupted. **UNEXPECTED:** Dimpling, retraction, or peau d'orange appearance. Changes or asymmetric appearance.
• *Skin color*	**EXPECTED:** Consistent color. **UNEXPECTED:** Areas of discoloration, erythema, or asymmetric appearance.
• *Venous patterns*	**EXPECTED:** Bilateral venous networks, although usually pronounced only in pregnant patients. **UNEXPECTED:** Unilateral network.
• *Markings*	**EXPECTED:** Long-standing nevi. Supernumerary nipples possible (but could signal other congenital abnormalities). **UNEXPECTED:** Changing or tender nevi. Lesions.
Inspect areolae and nipples	
• *Size/shape/symmetry*	**EXPECTED:** Areolae round or oval, bilaterally equal, or nearly equal. Nipples bilaterally equal or nearly equal in size and usually everted; long-standing inversion in one or both nipples. **UNEXPECTED:** Recent unilateral nipple inversion or retraction.

TECHNIQUE	FINDINGS
• *Color*	**EXPECTED:** Areolae and nipples pink to brown. **UNEXPECTED:** Nonhomogeneous in color.
• *Texture/contour*	**EXPECTED:** Areolae smooth, except for Montgomery tubercles. Nipples smooth or wrinkled. **UNEXPECTED:** Areolae with suppurative or tender Montgomery tubercles or with peau d'orange appearance. Nipples crusting, cracking, or with discharge.

Patients With Substantial Breast Tissue

With patient in the following positions, reinspect both breasts

TECHNIQUE	FINDINGS
• *Arms extended overhead or flexed behind the neck* • *Hands pressed on hips with shoulders rolled forward or pushed together in front* • *Seated and leaning over* • *Recumbent*	**EXPECTED:** All positions breasts bilaterally symmetric with even contour. **UNEXPECTED:** Dimpling, retraction, deviation, or fixation of breasts.

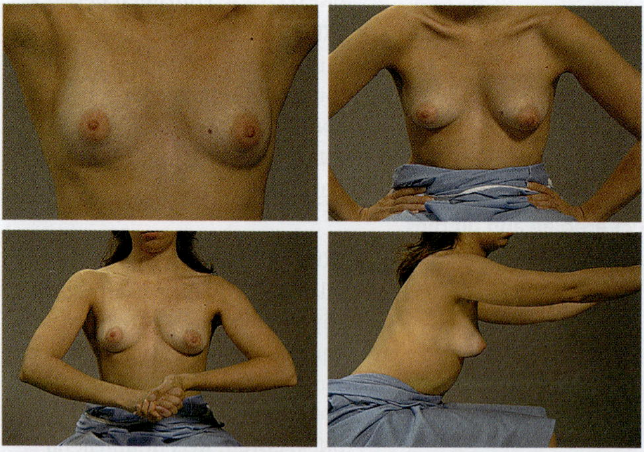

TECHNIQUE	FINDINGS

With patient seated and arms hanging loosely, palpate breasts

- *Chest wall sweep*
  Place the palm of your right hand at the patient's right clavicle at the sternum. Sweep downward from the clavicle to the nipple, feeling for superficial lumps. Repeat the sweep until you have covered the entire right chest wall. Repeat the procedure using your left hand for the left chest wall.

EXPECTED: Tissue smooth, free of lumps.

UNEXPECTED: Lumps or nodules. Reassess with additional palpation and characterize any masses by location, size, shape, consistency, tenderness, mobility, delineation of borders, and retraction. Use transillumination to assess presence of fluid in masses.

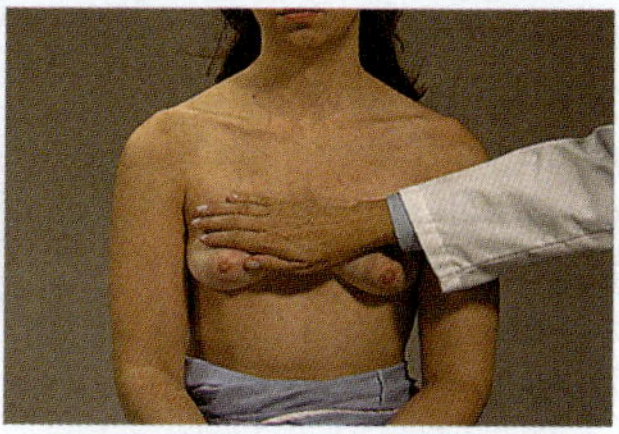

- *Bimanual digital palpation*
  Place one hand, palmar surface facing up, under the patient's right breast. Position your hand so that it acts as a flat surface against which to compress the breast tissue. Walk the fingers of the other hand across the breast tissue, feeling for lumps as you compress the tissue between your fingers and your flat hand. Repeat the procedure for the other breast.

EXPECTED: Tissue generally firm, nontender, and free of lumps. During menstrual cycle, cyclic pattern of breast enlargement, increased nodularity, and tenderness.

UNEXPECTED: Lumps or nodules. Reassess with additional palpation and characterize any masses by location, size, shape, consistency, tenderness, mobility, delineation of borders, and retraction. Use transillumination to assess presence of fluid in masses.

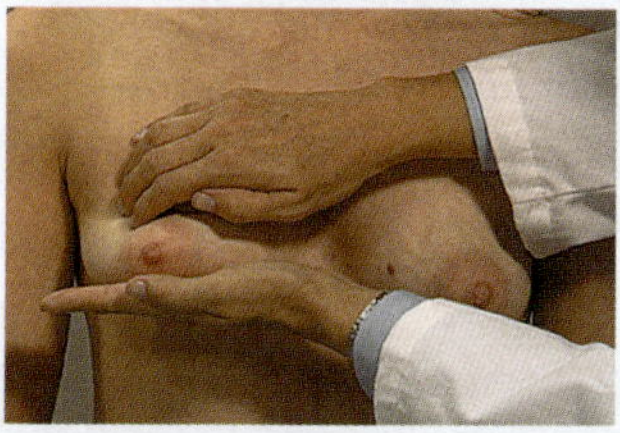

TECHNIQUE	FINDINGS

All Patients

With patient seated, palpate for lymph nodes

- *Axillary*
  Support patient's forearm with your contralateral arm and bring palm of examining hand flat into axilla. With palmar surface of fingers, reach deep into hollow, pushing firmly upward, then bring fingers down, rotating your fingers and gently rolling soft tissue against chest wall and axilla. Explore apex, medial, lateral aspects along rib cage; lateral aspects along upper surface of arm; and anterior and posterior walls of axilla. Repeat mirror image of this maneuver for the other axilla.

  EXPECTED: Nodes not palpable.
  UNEXPECTED: Nodes, especially in supraclavicular area. Describe nodes by location, size, shape, consistency, tenderness, fixation, delineation of borders.

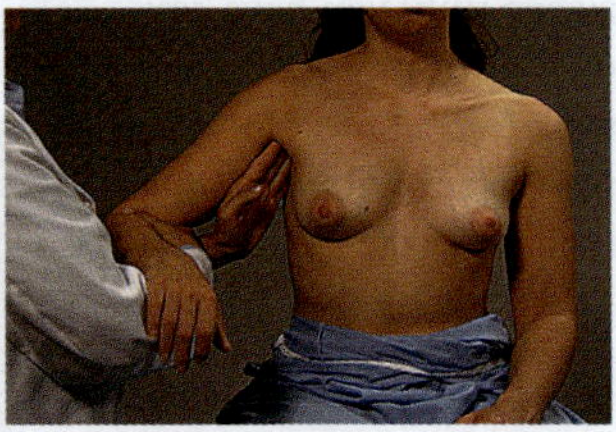

- *Supraclavicular area*
  Hook fingers over clavicle and rotate over supraclavicular fossa while patient turns head toward same side and raises shoulder.
- *Infraclavicular area*
  Palpate along the clavicle using a rotary motion with your fingers.

TECHNIQUE	FINDINGS
With patient supine, palpate breast tissue	
Have patient put one hand behind head. Place a towel under shoulder on same side. Compress breast tissue between fingers and chest wall using rotary motion of fingers. Using finger pads, systematically palpate each breast in all four quadrants, including tail of Spence and over areolae. Push gently but firmly toward chest while rotating fingers clockwise or counterclockwise, following a vertical strip, concentric circle, or wedge pattern. Press inward at each point using three depths of palpation: light, medium, and deep.	**EXPECTED:** Breast composition in people assigned female at birth: generally dense, firm, elastic, but sometimes lobular. May be fine and granular in older patients. Inframammary ridge may be felt along lower edge of breast. During menstrual cycle, cyclic pattern of breast enlargement, increased nodularity, and tenderness. Implants may be present. Breast composition in people assigned male at birth: Thin layer of fatty tissue overlying muscle. A thick layer in obesity may give appearance of breast enlargement. Firm disk of glandular tissue sometimes evident. **UNEXPECTED:** Lumps or nodules, hardened tissue. Characterize any masses by location, size, shape, consistency, tenderness, mobility, delineation of borders, and retraction. Use transillumination to assess presence of fluid in masses. Implants that have ruptured or contracted.
Return to the nipple and, with two fingers, gently depress the tissue inward into the well behind the areola. Repeat palpation maneuvers for other breast.	**EXPECTED:** Fingers and tissue move easily inward. **UNEXPECTED:** Lump, mass; absence of well behind areola.

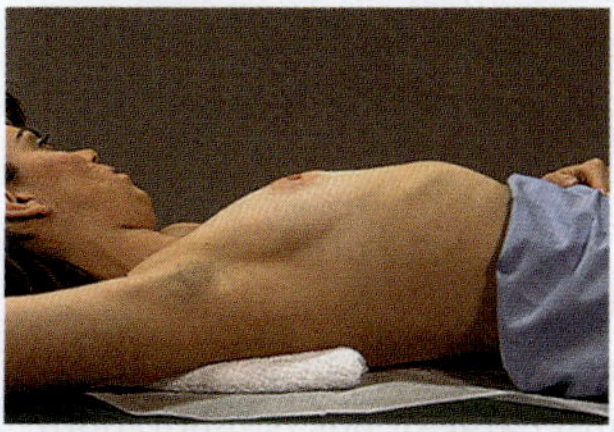

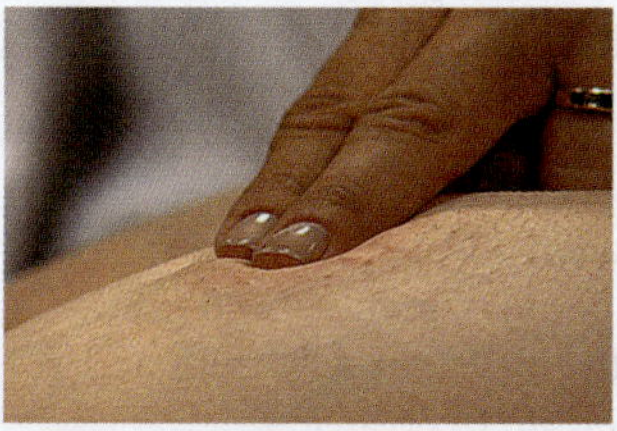

AIDS TO DIFFERENTIAL DIAGNOSIS

SUBJECTIVE DATA	OBJECTIVE DATA
Fibrocystic Changes	
Tender and painful breasts and/or palpable lumps that fluctuate with menses; usually worse premenstrually.	Round, soft to firm, tense, mobile masses with well-delineated borders; usually tender; usually bilateral; multiple or single.
Fibroadenoma	
Painless lumps that do not fluctuate with the menstrual cycle; may be asymptomatic with discovery on clinical breast examination or mammogram.	Round or discoid, firm, rubbery, mobile masses with well-delineated borders; usually nontender, bilateral, single; may be multiple; biopsy often performed to rule out carcinoma.
Malignant Breast Tumors	
Painless lump, change in size, shape, or contour of breast; axilla may be tender if lymph nodes involved; may be asymptomatic with discovery on clinical breast examination or mammogram.	Palpable mass that is usually single, unilateral, irregular, or stellate in shape; poorly delineated borders; fixed, hard, stonelike, and nontender; breast may have dimpling, retraction, prominent vasculature; skin may have peau d'orange or thickened appearance; nipple may be inverted or deviate in position.
Intraductal Papillomas and Papillomatosis	
Spontaneous nipple discharge, usually unilateral; usually serous or bloody.	Single-duct unilateral nipple discharge provoked on physical examination.
Gynecomastia	
Breast enlargement in male individuals.	Smooth, firm, mobile, tender disk of breast tissue behind areola, unilaterally or bilaterally.
Mastitis	
Sudden onset of swelling, tenderness, redness, and heat in the breast; usually chills and fever.	Tender, hard breast mass, with an area of fluctuation, erythema, and heat; may have discharge of pus (suppuration).

PEDIATRIC VARIATIONS

EXAMINATION

TECHNIQUE	FINDINGS
Palpate and compress nipples	
	EXPECTED: Breast enlargement is not unusual in newborns. "Witch's milk" may be expressed.
Assess stage of pubertal development	
In patients assigned female at birth assess the stage of breast development.	**EXPECTED:** The duration and tempo of each stage and sequence are quite variable between individuals. Findings may vary in transgender patients taking puberty blockers. **UNEXPECTED:** Failure to mature or premature maturation.

M_1—Tanner 1 (preadolescent). Only the nipple is raised above the level of the breast, as in the child.

M_2—Tanner 2. Budding stage; bud-shaped elevation of the areola; areola increased in diameter and surrounding area slightly elevated.

M_3—Tanner 3. Breast and areola enlarged. No contour separation.

M_4—Tanner 4. Increasing fat deposits. The areola forms a secondary elevation above that of the breast. This secondary mound occurs in approximately half of all girls and in some cases persists in adulthood.

M_5—Tanner 5 (adult stage). The areola is (usually) part of general breast contour and is strongly pigmented. Nipple projects.

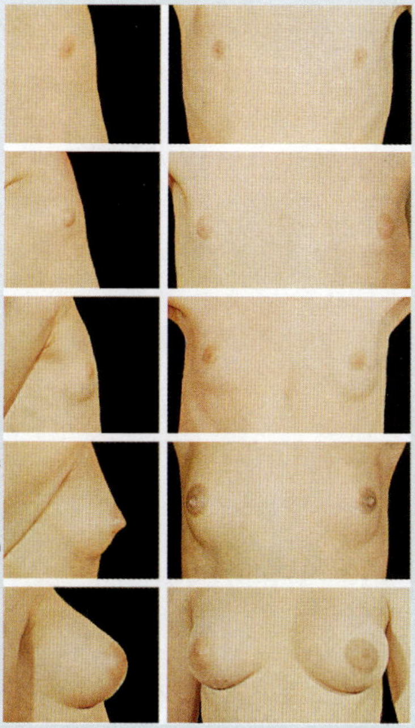

Five stages of breast development in females. (Growth diagrams from Van Wieringen JC, Wafelbakker F, Verbrugge HP, DeHaas JH: Netherlands: Second National Survey on 0-24-Year-Olds, *Groningen, The Netherlands, 1965, Noordhoff Uitgevers BV)*

AIDS TO DIFFERENTIAL DIAGNOSIS

SUBJECTIVE DATA	OBJECTIVE DATA
Premature thelarche	
Breast enlargement before onset of puberty.	Degree of enlargement varies from very slight to fully developed breasts. Usually bilateral. Other signs of sexual maturation may be absent.

CHAPTER 15

Abdomen

Equipment

- Stethoscope
- Centimeter measuring tape
- Marking pen

EXAMINATION

Have patient in the supine position to start examination. Approach the patient from the right side.

TECHNIQUE	FINDINGS
Inspect abdomen	
• *Skin color/surface characteristics*	**EXPECTED:** Same expected variations as rest of the body. May be paler if not exposed to the sun. Fine venous network (venous return toward head above umbilicus, toward feet below umbilicus). **UNEXPECTED:** Generalized color changes, such as jaundice or cyanosis. Glistening, taut appearance. Bluish periumbilical discoloration, bruises, other localized discoloration. Striae, lesions or nodules, a pearl-like enlarged umbilical node, scars.
• *Contour/symmetry* Begin seated to patient's right to enhance shadows and contouring. Inspect while patient breathes comfortably and while patient holds a deep breath. Assess symmetry, first seated at patient's side, then standing behind patient's head.	**EXPECTED:** Flat, rounded, or scaphoid. Contralateral areas are symmetric. Maximum height of convexity at umbilicus. Abdomen remains smooth and symmetric while patient holds breath.

TECHNIQUE	FINDINGS
	UNEXPECTED: Umbilicus displaced upward, downward, or laterally or is inflamed, swollen, or bulging. Any distention (symmetric or asymmetric), bulges, or masses while breathing comfortably or holding breath.
• *Surface motion*	**EXPECTED:** Smooth, even motion with respiration. Individuals with a greater inclination of the ribs show mostly costal movement, while others exhibit abdominal movement. Pulsations are often visible in upper midline in thin adults. **UNEXPECTED:** Limited motion with respiration in adults. Rippling movement (peristalsis) or marked pulsations.

Anatomic Correlates of the Four Quadrants of the Abdomen

Right Upper Quadrant	Left Upper Quadrant
Liver and gallbladder	Left lobe of liver
Pylorus	Spleen
Duodenum	Stomach
Head of pancreas	Body of pancreas
Right adrenal gland	Left adrenal gland
Portion of right kidney	Portion of left kidney
Hepatic flexure of colon	Splenic flexure of colon
Portions of ascending and transverse colon	Portions of transverse and descending colon
Right Lower Quadrant	**Left Lower Quadrant**
Lower pole of right kidney	Lower pole of left kidney
Cecum and appendix	Sigmoid colon
Portion of ascending colon	Portion of descending colon
Bladder (if distended)	Bladder (if distended)
Ovary and salpinx	Ovary and salpinx
Uterus (if enlarged)	Uterus (if enlarged)
Right spermatic cord	Left spermatic cord
Right ureter	Left ureter

TECHNIQUE	FINDINGS
Inspect abdominal muscles as patient raises head	
	EXPECTED: No masses or protrusions. **UNEXPECTED:** Masses, protrusion of the umbilicus and other hernia signs, or separation of rectus abdominis.
Auscultate with stethoscope diaphragm	
• *Frequency and character of bowel sounds* Warm up stethoscope diaphragm and hold with light pressure. May auscultate at a single site because bowel sounds generalize, but auscultate in all quadrants if there is cause for concern.	**EXPECTED:** 5–35 clicks and gurgles per minute. Borborygmi, or loud prolonged gurgles, may be because of hunger. **UNEXPECTED:** Increased sounds unrelated to hunger and high-pitched tinkling sounds may be caused by early intestinal obstruction; decreased or absent sounds after 3–5 minutes of listening may be associated with abdominal pain and rigidity and indicate a surgical emergency.
• *Liver and spleen*	**EXPECTED:** Silent. **UNEXPECTED:** Friction rubs (high-pitched grating sound in association with respiration).
Auscultate with stethoscope bell	
• *Vascular sounds* Listen with stethoscope bell in epigastric region, over aorta, and over renal, iliac, and femoral arteries.	**EXPECTED:** No bruits (harsh or musical sound indicating blood flow turbulence), venous hum (soft, low-pitched, and continuous sound), or friction rubs. **UNEXPECTED:** Bruits in aortic, renal, iliac, or femoral arteries.
• *Epigastric region and around umbilicus*	**EXPECTED:** No venous hum. **UNEXPECTED:** Venous hum.

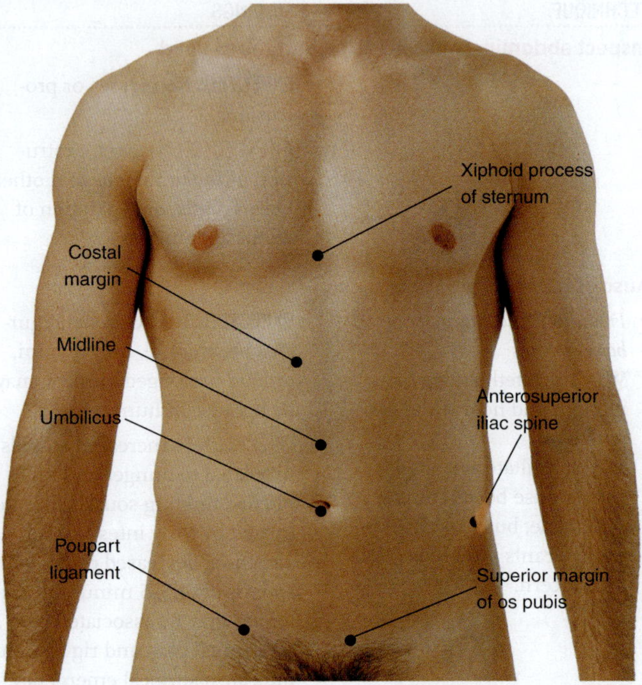

(From Wilson SF, Giddens J: Health assessment for nursing practice, *ed 4, St. Louis, 2009, Mosby.)*

Percussion Notes of the Abdomen

NOTE	DESCRIPTION	LOCATION
Tympany	Musical note of higher pitch than resonance	Over air-filled viscera
Hyperresonance	Pitch lies between tympany and resonance	Base of left lung
Resonance	Sustained note of moderate pitch	Over lung tissue and sometimes over abdomen
Dullness	Short, high-pitched note with little resonance	Over solid organs adjacent to air-filled structures

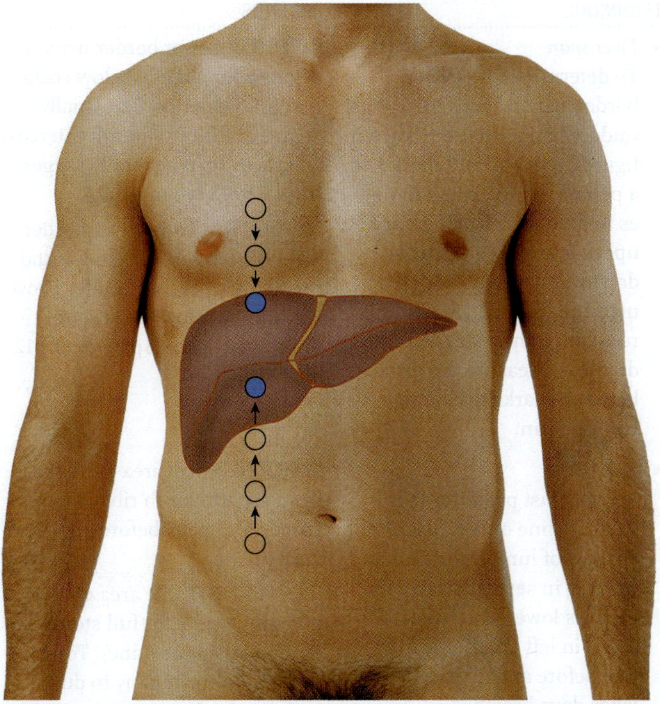

(From Wilson SF, Giddens J: Health assessment for nursing practice, ed 4, St. Louis, 2009, Mosby.)

TECHNIQUE	FINDINGS

Percuss abdomen

NOTE: Percussion can be done independently or concurrently with palpation.

- *Tone*
  Percuss in all four quadrants or nine regions.

EXPECTED: Tympany predominant. Dullness over organs and solid masses. Dullness in suprapubic area from distended bladder. See table on p. 143 for percussion notes.

UNEXPECTED: Dullness predominant.

TECHNIQUE	FINDINGS
• *Liver span* To determine lower liver border, percuss upward at right midclavicular line, as shown in figure on p. 144, and mark with a pen where tympany changes to dullness. To determine upper liver border, percuss downward at right midclavicular line from an area of lung resonance and mark change to dullness. Measure the distance between marks to estimate vertical span.	**EXPECTED:** Lower border usually begins at or slightly below costal margin. Upper border usually begins at fifth to seventh intercostal space. Span generally ranges from 6 to 12 cm in adults. **UNEXPECTED:** Lower liver border >2–3 cm (0.75–1 in) below costal margin. Upper liver border above the fifth or below the seventh intercostal space. Span <6 or >12 cm (2.5–4.5 in).
• *Spleen* Percuss just posterior to midaxillary line on left, beginning at areas of lung resonance and moving in several directions. Percuss lowest intercostal space in left anterior axillary line before and after patient takes deep breath.	**EXPECTED:** Small area of dullness from sixth to ninth rib (Traube's space). Tympany before and after deep breath. **UNEXPECTED:** Large area of dullness (check for full stomach or feces-filled intestine). Tone change from tympany to dullness with inspiration.
• *Stomach* Percuss in area of left lower anterior rib cage and left epigastric region.	**EXPECTED:** Tympany of gastric air bubble (lower than intestine tympany). **UNEXPECTED:** Dullness.

TECHNIQUE	FINDINGS
Lightly palpate abdomen	
Stand at patient's right side. Systematically palpate all quadrants, avoiding areas previously identified as problem spots. With palmar surface of fingers, depress abdominal wall up to 1 cm with light, even, circular motion.	**EXPECTED:** Abdomen smooth with consistent softness. Possible tension from palpating too deeply, cold hands, or ticklishness. **UNEXPECTED:** Muscular tension or resistance, tenderness, or masses. If resistance is present, place pillow under patient's knees and ask patient to breathe slowly through mouth. Feel for relaxation of rectus abdominis muscles on expiration. Continuing tension signals involuntary response to localized or generalized rigidity from underlying peritoneal irritation.
Palpate abdomen with moderate pressure	
Using same hand position as above, palpate all quadrants again, this time with moderate pressure.	**EXPECTED:** Soft, nontender. **UNEXPECTED:** Tenderness.
Deeply palpate abdomen	
With same hand position as above, repeat palpation in all quadrants or regions, pressing deeply and evenly into abdominal wall. Move fingers back and forth over abdominal contents. Use bimanual technique—exerting pressure with top hand and concentrating on sensation with bottom hand, as shown in the following figure—if obesity or muscular resistance makes deep palpation difficult. To help determine whether masses are superficial or intraabdominal, have patient lift head from examining table to contract abdominal muscles and obscure intraabdominal masses.	**EXPECTED:** Possible sensation of abdominal wall sliding back and forth. Possible awareness of borders of rectus abdominis muscles, aorta, and portions of colon. Possible tenderness over cecum, sigmoid colon, and aorta and in midline near xiphoid process. **UNEXPECTED:** Bulges, masses, tenderness unrelated to deep palpation of cecum, sigmoid colon, aorta, xiphoid process. Note location, size, shape, consistency, tenderness, pulsation, mobility, movement (with respiration) of any masses.

TECHNIQUE	FINDINGS
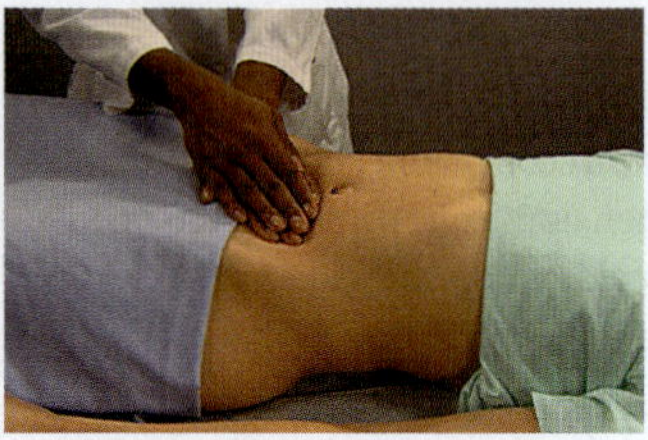	
• *Umbilical ring and umbilicus* Palpate umbilical ring and around umbilicus. Note whether ring is incomplete or soft in center.	**EXPECTED:** Umbilical ring circular and free of irregularities. Umbilicus either slightly inverted or everted. **UNEXPECTED:** Bulges, nodules, granulation. Protruding umbilicus.
• *Liver* Place left hand under patient at 11th and 12th ribs, lifting to elevate liver toward abdominal wall. Place right hand on abdomen, fingers extended toward head with tips on right midclavicular line below level of liver dullness, as shown in figure at right. Alternatively, place right hand parallel to right costal margin, as shown in bottom figure at right. Press right hand gently but deeply in and up. Ask patient to breathe comfortably a few times and then take a deep breath. Feel for liver edge as diaphragm pushes it down. If palpable, repeat maneuver medially and laterally to costal margin.	**EXPECTED:** Usually liver is not palpable, though may be felt in thin persons. If felt, liver edge should be firm, smooth, even. **UNEXPECTED:** Tenderness, nodules, or irregularity. 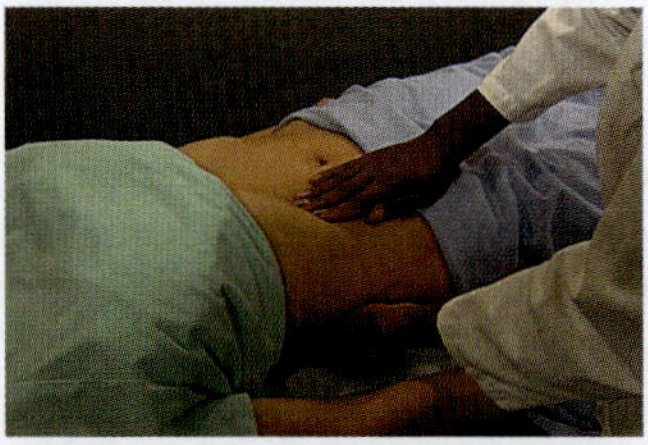 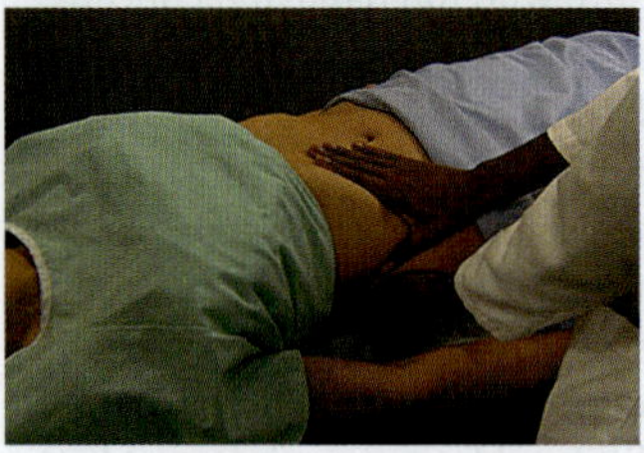

TECHNIQUE	FINDINGS
• *Gallbladder* Palpate below liver margin at lateral border of rectus abdominis muscle.	**EXPECTED:** Gallbladder not palpable. **UNEXPECTED:** Palpable, tender. If tender (possible cholecystitis), palpate deeply during inspiration and observe for pain (Murphy's sign).
• *Spleen* Still standing on right side, reach across patient with left hand, place it beneath patient over left costovertebral angle (CVA), and lift spleen anteriorly toward abdominal wall. As shown in figure at right, place right hand on abdomen below left costal margin and, using findings from percussion, gently press fingertips inward toward spleen while asking patient to take a deep breath. Feel for spleen as it moves downward, toward fingers. Repeat with patient lying on right side, as shown in figure at right, with hips and knees flexed. Press inward with left hand while using fingertips of right hand to feel edge of spleen.	**EXPECTED:** Spleen usually not palpable by either method. **UNEXPECTED:** Palpable spleen. 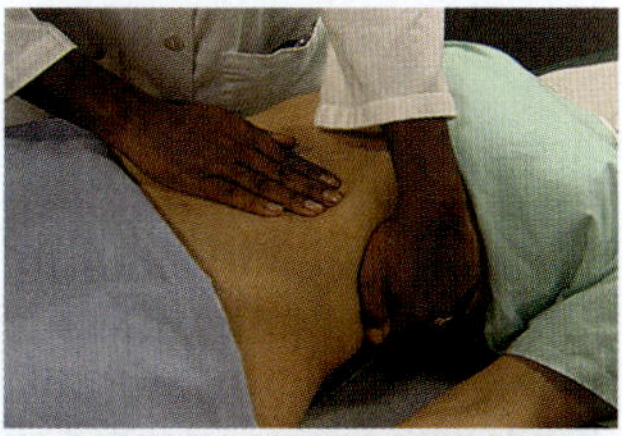 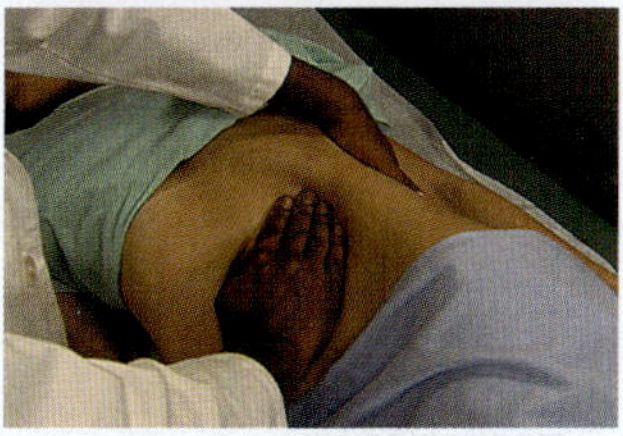
• *Left kidney* Standing on patient's right, reach across with left hand and place over left flank; then place right hand at patient's left costal margin. Ask patient to inhale deeply while you elevate left flank and palpate deeply with right hand.	**EXPECTED:** Left kidney usually not palpable. **UNEXPECTED:** Tenderness. 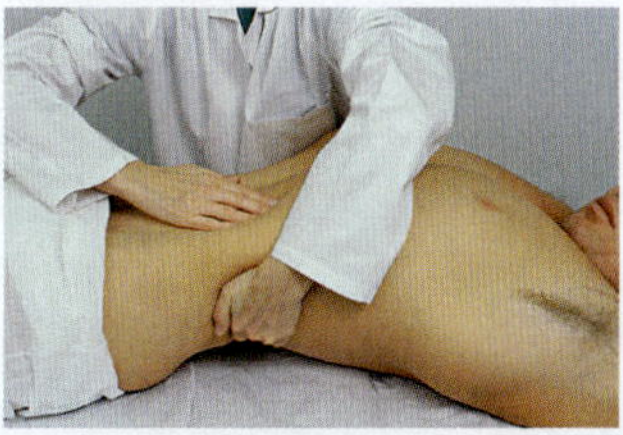

TECHNIQUE	FINDINGS
• *Right kidney* Standing on patient's right, place left hand under right flank, then place right hand at patient's right costal margin. Ask patient to inhale deeply while you elevate right flank and palpate deeply with right hand.	**EXPECTED:** If palpable, right kidney should be smooth and firm with rounded edges. **UNEXPECTED:** Tenderness. 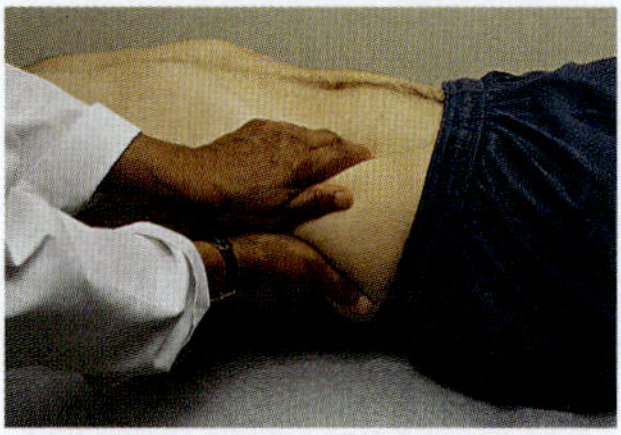
• *Aorta* Palpate deeply slightly to left of midline and feel for aortic pulsation. As an alternative technique, place palmar surface of hands with fingers extended on midline; press fingers deeply inward on each side of aorta and feel for pulsation. For thin patients, use one hand, placing thumb, and fingers on either side of aorta.	**EXPECTED:** If prominent, pulsation should be anterior in direction. **UNEXPECTED:** Prominent lateral pulsation (suggests aortic aneurysm). 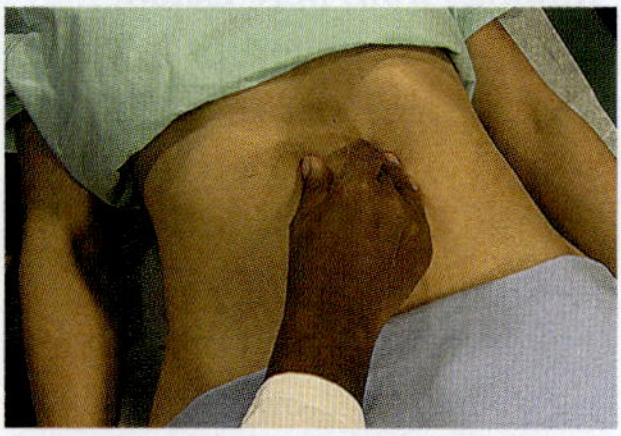
• *Urinary bladder* Percuss distended bladder to help determine outline, then palpate.	**EXPECTED:** Ordinarily not palpable unless distended with urine. If distended, bladder should be smooth, round, and tense and on percussion will elicit lower note than surrounding air-filled intestines. **UNEXPECTED:** Palpable when not distended with urine.

TECHNIQUE	FINDINGS
With patient sitting, percuss CVAs	
Stand behind patient. Right side: Place left hand over right CVA and strike with ulnar surface of right fist. Left side: Repeat with hands reversed.	EXPECTED: No tenderness. UNEXPECTED: Kidney tenderness or pain.
Pain assessment	
Keep eyes on patient's face while examining abdomen. To help characterize pain, have patient cough, take a deep breath, stand up, walk, or jump. Ask if patient is hungry.	UNEXPECTED: Unwillingness to move, nausea, vomiting, areas of localized tenderness. Lack of hunger. See box and table on following page.
Iliopsoas muscle test	
Use test for suspected appendicitis. With patient supine, place hand over right lower thigh. Ask patient to raise leg, flexing at hip, while you push downward.	UNEXPECTED: Right lower quadrant (RLQ) pain. 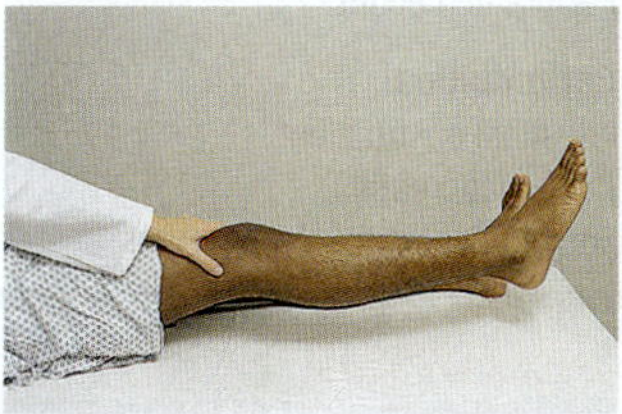
Obturator muscle test	
Use test for suspected ruptured appendix or pelvic abscess. With patient supine, ask them to flex right leg at hip and bend knee to 90 degrees. Hold leg just above knee, grasp ankle, and rotate leg laterally and medially, as shown in figure.	UNEXPECTED: Pain in right hypogastric region. 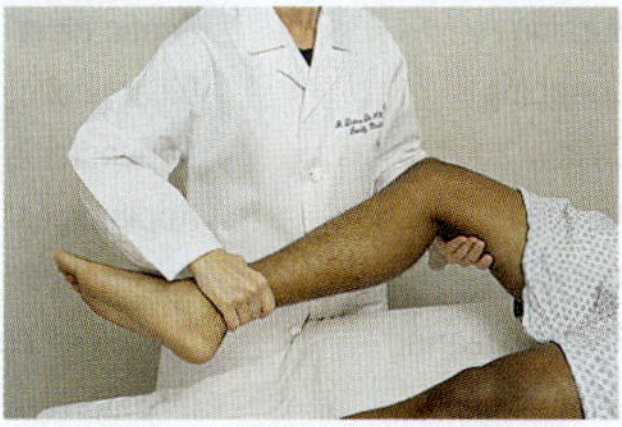

Some Causes of Pain Perceived in Anatomic Regions

Right Upper Quadrant
Duodenal ulcer
Hepatitis
Hepatomegaly
Lower lobe pneumonia
Cholecystitis

Right Lower Quadrant
Appendicitis
Salpingitis
Ovarian cyst
Tuboovarian abscess
Ruptured ectopic pregnancy
Renal/ureteral stone
Strangulated hernia
Meckel diverticulitis
Regional ileitis
Perforated cecum

Periumbilical
Intestinal obstruction
Acute pancreatitis
Early appendicitis
Mesenteric thrombosis
Aortic aneurysm
Diverticulitis

Left Upper Quadrant
Ruptured spleen
Gastric ulcer
Aortic aneurysm
Perforated colon
Lower lobe pneumonia

Left Lower Quadrant
Sigmoid diverticulitis
Salpingitis
Ovarian cyst
Ruptured ectopic pregnancy
Tuboovarian abscess
Renal/ureteral stone
Strangulated hernia
Perforated colon
Regional ileitis
Ulcerative colitis

Quality and Onset of Abdominal Pain

CHARACTERISTIC	POSSIBLE RELATED CONDITION
Burning	Peptic ulcer
Cramping	Biliary colic, gastroenteritis
Colic	Appendicitis with impacted feces; renal stone
Aching	Appendiceal irritation
Knifelike	Pancreatitis
Ripping, tearing	Aortic dissection
Gradual onset	Infection
Sudden onset	Duodenal ulcer, acute pancreatitis, obstruction, perforation

AIDS TO DIFFERENTIAL DIAGNOSIS

SUBJECTIVE DATA	OBJECTIVE DATA
Hiatal Hernia With Esophagitis	
Epigastric pain and/or heartburn that worsens with lying down and is relieved by sitting up or antacids; water brash (mouth fills with fluid); dysphagia; sudden onset of vomiting, pain, complete dysphagia are symptoms of hernia incarceration.	Generally unremarkable exam; with severe disease, may have erythema of the posterior pharynx and edematous vocal cords.
Gastroesophageal Reflux Disease	
Heartburn or acid indigestion (burning chest pain, located behind breastbone that moves up toward the neck and throat); sour taste of acid in the back of the throat or hoarseness; symptoms in infants and children include back arching or fussiness with feeding, regurgitation, and vomiting; can precipitate acute asthma exacerbation, can cause respiratory problems from aspiration, and can lead to esophageal bleeding.	Generally unremarkable exam; with severe disease, may have erythema of the posterior pharynx and edematous vocal cords; when frequent emesis occurs, may cause failure to thrive in an infant.
Stomach and Duodenal Ulcers	
Localized epigastric pain that occurs when the stomach is empty and is relieved with food or antacids; with upper gastrointestinal bleeding, may have hematemesis, melena, dizziness, syncope.	Anterior stomach wall ulcers may produce tenderness on palpation of the abdomen; with significant upper gastrointestinal bleeding, may have decreased blood pressure, increased pulse rate, and decreased hematocrit level; signs of an acute abdomen could indicate perforation of duodenum, a life-threatening event.

SUBJECTIVE DATA	OBJECTIVE DATA
Acute Diarrhea	
Abrupt onset, three or more loose stools per day, lasts <2 weeks; abdominal pain, diarrhea, nausea, vomiting, fever, tenesmus (feeling of incomplete defecation); if symptoms occur in two or more persons after ingestion of the same food, suspect food poisoning.	Diffuse abdominal tenderness; can mimic peritoneal inflammation with RLQ pain or guarding; when severe, may develop moderate to severe dehydration (decreased blood pressure, increased heart rate).
Crohn's Disease	
Chronic diarrhea (can be bloody) with malabsorption, cramping characterized by unpredictable flares and remissions.	Abdominal mass may be palpated from thickened or inflamed bowel; perianal skin tags, fistulae, and abscess formation; extraintestinal findings include arthritis of large joints, erythema nodosum, pyoderma gangrenosum.
Ulcerative Colitis	
Bloody, frequent (up to 20–30 stools/day), watery diarrhea; mild to severe symptoms based on degree of colon involvement; weight loss, fatigue, general debilitation.	Generally do not have fistulae or perianal disease; cholestatic pattern of elevated transaminases suggests sclerosing cholangitis.
Irritable Bowel Syndrome	
Cluster of symptoms consisting of abdominal pain, bloating, constipation, and diarrhea; some patients have alternating diarrhea and constipation; mucus may be present around or within the stool.	Generally unremarkable examination.
Colon Cancer (Colorectal Cancer)	
May have abdominal pain, gross blood in stool, but more often presents with occult blood in stool on fecal occult blood test; may have change in frequency or character of stool.	With progressive disease, may have palpable mass in right (RLQ) or left lower quadrant (LLQ); rectal mass may be palpable on digital rectal examination.

SUBJECTIVE DATA	OBJECTIVE DATA
Hepatitis	
Some asymptomatic; others experience jaundice, anorexia, abdominal pain, clay-colored stools, tea-colored urine, fatigue.	Abnormal liver function tests; jaundice; hepatomegaly.
Cirrhosis	
Some asymptomatic; others experience jaundice, anorexia, abdominal pain, clay-colored stools, tea-colored urine, fatigue; may report prominent abdominal vasculature, cutaneous spider angiomas, hematemesis, abdominal fullness.	Abnormal liver function tests; jaundice; initially with firm, nontender enlarged liver; in severe disease, liver size decreases, portal hypertension and esophageal varices may develop, and muscle wasting and nutritional deficiencies may occur.
Cholecystitis	
Acute: Right upper quadrant (RUQ) pain with radiation around mid-torso to right scapular region; pain is abrupt and severe, lasting 2–4 hours; may have fever, jaundice, anorexia. *Chronic:* Repeated acute attacks; fat intolerance, flatulence, nausea, anorexia, nonspecific abdominal pain.	Marked tenderness in the RUQ or epigastrium; involuntary guarding or rebound tenderness; some with full palpable gallbladder in RUQ.
Chronic Pancreatitis	
Unremitting abdominal pain, weight loss, steatorrhea.	Diffuse abdominal tenderness to palpation; involuntary guarding and abdominal distention can occur; elevated pancreatic enzymes (amylase and lipase); may develop pseudocyst formation; with advanced disease, may show subcutaneous fat and temporal wasting from malnutrition.

SUBJECTIVE DATA	OBJECTIVE DATA
Pyelonephritis	
Flank pain, dysuria, fever; may have rigors, urinary frequency, urgency, and hematuria.	Ill appearing with CVA tenderness; pyuria and bacteria.
Renal Calculi	
Fever, dysuria, hematuria; severe cramping and flank pain with nausea and vomiting; as the stone passes, pain typically moves from flank to groin to scrotal or labial area.	Ill appearing with severe cramping pain; may have CVA tenderness or abdominal tenderness on palpation; microscopic hematuria.
Appendicitis	
Initially periumbilical or epigastric pain; colicky; later becomes localized to RLQ; anorexia, nausea, or vomiting after onset of pain; low-grade fever.	Guarding, tenderness, positive iliopsoas and/or obturator signs, RLQ pain on palpation (McBurney's sign).

Abdominal Signs Associated With Common Abnormal Conditions

SIGN	DESCRIPTION	ASSOCIATED CONDITIONS
Aaron	Pain or distress occurs in the area of patient's heart or stomach on palpation of McBurney point	Appendicitis
Ballance	Fixed dullness to percussion in left flank and dullness in right flank disappearing on change of position	Peritoneal irritation
Blumberg	Rebound tenderness	Peritoneal irritation, appendicitis
Cullen	Ecchymosis around umbilicus	Hemoperitoneum, pancreatitis, ectopic pregnancy
Dance	Absence of bowel sounds in RLQ	Intussusception
Grey Turner	Ecchymosis of flanks	Hemoperitoneum, pancreatitis

Abdominal Signs Associated With Common Abnormal Conditions—cont'd

SIGN	DESCRIPTION	ASSOCIATED CONDITIONS
Kehr	Abdominal pain radiating to left shoulder	Spleen rupture, renal calculi, ectopic pregnancy
Markle (heel jar)	Patient stands with straightened knees, then raises up on toes, relaxes, and allows heels to hit floor, thus jarring body; action will cause abdominal pain if positive	Peritoneal irritation, appendicitis
McBurney	Rebound tenderness and sharp pain when McBurney point is palpated (2/3 the distance from the umbilicus to the anterior superior iliac spine)	Appendicitis
Murphy	Abrupt cessation of inspiration on palpation of gallbladder	Cholecystitis
Romberg-Howship	Pain down medial aspect of thigh to knees	Strangulated obturator hernia
Rovsing	RLQ pain intensified by LLQ abdominal palpation	Peritoneal irritation, appendicitis

Conditions Producing Acute Abdominal Pain

CONDITION	USUAL PAIN CHARACTERISTICS	POSSIBLE ASSOCIATED FINDINGS
Appendicitis	Initially periumbilical or epigastric; colicky; later becomes localized to RLQ, often at McBurney point	Guarding, tenderness; positive iliopsoas and positive obturator tests, RLQ skin hyperesthesia; anorexia, nausea, or vomiting after onset of pain; low-grade fever; positive Aaron, Rovsing, Markle, and McBurney signs*
Peritonitis	Onset sudden or gradual; pain generalized or localized, dull or severe and unrelenting; guarding; pain on deep inspiration	Shallow respiration; positive Blumberg, Markle, and Ballance signs; reduced bowel sounds, nausea and vomiting; positive obturator and iliopsoas tests

Continued

Conditions Producing Acute Abdominal Pain—cont'd

CONDITION	USUAL PAIN CHARACTERISTICS	POSSIBLE ASSOCIATED FINDINGS
Cholecystitis	Severe, unrelenting RUQ or epigastric pain; may be referred to right subscapular area	RUQ tenderness and rigidity, positive Murphy sign, palpable gallbladder, anorexia, vomiting, fever, possible jaundice
Pancreatitis	Dramatic, sudden, excruciating left upper quadrant (LUQ), epigastric, or umbilical pain; may be present in one or both flanks; may be referred to left shoulder	Epigastric tenderness, vomiting, fever, shock; positive Grey Turner sign; positive Cullen sign; both signs may occur 2–3 days after onset
Salpingitis	Lower quadrant, worse on left	Nausea, vomiting, fever, suprapubic tenderness, rigid abdomen, pain on pelvic examination
Pelvic inflammatory disease	Lower quadrant, increases with activity	Tender adnexa and cervix, cervical discharge, dyspareunia
Diverticulitis	Epigastric, radiating down left side of abdomen, especially after eating; may be referred to back	Flatulence, borborygmi, diarrhea, dysuria, tenderness on palpation
Perforated gastric or duodenal ulcer	Abrupt RUQ; may be referred to shoulders	Abdominal free air and distention with increased resonance over liver; tenderness in epigastrium or RUQ; rigid abdominal wall, rebound tenderness
Intestinal obstruction	Abrupt, severe, spasmodic; referred to epigastrium, umbilicus	Distention, minimal rebound tenderness, vomiting, localized tenderness, visible peristalsis; bowel sounds absent (with paralytic obstruction) or hyperactive high-pitched (with mechanical obstruction)
Volvulus	Referred to hypogastrium and umbilicus	Distention, nausea, vomiting, guarding; sigmoid loop volvulus may be palpable

Conditions Producing Acute Abdominal Pain—cont'd

CONDITION	USUAL PAIN CHARACTERISTICS	POSSIBLE ASSOCIATED FINDINGS
Leaking abdominal aneurysm	Steady throbbing midline over aneurysm; may penetrate to back, flank	Nausea, vomiting, abdominal mass, bruit
Biliary stones, colic	Episodic, severe, RUQ, or epigastrium lasting 15 minutes to several hours; may be referred to subscapular area, especially right	RUQ tenderness, soft abdominal wall, anorexia, vomiting, jaundice, subnormal temperature
Renal calculi	Intense; flank, extending to groin and genitals; may be episodic	Fever, hematuria; positive Kehr sign
Ectopic pregnancy	Lower quadrant; referred to shoulder; with rupture is agonizing	Hypogastric tenderness, symptoms of pregnancy, spotting, irregular menses, soft abdominal wall, mass on bimanual pelvic examination; ruptured: shock, rigid abdominal wall, distention; positive Kehr, Cullen signs
Ruptured ovarian cyst	Lower quadrant, steady, increases with cough or motion	Vomiting, low-grade fever, anorexia, tenderness on pelvic examination
Splenic rupture	Intense; LUQ, radiating to left shoulder; may worsen if foot of bed is elevated	Shock, pallor, lowered temperature

*See table on pp. 155–156 for explanation of signs.

Conditions Producing Chronic Abdominal Pain

CONDITION	USUAL PAIN CHARACTERISTICS	POSSIBLE ASSOCIATED FINDINGS
Irritable bowel syndrome	Hypogastric pain; crampy, variable, infrequent; associated with bowel function	Unremarkable physical examination; pain associated with gas, bloating, distention; relief with passage of flatus, feces
Lactose intolerance	Crampy pain after drinking milk or eating milk products	Associated diarrhea; unremarkable physical examination

Continued

Conditions Producing Chronic Abdominal Pain—cont'd

CONDITION	USUAL PAIN CHARACTERISTICS	POSSIBLE ASSOCIATED FINDINGS
Diverticular disease	Localized pain	Abdominal tenderness, fever
Constipation	Colicky or dull and steady pain that does not progress or worsen	Fecal mass palpable, stool in rectum
Uterine fibroids	Pain related to menses, intercourse	Palpable myoma(s)
Hernia	Localized pain that increases with exertion or lifting	Hernia on physical examination
Esophagitis/gastroesophageal reflux disease	Burning, gnawing pain in midepigastrium, worsens with recumbency	Unremarkable physical examination
Peptic ulcer	Burning or gnawing pain	May have epigastric tenderness on palpation
Gastritis	Constant burning pain in epigastrium	May be accompanied by nausea, vomiting, diarrhea, or fever; unremarkable physical examination

Modified from Dains JE, Baumann LC, Dains PS: *Advanced health assessment & clinical diagnosis in primary care*, St. Louis, 2011, Mosby.

PEDIATRIC VARIATIONS

EXAMINATION

TECHNIQUE | **FINDINGS**

Inspect abdomen in all four quadrants

Infant's abdomen should be examined, if possible, during a time of relaxation and quiet. Sucking on a pacifier may help relax infant. The parent's lap can serve as the best examining surface for toddlers through ages 2–3 years.

- *Contour/symmetry* — **EXPECTED:** Until the age of 3 years, abdomen will protrude when standing.

  UNEXPECTED: Distention can indicate organ enlargement, fecal impaction, or abdominal mass.

TECHNIQUE	FINDINGS
• *Surface motion*	**EXPECTED:** Pulsation in epigastric area in newborns and infants. **UNEXPECTED:** Peristaltic waves associated with pyloric stenosis.
Percuss abdomen	
• *Tone*	**EXPECTED:** More tympany is present in infants than adults because of air swallowing during crying and feeding.
Lightly and deeply palpate abdomen	
• *Umbilical ring*	**EXPECTED:** Infants and children may have a small umbilical hernia (typically closes spontaneously by 1–2 years of age).
• *Liver*	**EXPECTED:** Liver may be palpable in young children 2–3 cm below costal margin.

Age	*Liver Span (cm)*
0–2 months	4.0–6.3
2–12 months	4.0–7.9
1–5 years	6.3–10.5
5–10 years	6.9–11.4
10–15 year	7.4–12.3

From Amatya P, Shah D, Gupta N, Bhatta NK: Clinical and ultrasonographic measurement of liver size in normal children. *Indian J Pediatr*, 81(5):441–5, 2014.

CHAPTER

16 Female Genitalia

For ease of communication, the term "female genitalia" within this handbook refers to the following internal and external anatomic structures: mons pubis, labia, clitoris, vestibular glands, vagina, cervix, uterus, fallopian tubes, ovaries, and bony pelvis, regardless of the gender identity of the patient.

Equipment

- Lamp or light source
- Drapes
- Speculum
- Gloves
- Water-soluble lubricant
- Papanicolaou (Pap) smear/human papillomavirus (HPV) collection equipment:
  - Collection device (wooden or plastic spatula; cervical brush or broom)
  - Glass slides and cytologic fixative or fluid collection media
- Other specimen collection equipment as needed:
  - Cotton swabs
  - Culture plates or media
  - DNA tests for organisms

Examination

Have patient in lithotomy position, draped for minimal exposure.

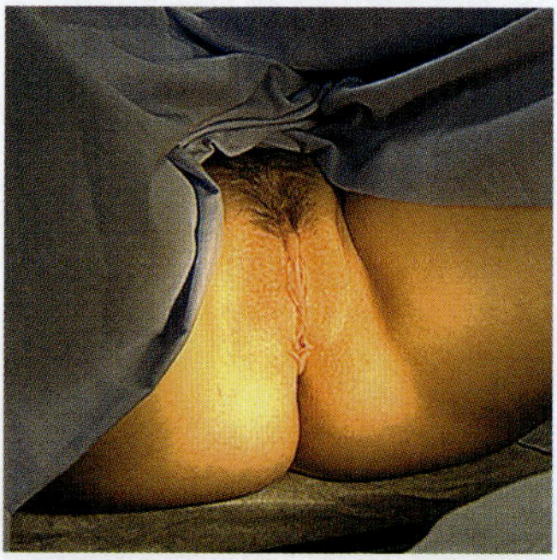

TECHNIQUE	FINDINGS

External Genitalia

Wash or sanitize hands and wear gloves on both hands

Ask patient to separate or drop open the knees. Tell patient you are beginning the examination, then touch lower thigh and—without breaking contact—move hand along thigh to external genitalia.

Inspect and palpate mons pubis

- *Characteristics*

  EXPECTED: Skin smooth and clean.

  UNEXPECTED: Inadequate hygiene.

- *Pubic hair*

  EXPECTED: In patients assigned female at birth, triangle shape distribution: pointing downward, with horizontal border at the level of the pubic symphysis.

  UNEXPECTED: Nits or lice.

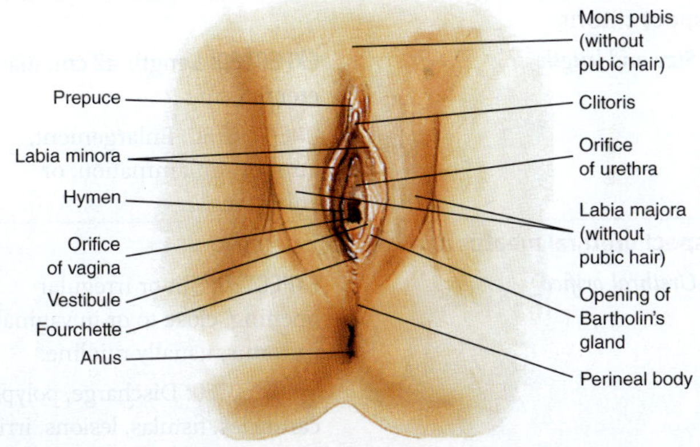

(From Lowdermilk DL, Perry SE: Maternity and women's health care, *ed 8, St. Louis, 2007, Mosby.)*

Inspect and palpate labia

- *Labia majora*

  EXPECTED: Gaping or closed, dry or moist, shriveled or full, tissue soft and homogeneous, usually symmetric.

TECHNIQUE	FINDINGS
	UNEXPECTED: Swelling, redness, tenderness, discoloration, varicosities, obvious stretching, or signs of trauma or scarring. If excoriation, rashes, or lesions are present, ask patient about scratching.
• *Labia minora* Separate labia majora with fingers of one hand. With other hand, palpate labia minora between thumb and second finger.	**EXPECTED:** Moist, dark pink inner surface. Tissue soft and homogeneous. **UNEXPECTED:** Tenderness, inflammation, irritation, excoriation, caking of discharge in tissue folds, discoloration, ulcers, vesicles, irregularities, or nodules. Hyperemia of fourchette not related to recent sexual activity.
Inspect clitoris	
• *Size and length*	**EXPECTED:** Length ≤2 cm; diameter 0.5 cm. **UNEXPECTED:** Enlargement, atrophy, inflammation, or adhesions.
Inspect urethral meatus and vaginal opening	
• *Urethral orifice*	**EXPECTED:** Slit or irregular opening, close to or in vaginal introitus, usually midline. **UNEXPECTED:** Discharge, polyps, caruncles, fistulas, lesions, irritation, inflammation, or dilation.
• *Vaginal introitus*	**EXPECTED:** Thin vertical slit or large orifice with irregular edges. Tissue moist. **UNEXPECTED:** Swelling, discoloration, discharge, lesions, fistulas, or fissures.

TECHNIQUE	FINDINGS
Milk Skene glands	
Tell patient you will be inserting one finger into the vagina and pressing forward with it. With palm up, insert index finger to second joint, press upward, and milk Skene glands by moving finger outward. Perform on both sides of urethra and directly on urethra.	**UNEXPECTED:** Discharge or tenderness. Note color, consistency, odor of any discharge; obtain culture. 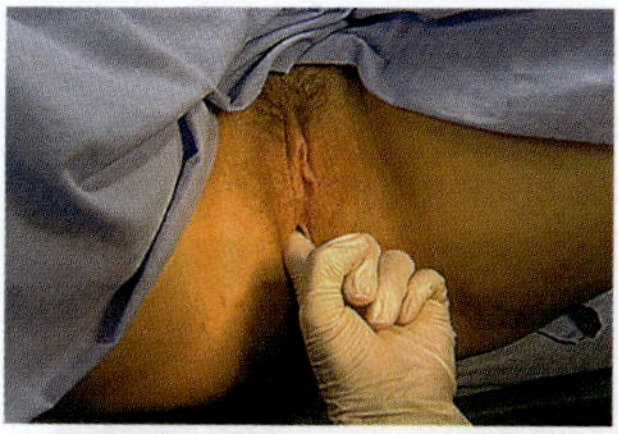
Palpate Bartholin glands	
Tell patient to expect to feel you pressing around the entrance to the vagina. Palpate lateral tissue between index finger and thumb, then palpate entire area bilaterally, particularly posterolateral portion of labia majora.	**EXPECTED:** No swelling. **UNEXPECTED:** Swelling, tenderness, masses, heat, fluctuation, or discharge. Note color, consistency, odor of any discharge; obtain culture.
Test vaginal muscle tone if indicated	
Ask patient to squeeze vaginal opening around your finger.	**EXPECTED:** Fairly tight squeezing by some nulliparous patients, less so by some multiparous patients. **UNEXPECTED:** Protrusion of cervix or uterus.
Locate the cervix	
With your finger still in place, reach in farther to locate the cervix and note the direction in which it points. This may help you locate the cervix when you insert the speculum.	**EXPECTED:** Midline may point horizontally, anteriorly, or posteriorly. May be surgically absent. The neovagina in a transgender woman will not have a cervix. **UNEXPECTED:** Deviates to right or left.

TECHNIQUE	FINDINGS
Inspect for bulging and urinary incontinence if indicated	
Ask patient to bear down.	EXPECTED: No bulging. UNEXPECTED: Bulging of anterior or posterior wall, or urinary incontinence.
Inspect and palpate perineum	
Compress perineal tissue between finger and thumb. 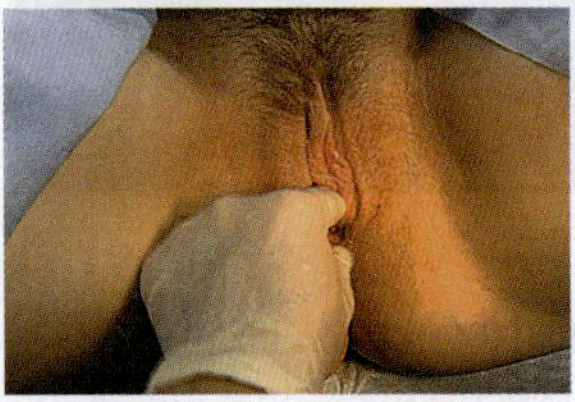	EXPECTED: Perineum surface smooth—generally thick and smooth in a nulliparous patient, thinner and rigid in a multiparous patient. Possible episiotomy scarring from childbirth. UNEXPECTED: Tenderness, inflammation, fistulas, lesions, or growths.
Inspect anus	
• *Skin characteristics*	EXPECTED: Skin darkly pigmented and possibly coarse. UNEXPECTED: Scarring, lesions, inflammation, fissures, lumps, skin tags, or excoriation.

Internal Genitalia—Speculum Examination

If you touched the perineum or anal skin while examining the external genitalia, change gloves before beginning internal examination. Lubricate speculum and gloved fingers with water or water-soluble gel lubricant. Water is preferred if obtaining a Pap smear.

Insert speculum	
Tell patient you will be touching again; then, insert two fingers of hand not holding the speculum just inside vaginal introitus and gently press downward. Ask patient to breathe slowly and to try consciously relaxing pelvic and buttock muscles.	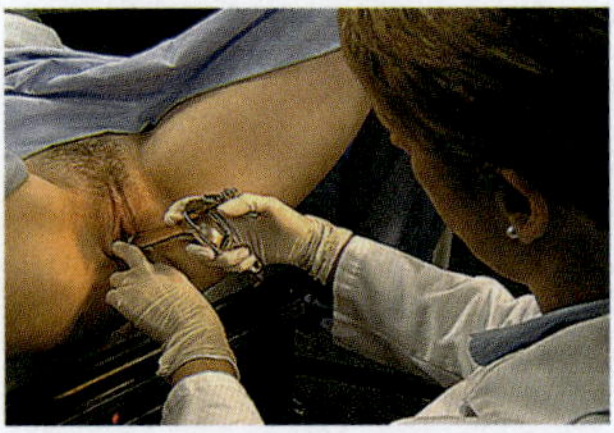

TECHNIQUE	FINDINGS
Use fingers of that hand to separate labia minora widely so that the vaginal opening becomes clearly visible. Then slowly insert speculum along path of least resistance, often slightly downward, avoiding trauma to urethra and vaginal walls. Some clinicians insert speculum blades at an oblique angle; others prefer to keep blades horizontal.	
Avoid touching clitoris, catching pubic hair, or pinching labial skin. Insert speculum the length of the vaginal canal. Maintaining downward pressure, open speculum by pressing on thumb piece. Sweep speculum slowly upward until cervix comes into view. Adjust light, then manipulate speculum farther into vagina to fully expose the cervix between anterior and posterior blades. Stabilize distal spread of blades and adjust proximal spread as needed.	

Inspect cervix

- *Color*

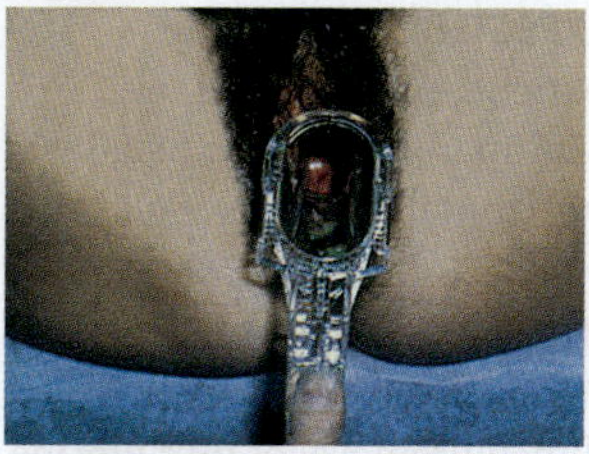

(From Edge V, Miller M: Women's health care, *St. Louis, 1994, Mosby.)*

EXPECTED: Evenly distributed pink. Symmetric, circumscribed erythema around os can be expected.

UNEXPECTED: Bluish, pale, or reddened cervix (especially if patchy or with irregular borders).

TECHNIQUE	FINDINGS
• *Position*	**EXPECTED:** In midline, horizontal, or pointing anteriorly or posteriorly. Protruding into vagina 1–3 cm. **UNEXPECTED:** Deviation to right or left. Protrusion into vagina >1–3 cm.
• *Size*	**EXPECTED:** 3 cm in diameter. **UNEXPECTED:** >3 cm.
• *Shape*	**EXPECTED:** Uniform. **UNEXPECTED:** Distorted.
• *Surface characteristics*	**EXPECTED:** Surface smooth. Possible symmetric, reddened circle around os (squamocolumnar epithelium). Possible small, white, or yellow raised round areas on cervix (nabothian cysts). **UNEXPECTED:** Friable tissue, red patchy areas, granular areas, or white patches.
• *Discharge* Note any discharge. Determine origin (cervix or vagina).	**EXPECTED:** Odorless; creamy or clear; thick, thin, or stringy (often heavier at midcycle or immediately before menstruation). **UNEXPECTED:** Odorous and white to yellow, green, or gray.
• *Size and shape of os* Follow standard precautions for safe collection of human secretions.	**EXPECTED:** Nulliparous patient: small, round, oval. Multiparous patient: usually a horizontal slit or irregular and stellate. **UNEXPECTED:** Slit resulting from trauma from induced abortion, difficult removal of intrauterine device, or sexual abuse.

TECHNIQUE	FINDINGS
Withdraw speculum and inspect vaginal walls	
Unlock speculum and remove it slowly, rotating it so vaginal walls can be inspected. Maintain downward pressure and hook index finger over anterior blade as it is removed. Note odor of any discharge pooled in posterior blade and obtain specimen if not already obtained.	EXPECTED: Vaginal wall color same pink as cervix or lighter; moist, smooth or rugated; and homogeneous. Thin, clear or cloudy, odorless secretions. UNEXPECTED: Reddened patches, lesions, pallor, cracks, bleeding, nodules, swelling. Secretions that are profuse; thick, curdy, or frothy; gray, green, or yellow; or malodorous.

Internal Genitalia—Bimanual Examination

Change gloves, then lubricate index and middle fingers of examining hand. Tell patient you are going to examine internally with your fingers. Prevent thumb from touching clitoris during examination.

Obtaining Vaginal Smears and Cultures

Vaginal specimens for smears and cultures are often obtained during the speculum examination. Vaginal specimens are obtained while the speculum is in place but after the cervix and its surrounding tissue have been inspected. Collect specimens as indicated for Pap smear, HPV testing, sexually transmitted infection screening, and wet mount. Be sure to follow Standard Precautions for the safe collection of human secretions. Label the specimen with the patient's name, date, and a description of the specimen (e.g., cervical smear, vaginal smear, culture). If the Pap smear cervical specimen is from a transgender man, it is essential to make clear to the laboratory that the sample is a cervical Pap smear (especially if the listed gender marker is "male") to avoid the sample being run incorrectly as an anal Pap smear or discarded. The use of testosterone or the presence of amenorrhea should be indicated on the requisition.

Conventional Papanicolaou Smear

Brushes and brooms used in conjunction with or instead of the conventional spatula improve the quality of cells obtained. The cylindric-type brush (e.g., a cytobrush) collects endocervical cells only. First, collect a sample from the ectocervix with a spatula. Insert the longer projection of the spatula into the cervical os. Rotate it 360 degrees, keeping it flush against the cervical tissue. Withdraw

Continued

the spatula and spread the specimen on a glass slide. A single light stroke with each side of the spatula is sufficient to thin out the specimen over the slide. Fix the specimen and label as ectocervical. Then, introduce the brush device into the vagina and insert it into the cervical os until only the bristles closest to the handle are exposed. Slowly rotate one-half to one full turn. Remove it, and prepare the slide. A single light stroke with each side of the spatula is sufficient to thin out the specimen over the slide. Fix the specimen and label it as ectocervical. Then, introduce the brush device into the vagina, and insert it into the cervical os until only the bristles closest to the handle are exposed. Slowly rotate one-half to one full turn. Remove it, and prepare the endocervical smear by rolling the brush with moderate pressure across a glass slide. Fix the specimen, and label it as endocervical. Alternatively, both specimens can be placed on a single slide.

The broom-type brush is used for collecting ectocervical and endocervical cells at the same time. The broom has flexible plastic bristles, which are reported to cause less blood spotting after the examination. Introduce the brush into the vagina and insert the central long bristles into the cervical os until the lateral bristles bend fully against the ectocervix. Maintain gentle pressure and rotate the brush by rolling the handle between the thumb and forefinger three to five times to the left and right. Withdraw the brush and transfer the sample to a glass slide with two single "paint" strokes. Apply first one side of the bristle, then turn the brush over and paint the slide again in exactly the same area. Apply fixative, then label the specimen as ectocervical and endocervical.

Liquid-Based Testing

The liquid-based cytology replaces the use of a glass slide and fixative spray. Use a brush and/or the broom-type device to collect the specimen, following the same collection steps as with the conventional Pap smear. Rinse the brush in the solution by swirling. Deposit the broom end of the device directly into the collection vial. With any collection device, be sure to follow both the manufacturer and laboratory instructions to appropriately collect and preserve the specimen. Close the vial tightly to prevent leakage and loss of the sample during transport. Label it with the patient's name, the date, and the origin of the specimen (ectocervical only or ectocervical and endocervical). The liquid sample is also used to test for HPV.

Gonococcal Culture Specimen

Immediately after the Pap smear is obtained, introduce a sterile cotton swab into the vagina and insert it into the cervical os. Hold it in place for 10–30 seconds. Withdraw the swab and spread the specimen in a large z pattern over the culture medium, rotating the swab at the same time. Label the tube or plate, then follow agency routine for transporting and warming the specimen. If indicated, an anal culture can be obtained after the vaginal speculum has been removed. Insert a fresh, sterile cotton swab about 2.5 cm into the rectum and rotate it in a full circle. Hold it in place for 10–30 seconds. Withdraw the swab and prepare the specimen as described for the vaginal culture. Gonococcal cultures are now used less frequently than DNA testing for chlamydia and gonorrhea.

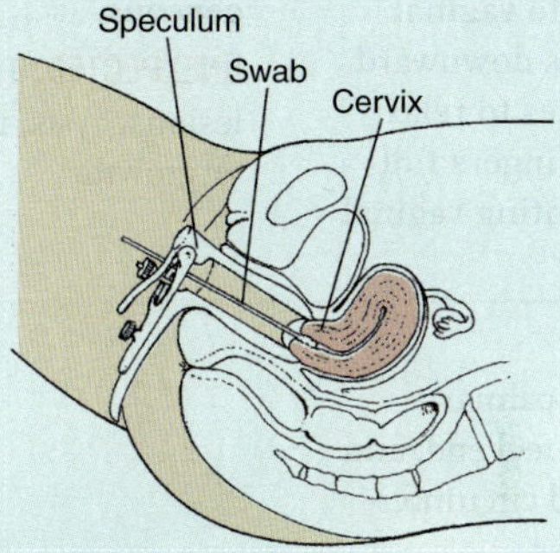

(From Grimes D: Infectious diseases, St. Louis, 1991, Mosby.)

DNA Testing for Organisms

Use a Dacron swab (with a plastic or wire shaft) when collecting the specimen; wooden, cotton-tipped applicators may interfere with test results. Also be sure to check the expiration date so as not to use out-of-date materials. Insert the swab into the cervical os, then rotate the swab in the endocervical canal for 30 seconds to ensure adequate sampling and absorption by the swab. Avoid contact with the vaginal mucous membranes, which would contaminate the specimen. Remove the swab and place it in the tube containing the specimen reagent. Single- or dual-organism tests are available for *Chlamydia trachomatis* and *Neisseria gonorrhoeae*. Multiorganism tests are available for *Trichomonas vaginalis, Gardnerella vaginalis*, and *Candida* species.

Wet Mount and Potassium Hydroxide Procedures

In a patient with vaginal discharge, these microscope examinations can demonstrate the presence of *T. vaginalis*, bacterial vaginosis, or candidiasis. For the wet mount, obtain a specimen of vaginal discharge using a swab. Smear the sample on a glass slide and add a drop of normal saline solution. Place a coverslip on the slide and view under the microscope. The presence of trichomonads indicates *T. vaginalis*. The presence of bacteria-filled epithelial cells (clue cells) indicates bacterial vaginosis. On a separate glass slide, place a specimen of vaginal discharge, apply a drop of aqueous 10% potassium hydroxide (KOH), and put a coverslip in place. The presence of a fishy odor (the "whiff test") suggests bacterial vaginosis. The KOH dissolves epithelial cells and debris and facilitates visualization of the mycelia of a fungus. View the specimen under the microscope for the presence of mycelial fragments, hyphae, and budding yeast cells, which indicate candidiasis.

TECHNIQUE	FINDINGS
Palpate vaginal wall while inserting fingers into vagina	
Insert tips of index and middle fingers into vaginal opening and press downward, waiting for muscles to relax. Gradually insert fingers full length while palpating vaginal wall.	**EXPECTED:** Smooth and homogeneous. **UNEXPECTED:** Tenderness, lesions, cysts, nodules, masses, or growths.
Palpate cervix	
Locate cervix with palmar surface of fingers, feel end, and run fingers around circumference to feel fornices.	
• *Size, shape, length*	**EXPECTED:** Consistent with speculum examination. The neovagina in a transgender woman is a blind cuff without a cervix or fornices.
• *Consistency*	**EXPECTED:** Firm in nonpregnant patient; softer in pregnant patient. **UNEXPECTED:** Nodules, hardness, or roughness.
• *Position*	**EXPECTED:** In midline, horizontal, or pointing anteriorly or posteriorly. Protruding into vagina 1–3 cm. **UNEXPECTED:** Deviation to right or left. Protrusion into vagina >1–3 cm.
• *Mobility* Grasp cervix gently between fingers and move from side to side. Observe patient's facial expression.	**EXPECTED:** 1–2-cm movement in each direction. Minimal discomfort. **UNEXPECTED:** Pain on movement (cervical motion tenderness).

TECHNIQUE	FINDINGS
Palpate uterus	
• *Location and position* Place palmar surface of outside hand on abdominal midline, halfway between umbilicus and symphysis pubis, and place intravaginal fingers in anterior fornix. Slowly slide outside hand toward pubis while pressing down and forward with flat surface of fingers; at the same time, push inward and up with fingertips of intravaginal hand while pushing down on cervix with backs of fingers. If uterus is anteverted or anteflexed, you should feel fundus between fingers of two hands at level of pubis. If uterus cannot be felt with this maneuver, place intravaginal fingers together in posterior fornix and outside hand immediately above symphysis pubis. Press down firmly with outside hand while pressing inward against cervix with intravaginal hand. If uterus is retroverted or retroflexed, you should feel fundus. If uterus cannot be felt with either of these maneuvers, move intravaginal fingers to each side of cervix, press inward, and feel as far as possible while keeping contact with cervix.	**EXPECTED:** In midline, horizontal, or pointing anteriorly or posteriorly. Protruding into vagina 1–3 cm. May be surgically absent. **UNEXPECTED:** Deviation to right or left. Protrusion into vagina >1–3 cm. 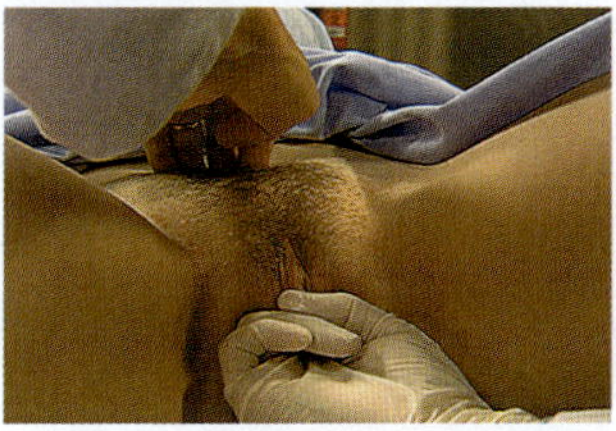

TECHNIQUE	FINDINGS
Slide fingers so they are on top and bottom of cervix, and continue pressing in while moving fingers to feel as much of uterus as possible (when uterus is in midposition, you will not be able to feel it with outside hand).	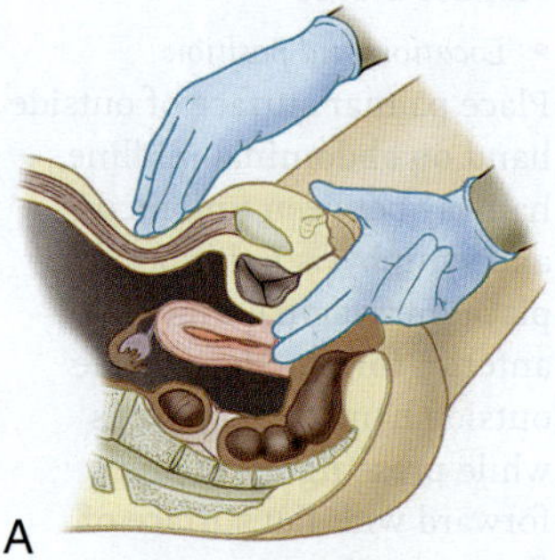

A

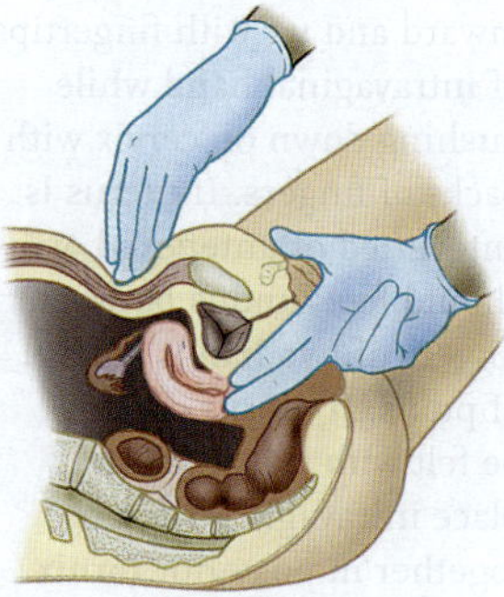

B

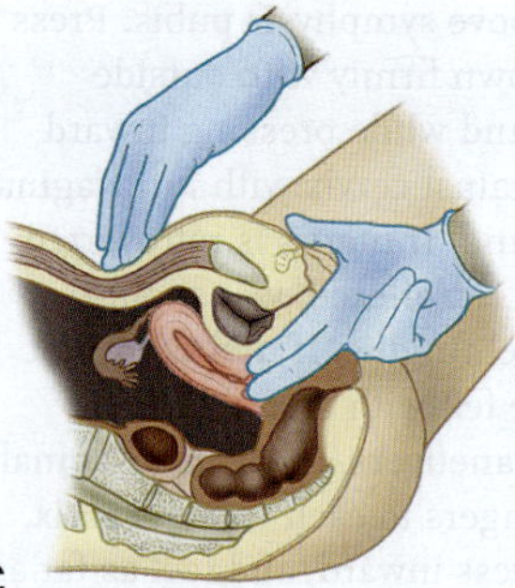

C

TECHNIQUE	FINDINGS

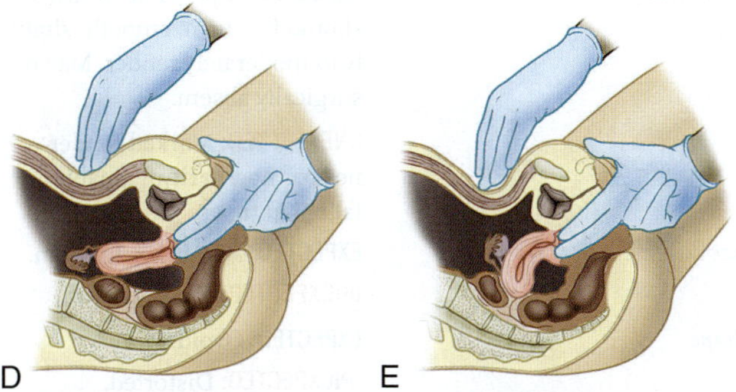

D E

(A) Retroverted. (B) Anteflexed. (C) Anteverted. (D) Midline. (E) Retroflexed.

TECHNIQUE	FINDINGS
• *Size, shape, contour*	**EXPECTED:** Pear-shaped and 5.5–8 cm long (larger in all dimensions in multiparous patients). Contour rounded and, in nonpregnant patients, walls firm and smooth. **UNEXPECTED:** Larger than expected or interrupted contour or smoothness.
• *Mobility* Gently move uterus between intravaginal fingers and outside hand.	**EXPECTED:** Mobile in anteroposterior plane. **UNEXPECTED:** Fixed uterus or tenderness on movement.

Palpate ovaries

Place fingers of outside hand on lower right quadrant. With intravaginal hand facing up, place both fingers in right lateral fornix. Press intravaginal fingers deeply in and up toward abdominal hand while sweeping flat surface of fingers of outside hand deeply in and obliquely down toward symphysis pubis. Palpate entire area by firmly pressing outside hand and intravaginal fingers together. Repeat on left side.

TECHNIQUE	FINDINGS
• *Consistency*	**EXPECTED:** If palpable, ovaries should feel firm, smooth, slightly to moderately tender. May be surgically absent. **UNEXPECTED:** Marked tenderness or nodularity. Palpable fallopian tubes.
• *Size*	**EXPECTED:** About 3 × 2 × 1 cm. **UNEXPECTED:** Enlargement.
• *Shape*	**EXPECTED:** Ovoid. **UNEXPECTED:** Distorted.

Palpate adnexal areas

Use hand positions for palpating ovaries.	**EXPECTED:** Adnexa difficult to palpate. **UNEXPECTED:** Masses and tenderness. If adnexal masses are found, characterize by size, shape, location, consistency, tenderness.

Internal Genitalia—Rectovaginal Examination

Change gloves. This examination may be uncomfortable for the patient. Assure them that the urgent feeling of a bowel movement will pass. Ask the patient to breathe slowly and try to relax the sphincter, rectum, and buttocks.

Insert index finger into vagina and middle finger into anus

To insert middle finger into anus, press against anus and ask patient to bear down; slip tip of finger into rectum just past sphincter.

Assess sphincter tone

Palpate area of anorectal junction and just above it. Ask patient to tighten and relax anal sphincter.	**EXPECTED:** Even sphincter tightening. **UNEXPECTED:** Extremely tight, lax, or absent sphincter.

TECHNIQUE	FINDINGS
Palpate anterior rectal wall and rectovaginal septum	
Slide both fingers in as far as possible, then ask patient to bear down. Rotate rectal finger to explore anterior rectal wall and palpate rectovaginal septum.	**EXPECTED:** Smooth and uninterrupted. Uterine body and uterine fundus sometimes felt with retroflexed uterus. **UNEXPECTED:** Masses, polyps, nodules, strictures, irregularities, tenderness.
Palpate posterior aspect of uterus	
Place outside hand just above symphysis pubis and press down firmly and deeply while positioning intravaginal finger in posterior vaginal fornix and pressing strongly upward against posterior side of cervix, as shown in the following figure. Palpate as much of posterior side of uterus as possible.	**EXPECTED:** Consistent with bimanual examination regarding location, position, size, shape, contour. **UNEXPECTED:** Tenderness.

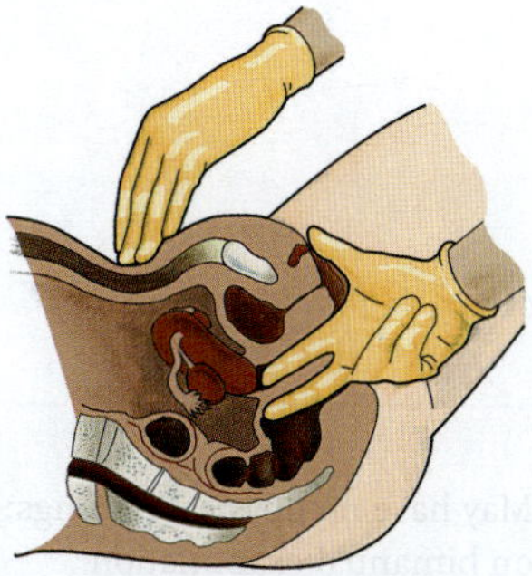

(From Lowdermilk DL, Perry SE: Maternity and women's health care, *ed 8, St. Louis, 2007, Mosby.)*

TECHNIQUE	FINDINGS
Palpate posterior rectal wall	
As you withdraw fingers, rotate intrarectal finger to evaluate posterior rectal wall.	**EXPECTED:** Smooth and uninterrupted. **UNEXPECTED:** Masses, polyps, nodules, strictures, irregularities, tenderness.
Note characteristics of feces when gloved finger removed	
	EXPECTED: Light to dark brown. **UNEXPECTED:** Blood. Note color and prepare specimen for fecal occult blood test if indicated.
Unless they are unable to do so, let patient wipe off the lubricating gel	

AIDS TO DIFFERENTIAL DIAGNOSIS

SUBJECTIVE DATA	OBJECTIVE DATA
Premenstrual Syndrome	
Breast swelling and tenderness, acne, bloating and weight gain, headache or joint pain, food cravings, irritability, difficulty concentrating, mood swings, crying spells, depression. Symptoms occur 5–7 days before menses (luteal phase) and subside with onset of menses.	None; diagnosis based on symptoms.
Endometriosis	
Pelvic pain, dysmenorrhea, heavy or prolonged menstrual flow.	May have no physical findings; on bimanual examination, tender nodules may be palpable along the uterosacral ligaments. Diagnosis confirmed by laparoscopy.

SUBJECTIVE DATA	OBJECTIVE DATA
Condylomata Acuminata (Genital Warts)	
Warty lesions on labia, within vestibule, or in perianal region.	Flesh-colored, whitish pink to reddish brown, discrete, soft growths on labia, vestibule, or perianal area; may occur singly or in clusters and may enlarge to cauliflower masses.
Genital Herpes	
Painful lesions in genital area; history of sexual contact; may report burning or pain with urination.	Small, red vesicles in genital area.
Vaginal Infections	
Vaginal discharge, possibly accompanied by urinary symptoms. Sometimes asymptomatic.	See table on pp. 183–184.
Cervical Carcinoma	
Often asymptomatic; sometimes vaginal bleeding.	Hard, granular surface at or near cervical os. Lesion can evolve to form extensive, irregular, easily bleeding cauliflower growth. Precancerous and early cancer changes detected by Pap smear, not by physical examination.
Abnormal Uterine Bleeding	
See table on p. 185. Irregularities in the menstrual cycle involving frequency, regularity, duration, and volume of flow outside of pregnancy. AUB also includes intermenstrual bleeding.	

SUBJECTIVE DATA	OBJECTIVE DATA
Pelvic Inflammatory Disease (PID)	
Painful intercourse, painful urination, irregular menstrual bleeding, pain in the right upper abdomen.	*Acute PID:* Very tender bilateral adnexal areas. *Chronic PID:* Bilateral tender, irregular, fairly fixed adnexal areas.
Ovarian Cancer	
Persistent and unexplained vague gastrointestinal symptoms such as generalized abdominal discomfort and/or pain, gas, indigestion, pressure, swelling, bloating, cramps, or feeling of fullness, even after a light meal.	May have no physical findings; on bimanual examination, an enlarged ovary in premenopausal patient or a palpable ovary in postmenopausal patients.

Differential Diagnosis of Vaginal Discharges and Infections

CONDITION	HISTORY	PHYSICAL FINDINGS	DIAGNOSTIC TESTS
Physiologic vaginitis	Increase in discharge; no foul odor, itching, or edema	Clear or mucoid discharge; pH < 4.5	Wet mount: up to 3–5 white blood cells (WBCs); epithelial cells
Bacterial vaginosis (*G. vaginalis*)	Foul-smelling discharge; has concern about "fishy odor"	Homogeneous, thin, white or gray discharge; pH ≥ 4.5	Positive KOH "whiff" test; wet mount: positive clue cells
Candida vulvovaginitis (*Candida albicans*)	Pruritic discharge, itching of labia; itching may extend to thighs	White, curdy discharge; pH 4.0–5.0; cervix may be red; may have erythema of perineum and thighs	KOH prep: Mycelia, budding, branching yeast, pseudohyphae
Trichomoniasis (*T. vaginalis*)	Watery discharge; foul odor; dysuria and dyspareunia with severe infection	Profuse, frothy, greenish discharge; pH 5.0–6.6; red friable cervix with petechiae ("strawberry" cervix)	Wet mount: Round or pear-shaped protozoa, motile "gyrating" flagella
Gonorrhea (*N. gonorrhoeae*)	Partner with sexually transmitted disease; often asymptomatic or may have symptoms of PID	Purulent discharge from cervix; Skene/Bartholin gland inflammation; cervix and vulva may be inflamed	Gram stain, culture, DNA probe
Chlamydia (*C. trachomatis*)	Partner with nongonococcal urethritis; often asymptomatic; may express concern about spotting after intercourse or urethritis	With or without purulent discharge; cervix may or may not be red or friable	DNA probe

Differential Diagnosis of Vaginal Discharges and Infections—cont'd

CONDITION	HISTORY	PHYSICAL FINDINGS	DIAGNOSTIC TESTS
Atrophic vaginitis	Dyspareunia; vaginal dryness; perimenopausal or postmenopausal	Pale, thin vaginal mucosa; pH > 4.5	Wet mount: Folded, clumped epithelial cells
Allergic vaginitis	New bubble bath, soap, douche, or other hygiene products	Foul smell, erythema; pH < 4.5	Wet mount: WBCs
Foreign body	Red and swollen vulva; vaginal discharge; history of tampon, condom, or diaphragm use	Bloody or foul-smelling discharge	Wet mount: WBCs

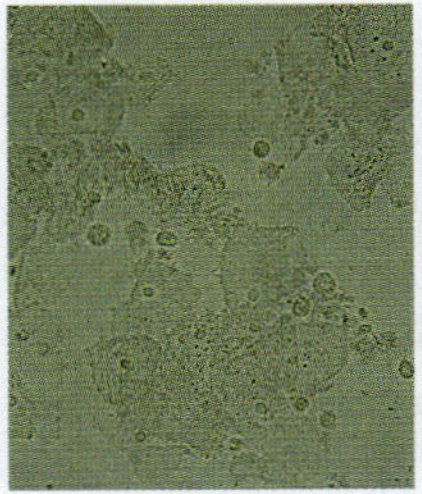

Bacterial vaginosis

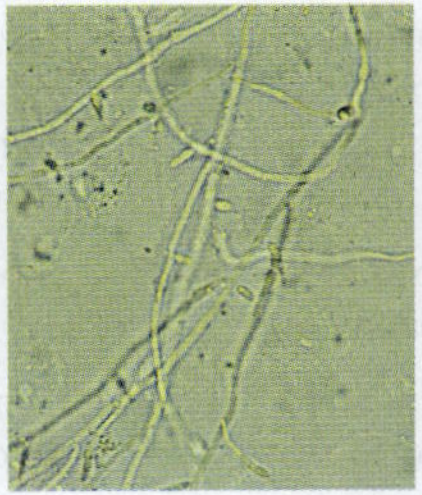

Candida vulvovaginitis

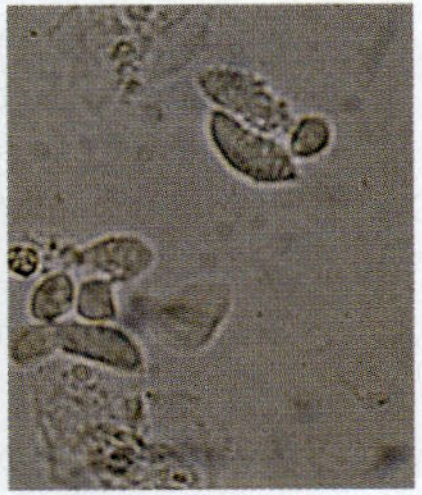

Trichomoniasis

Abnormal Uterine Bleeding: Parameters

PARAMETER	DESCRIPTION
Frequency	Absent (no bleeding) = amenorrhea Infrequent (>38 days) Normal (24 to ≤38 days) Frequent (<24 days)
Duration	Normal (≤8 days) Prolonged (>8 days)
Regularity	Normal or "Regular" (shortest to longest cycle variation: ≤7–9 days) Irregular (shortest to longest cycle variation: ≥8–10 days)
Flow Volume (patient determined)	Light Normal Heavy
Intermenstrual Bleeding	Bleeding between cyclically regular onset of menses Random or cyclical: early, mid or late cycle

Types of Uterine Abnormal Bleeding and Associated Causes

TYPE	COMMON CAUSES
Midcycle spotting	Midcycle estradiol fluctuation associated with ovulation
Delayed menstruation	Anovulation or threatened abortion with excessive bleeding
Frequent bleeding	Chronic PID, endometriosis, anovulation
Profuse menstrual bleeding	Endometrial polyps, adenomyosis, submucous leiomyomas, intrauterine device
Intermenstrual or irregular bleeding	Endometrial polyps, uterine or cervical cancer, oral contraceptives
Postmenopausal bleeding	Endometrial hyperplasia, estrogen therapy, endometrial cancer

PEDIATRIC VARIATIONS

EXAMINATION

TECHNIQUE	FINDINGS
Inspect external genitalia	
Examine infant using the frog-leg position.	**EXPECTED:** Genitalia of newborns reflect influence of maternal hormones. Labia majora and minora may be swollen, with labia minora often more prominent.
Inspect clitoris	
• *Size and length*	**EXPECTED:** The clitoris of a term infant is usually covered by labia minora and may appear relatively large.
Inspect urethral meatus and vaginal opening	
• *Inspect for discharge in infants and children*	**EXPECTED:** Mucoid whitish discharge is frequently seen during newborn period and sometimes as late as 4 weeks after birth. Discharge may be mixed with blood. **UNEXPECTED:** Mucoid discharge from irritation by diapers or powder; any discharge in children.
Assess pubertal development	
Assess Tanner stages of pubic hair development in patients assigned female at birth.	**EXPECTED:** Tanner stages of pubic hair development progress in the sequence shown. Findings may vary in transgender patients taking puberty blockers. **UNEXPECTED:** Failure to mature and premature maturation.

TECHNIQUE	FINDINGS

P_1—Tanner 1 (preadolescent). No growth of pubic hair.

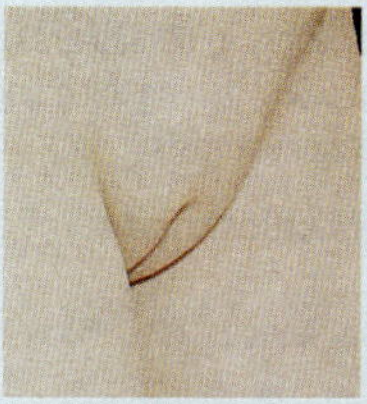

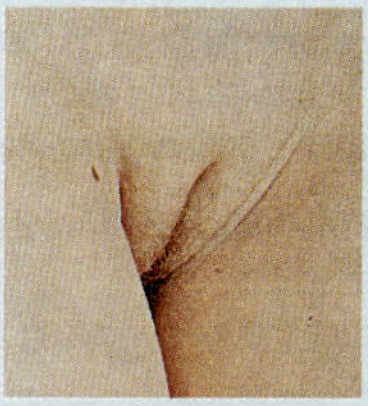

P_2—Tanner 2. Initial, scarcely pigmented straight hair, especially along medial border of the labia.

P_3—Tanner 3. Sparse, dark, visibly pigmented, curly pubic hair on labia.

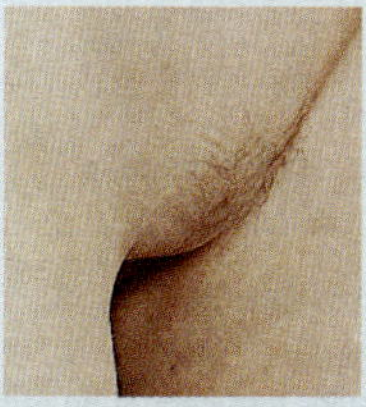

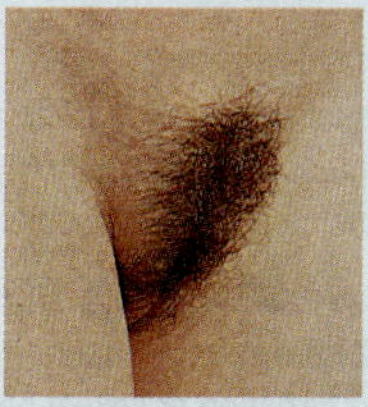

P_4—Tanner 4. Hair coarse and curly, abundant but less than adult.

P_5—Tanner 5. Lateral spreading; type and triangle spread of adult hair to medial surface of thighs.

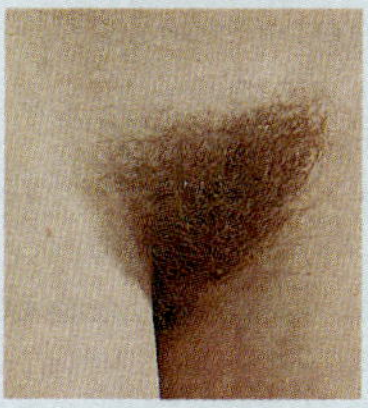

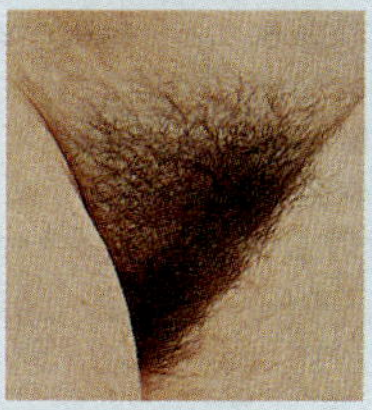

P_6—Tanner 6. Further extension laterally, upward, or dispersed (occurs in only 10% of women).

Six stages of public hair development in females. (Growth diagrams from Groningen J, Van Wieringen C, Wafelbakker F, Verbrugge HP, DeHaas JH: Second National Survey on 0-24-Year-Olds, *The Netherlands: Noordhoff Uitgevers BV, 1965.)*

"Red Flags" for Sexual Abuse

The following signs and symptoms in children or adolescents should raise your suspicion for sexual abuse. However, remember that any sign or symptom by itself is of limited significance; it may be related to sexual abuse, or it may be from another cause altogether. This is an area in which good clinical judgment is imperative. Each sign or symptom must be considered in context with the particular child's health status, stage of growth and development, and entire history.

Medical Concerns and Findings

- Evidence of general physical abuse or neglect
- Evidence of trauma and/or scarring in genital, anal, and perianal areas
- Unusual changes in skin color or pigmentation in genital or anal area
- Presence of sexually transmitted infection (oral, anal, genital)

Continued

- Anorectal problems such as itching, bleeding, pain, fecal incontinence, poor anal sphincter tone, bowel habit dysfunction
- Genitourinary problems, such as rash or sores in genital area, vaginal odor or discharge, pain (including abdominal pain), itching, bleeding, discharge, dysuria, hematuria, urinary tract infections, enuresis

Examples of Nonspecific Behavioral Manifestations

- Problems with school
- Dramatic weight changes or eating disturbances
- Depression
- Anxiety
- Sleep problems or nightmares
- Sudden change in personality or behavior
- Increased aggression and impulsivity or destructiveness
- Sudden avoidance of certain people or places

Examples of Sexual Behaviors That Are Concerning

- Use of sexually provocative mannerisms
- Excessive masturbation or sexual behavior that cannot be redirected
- Age-inappropriate sexual knowledge or experience
- Repeated object insertion into vagina and/or anus
- Child asking to be touched/kissed in genital area
- Sex play between children with 4 or more years of age difference
- Sex play that involves the use of force, threats, or bribes

Modified from Hornor (2004), Jenny et al. (2013); Kellogg (2010), Koop (1988), McClain et al. (2000).

Early Signs of Pregnancy

The following are physical signs that occur early in pregnancy. These signs, along with internal ballottement, palpation of fetal parts, and positive test results for urine or serum human chorionic gonadotropin, are probable indicators of pregnancy. They are considered "probable" because clinical conditions other than pregnancy may cause any one of them. However, their simultaneous occurrence creates a strong case for the presence of a pregnancy.

SIGN	FINDING	APPROXIMATE WEEKS OF GESTATION
Goodell	Softening of cervix	4–6
Hegar	Softening of uterine isthmus	6–8
McDonald	Easy flexing of fundus on cervix	7–8
Braun von Fernwald	Fullness and softening of fundus near site of implantation	7–8
Piskacek	Palpable lateral bulge or soft prominence of one uterine cornu	7–8
Chadwick	Bluish color of cervix, vagina, vulva	8–12

CHAPTER

17 Male Genitalia

For ease of communication, in this handbook the term “male genitalia” refers to the following anatomic structures: penis, testicles, epididymides, scrotum, and seminal vesicles, regardless of the gender identity of the patient.

Equipment

- Gloves
- Penlight

EXAMINATION

Have patient lying or standing to start examination.

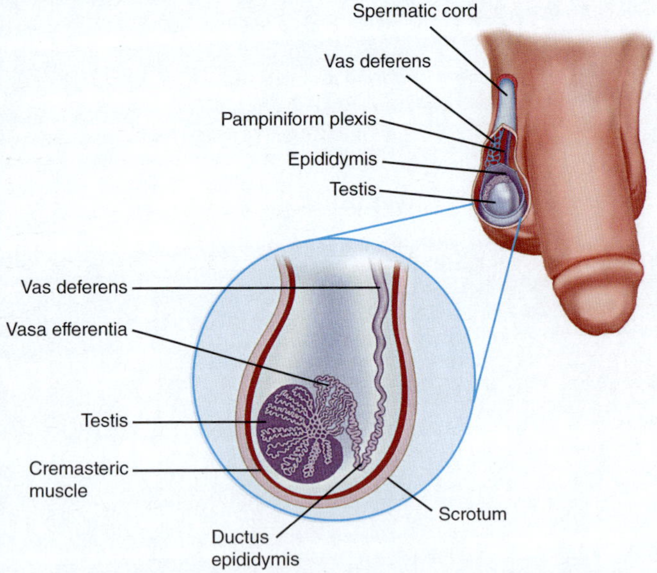

(From Phipps, et al.: Medical-surgical nursing, ed 8, St. Louis, 2007, Mosby.)

TECHNIQUE	FINDINGS
Wear gloves on both hands	
Inspect pubic hair	
• *Characteristics*	**EXPECTED:** Coarser than scalp hair.
• *Distribution*	**EXPECTED:** Diamond-shaped distribution in patients assigned male at birth: abundant in pubic region, continuing around scrotum to anal orifice, possibly continuing in narrowing midline to umbilicus. Penis without hair, scrotum with scant hair. **UNEXPECTED:** Alopecia. Nits or lice.
Inspect glans penis	
• *Uncircumcised patient* Retract foreskin or ask patient to do so.	**EXPECTED:** Dorsal vein apparent. Foreskin easily retracted. White, cheesy smegma visible over glans. **UNEXPECTED:** Tight foreskin (phimosis). Lesions or discharge.
• *Circumcised patient*	**EXPECTED:** Dorsal vein apparent. Exposed glans erythematous and dry. **UNEXPECTED:** Lesions or discharge.
Examine external meatus of urethra (foreskin retracted in uncircumcised patient)	
• *Shape*	**EXPECTED:** Slitlike opening. **UNEXPECTED:** Pinpoint or round opening.
• *Location*	**EXPECTED:** On ventral surface and only millimeters from tip of glans. **UNEXPECTED:** Anyplace other than tip of glans, or along shaft of penis.
• *Urethral orifice* Press glans between thumb and forefinger.	**EXPECTED:** Opening glistening and pink. **UNEXPECTED:** Bright erythema or discharge.

TECHNIQUE	FINDINGS
Palpate penis	
Palpate the shaft of the penis.	**EXPECTED:** Soft (flaccid penis). **UNEXPECTED:** Tenderness, induration, or nodularity. Prolonged erection (priapism).
Strip urethra	
Firmly compress base of penis with thumb and forefinger; move toward glans.	**EXPECTED:** No discharge. **UNEXPECTED:** Discharge.
Inspect scrotum and ventral surface of penis	
• *Color*	**EXPECTED:** Darker than body skin and often reddened in red-haired patients.
• *Texture*	**EXPECTED:** Surface possibly coarse. Small lumps on scrotal skin (sebaceous or epidermoid cysts) that sometimes discharge oily material.
• *Shape*	**EXPECTED:** Asymmetry. Thickness varying with temperature, age, emotional state. **UNEXPECTED:** Unusual thickening, often with pitting.
Palpate inguinal canal for direct or indirect hernia	
With patient standing, instruct to bear down as if for bowel movement. While patient strains, inspect area of inguinal canal and region of fossa ovalis. Ask patient to relax, and insert examining finger into lower part of scrotum and carry upward along vas deferens into inguinal canal, as shown in figure on p. 4. Ask patient to cough. Repeat examination on opposite side.	**EXPECTED:** Presence of oval external ring. **UNEXPECTED:** Feeling a viscus against examining finger with coughing. If hernia felt, note as indirect (felt within inguinal canal or even into scrotum) or direct (felt medial to external canal).

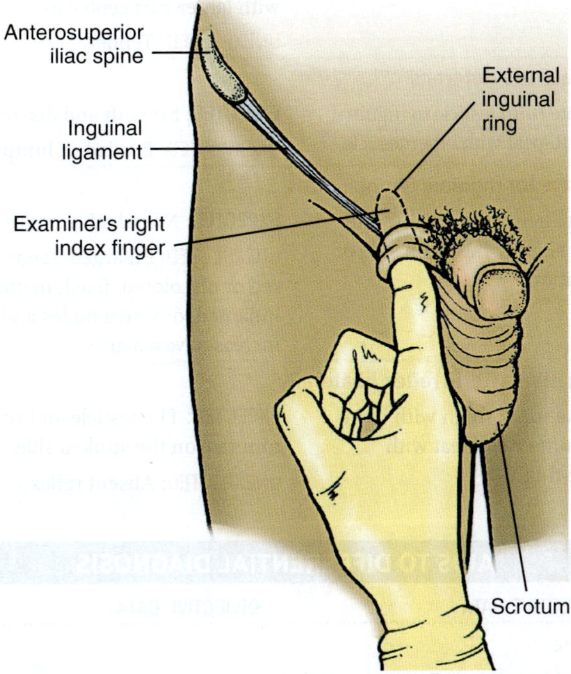

TECHNIQUE	FINDINGS
Palpate testes	
Use thumb and first two fingers. Compress gently.	
• *Descent*	**EXPECTED:** Both testes are present in scrotal sac. **UNEXPECTED:** Cryptorchidism.
• *Consistency*	**EXPECTED:** Smooth and rubbery. Sensitive to gentle compression. **UNEXPECTED:** Tenderness or nodules. Total insensitivity to painful stimuli.
• *Texture*	**UNEXPECTED:** Irregular texture.
• *Size*	**UNEXPECTED:** Irregular size; asymmetry in size <1 cm or >5 cm.

TECHNIQUE	FINDINGS
Palpate epididymides	
	EXPECTED: Smooth and discrete, with larger part cephalad. UNEXPECTED: Tender.
Palpate vas deferens	
Palpate from testicle to inguinal ring. Repeat with other testicle.	EXPECTED: Smooth and discrete. UNEXPECTED: Beaded or lumpy.
Palpate for inguinal lymph nodes	
Ask patient to lie supine with knee slightly flexed on side of palpation.	EXPECTED: No palpable nodes. UNEXPECTED: Enlarged, tender, red or discolored, fixed, matted, inflamed, or warm nodes and increased vascularity.
Elicit cremasteric reflex bilaterally	
Stroke inner thigh with blunt instrument. Repeat with other thigh.	EXPECTED: The testicle and scrotum rise on the stroked side. UNEXPECTED: Absent reflex.

AIDS TO DIFFERENTIAL DIAGNOSIS

SUBJECTIVE DATA	OBJECTIVE DATA
Hernia	
See table on pp. 6–7	
Genital Herpes	
Painful lesions on penis; sexually active; may report burning or pain with urination.	Superficial vesicles—located on glans, penile shaft, or base of penis; often associated with inguinal lymphadenopathy.
Condylomata Acuminata (Genital Warts)	
Soft, painless, wartlike lesions on penis. Sexually active.	Single or multiple papular lesions; may be pearly, filiform, fungating (ulcerating and necrotic), cauliflower-like, or plaquelike.
Hydrocele	
Painless enlargement or swelling of the scrotum.	Nontender, smooth, firm mass superior and anterior to the testis. Transilluminates.

SUBJECTIVE DATA	OBJECTIVE DATA
Varicocele	
Usually asymptomatic (and found during evaluation for infertility); may report scrotal pain or heaviness.	Abnormal tortuosity and dilated veins of pampiniform plexus within spermatic cord; described as "bag of worms."
Epididymitis	
Painful scrotum, urethral discharge, fever, pyuria, recent sexual activity.	Possible erythema of overlying scrotum, epididymis feels firm and lumpy and may be slightly tender, and vasa deferentia may be beaded.
Testicular Torsion	
Acute onset of scrotal pain, often accompanied by nausea and vomiting; absence of systemic symptoms such as fever and myalgia.	Testicle is exquisitely tender; scrotal discoloration often present.
Testicular Cancer	
Painless mass in testicle, scrotal enlargement or swelling; sensation of heaviness in the scrotum, dull ache in the lower abdomen, back, or groin.	Irregular, nontender mass fixed on the testis; does not transilluminate.
Paraphimosis	
Retraction of the foreskin during penile examination, cleaning, urethral catheterization, or cystoscopy; penile pain and swelling.	Glans penis congested and enlarged; foreskin edematous; constricting band of tissue directly behind the head of the penis.

Distinguishing Characteristics of Hernias

	INDIRECT INGUINAL	DIRECT INGUINAL	FEMORAL
Incidence	Most common type of hernia; often patients are children and young males	Less common than indirect inguinal; more common in those older than 40 years	Least common type of hernia; rare in children

Continued

Distinguishing Characteristics of Hernias—cont'd

	INDIRECT INGUINAL	DIRECT INGUINAL	FEMORAL
Pathway	Through internal inguinal ring; can remain in canal, exit external ring, or pass into scrotum; may be bilateral	Through femoral external inguinal ring; located in region of Hesselbach triangle; rarely enters scrotum	Through femoral ring, femoral canal, fossa ovalis
Presentation	Soft swelling in area of internal ring; pain on straining; hernia comes down canal and touches fingertip on examination	Bulge in area of Hesselbach triangle; usually painless; easily reduced; hernia bulges anteriorly, pushes against side of finger on examination	Right side presentation more common than left; pain may be severe; inguinal canal empty on examination

PEDIATRIC VARIATIONS

EXAMINATION

TECHNIQUE	FINDINGS
Inspect glans penis • *Uncircumcised patient* Retract foreskin.	**EXPECTED:** In children, foreskin is fully retractable by age 3–4 years. Before that age, forced retraction of foreskin may result in injury. Urethral meatus at tip of penis. **UNEXPECTED:** Foreskin adherent in children >4 years. Urethral meatus on dorsal or ventral surface or base of penis.
Palpate scrotum • *Descent* Palpate testes in children to determine whether testes have descended. If any mass other than testicles or spermatic cord is palpated in scrotum, determine whether it is filled with fluid, gas, or solid material.	**EXPECTED:** Bilaterally palpable; 1 cm. Considered descended if testis can be pushed into scrotum. **UNEXPECTED:** Not palpable unilaterally or bilaterally. If penlight transilluminates, most likely contains fluid (hydrocele). If no light transillumination, most likely a hernia.

TECHNIQUE	FINDINGS

Evaluate maturation in adolescence

Assess stage of pubertal development

In patients assigned male at birth, assess the stage of genital and pubic hair development.

EXPECTED: Tanner stages of pubic hair and external genital development progress in the sequence shown. Findings may vary in transgender patients taking puberty blockers.

UNEXPECTED: Failure to mature and premature maturation.

G_1—Tanner 1. Testes, scrotum, and penis are the same size and shape as in the young child.

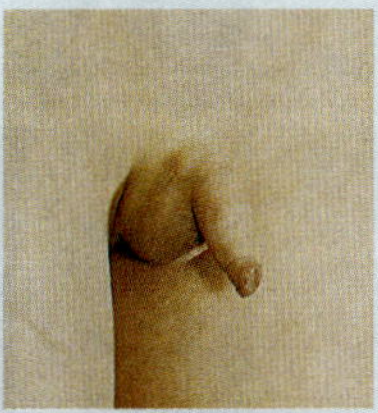

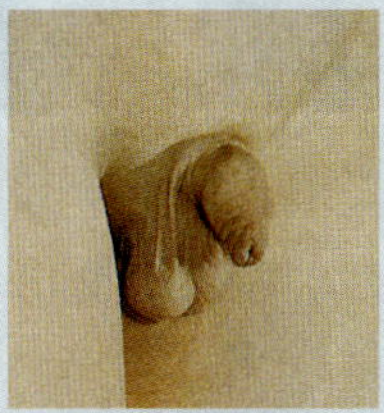

G_2—Tanner 2. Enlargement of scrotum and testes. The skin of the scrotum becomes redder, thinner, and wrinkled. Penis no larger or scarcely so.

G_3—Tanner 3. Enlargement of the penis, especially in length; further enlargement of testes; descent of scrotum.

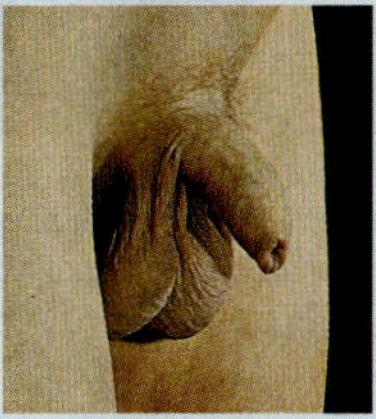

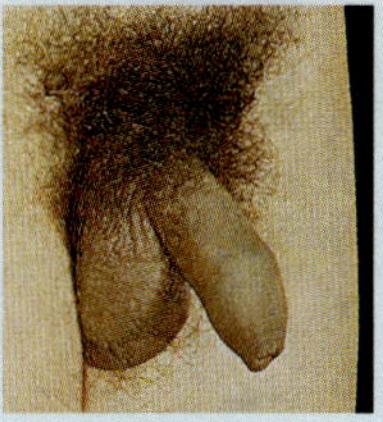

G_4—Tanner 4. Continued enlargement of the penis and sculpturing of the glans; increased pigmentation of scrotum.

G_5—Tanner 5 (adult stage). Scrotum ample, penis reaching nearly to bottom of scrotum.

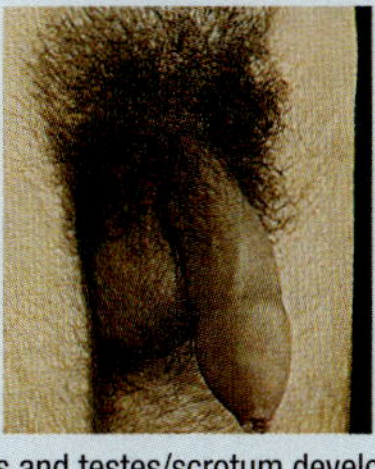

Five stages of penis and testes/scrotum development in people assigned male at birth. (Growth diagrams from Groningen J, Van Wieringen C, Wafelbakker F, Verbrugge HP, DeHaas JH: *Second national survey on 0–24-year-olds,* The Netherlands, 1965, Noordhoff Uitgevers BV.)

Continued

P_1—Tanner 1 (preadolescent). No growth of pubic hair; that is, hair in pubic area no different from that on the rest of the abdomen.

P_2—Tanner 2. Slightly pigmented, longer, straight hair, often still downy; usually at base of penis, sometimes on scrotum. Stage is difficult to photograph.

P_3—Tanner 3. Dark, definitely pigmented, curly pubic hair around base of penis. Stage 3 can be photographed.

P_4—Tanner 4. Pubic hair definitely adult in type but not in extent (no further than inguinal fold).

P_5—Tanner 5 (adult distribution). Hair spread to medial surface of thighs, but not upward.

P_6—Hair spread along linea alba (occurs in 80% of men).

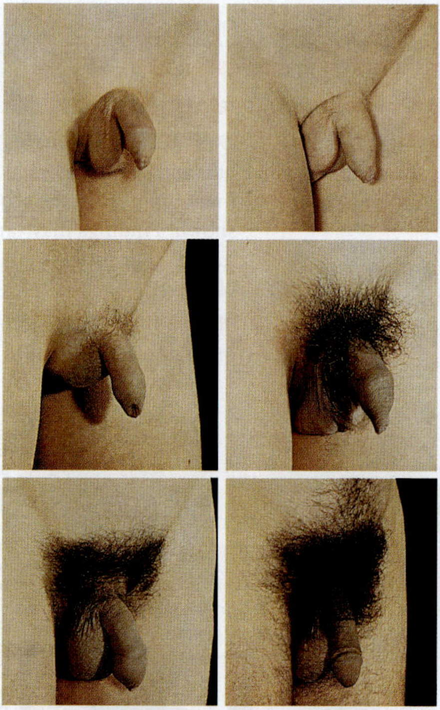

Six stages of pubic hair development in people assigned male at birth.
(Growth diagrams from Groningen J, Van Wieringen C, Wafelbakker F, Verbrugge HP, DeHaas JH: *Second national survey on 0–24-year-olds,* The Netherlands, 1965, Noordhoff Uitgevers BV.)

CHAPTER 18

Anus, Rectum, and Prostate

Equipment

- Gloves
- Water-soluble lubricant
- Light source
- Drapes
- Fecal occult blood testing materials if indicated

EXAMINATION

Rectal examination can be performed with the patient in any of these positions: knee-chest; lithotomy; left lateral with hips and knees flexed; or standing with the hips flexed and the upper body supported by the examining table. Patients should be examined in the position congruent with their identified gender and accounting for their comfort and anatomy. Drape patient appropriately. In patients with a prostate, the latter two positions are satisfactory and allow adequate visualization of the perianal and sacrococcygeal areas as well as positioning for the prostate examination. For transgender women who have had a vaginoplasty, the prostate is anterior to the vaginal wall. A digital neovaginal exam may be more effective.

TECHNIQUE	FINDINGS
Wear Gloves on Both Hands	
Inspect and palpate sacrococcygeal and perianal area	
• *Skin characteristics*	**EXPECTED:** Smooth and uninterrupted. **UNEXPECTED:** Lumps, rashes, tenderness, inflammation, excoriation, pilonidal dimpling, or tufts of hair.
Inspect anus Spread patient's buttocks. Examine, using penlight or lamp if needed, with patient relaxed and bearing down.	

TECHNIQUE	FINDINGS
• *Skin characteristics*	**EXPECTED:** Skin coarser and darker than on buttocks. **UNEXPECTED:** Skin lesions, skin tags or warts, external or internal hemorrhoids, fissures and fistulas, rectal prolapse, or polyps.

Inspect, palpate, and assess sphincter tone

TECHNIQUE	FINDINGS
Put water-soluble lubricant on index or middle finger; press pad against anal opening and ask patient to bear down to relax external sphincter. As relaxation occurs, slip tip of finger into anal canal, as shown in the following figure on p. 200. (Assure patient that although they may feel the urgency of a bowel movement, it will not occur.) Ask patient to tighten external sphincter around finger.	**EXPECTED:** Even sphincter tightening. **UNEXPECTED:** Patient discomfort. Lax or extremely tight sphincter, tenderness.

Palpate muscular anal ring

TECHNIQUE	FINDINGS
Rotate finger.	**EXPECTED:** Smooth, even with consistent pressure exerted. **UNEXPECTED:** Nodules or other irregularities.

Palpate lateral and posterior rectal walls

TECHNIQUE	FINDINGS
Insert finger farther and rotate to palpate lateral, then posterior, rectal walls. If helpful, perform bidigital palpation with thumb and finger by lightly pressing thumb against perianal tissue and bringing finger toward thumb.	**EXPECTED:** Smooth, even, uninterrupted. **UNEXPECTED:** Nodules, masses, polyps, tenderness, or irregularities. (Internal hemorrhoids not ordinarily felt unless thrombosed.)

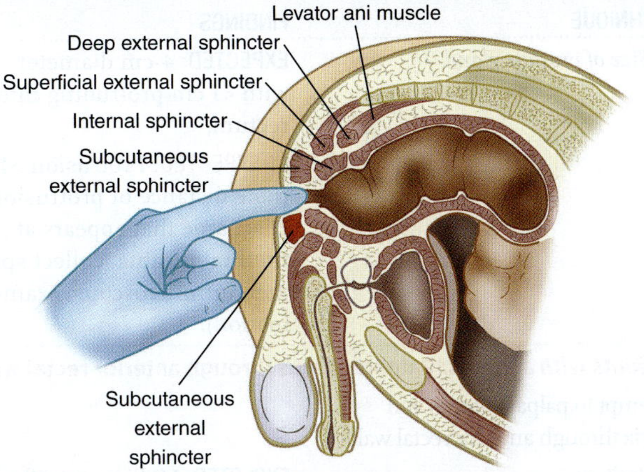

TECHNIQUE	FINDINGS
Patients with a prostate: **Palpate posterior surface of prostate gland through anterior rectal wall**	
For transgender women who have had a vaginoplasty, the prostate is anterior to the vaginal wall. A digital neovaginal exam may be more effective.	
Rotate finger and palpate anterior rectal wall and posterior surface of prostate gland. In transgender women with vaginoplasty, palpate the posterior surface of the prostate gland through the anterior neovaginal wall. Alert patient that the feeling of needing to urinate will pass.	
• *Consistency and characteristics of anterior rectal wall*	**EXPECTED:** Smooth, even, uninterrupted. **UNEXPECTED:** Nodules, masses, polyps, tenderness, or irregularities.
• *Consistency, contour, characteristics of prostate*	**EXPECTED:** Surface firm and smooth, lateral lobes symmetric, median sulcus palpable, seminal vesicles not palpable. **UNEXPECTED:** Rubberiness, bogginess, fluctuant softness, stony hard nodularity, tenderness, obliterated sulcus, or palpable seminal vesicles.

TECHNIQUE	FINDINGS
• *Size of prostate gland*	**EXPECTED:** 4-cm diameter with <1 cm protruding into rectum. **UNEXPECTED:** Protrusion >1 cm (note distance of protrusion). Discharge that appears at urethral meatus (collect specimen for microscopic examination).

Patients with a uterus: Palpate uterus through anterior rectal wall

Attempt to palpate uterus and cervix through anterior rectal wall.	
• *Position*	**EXPECTED:** Midline, retroflexed, or retroverted. **UNEXPECTED:** Deviation to right or left.
• *Surface characteristics*	**EXPECTED:** Smooth. **UNEXPECTED:** Irregular.

Have patient bear down, and palpate deeper

Ask patient to bear down while you reach farther into rectum.	**UNEXPECTED:** Tenderness of peritoneal area or nodules.

Withdraw finger and examine fecal material

• *Color and consistency*	**EXPECTED:** Soft and brown. **UNEXPECTED:** Blood, pus, or light tan, gray, or tarry black stool. If indicated, fecal material can be tested for blood using a chemical guaiac procedure.

AIDS TO DIFFERENTIAL DIAGNOSIS

SUBJECTIVE DATA	OBJECTIVE DATA
Anal warts (Condyloma acuminata)	
Growths on the anus and genitalia.	Single or multiple papular lesions; may be pearly, filiform, fungating (ulcerating and necrotic), cauliflower-like, or plaquelike.

SUBJECTIVE DATA	OBJECTIVE DATA
Perianal and Perirectal Abscesses	
Pain and tenderness in anal area.	Tender, swollen, fluctuant mass; may be draining.
Enterobius Infestation in Children	
Intense perianal itching, especially at night.	Positive tape test. Press the sticky side of cellulose tape against the perianal folds and then press the tape on a glass slide. Nematodes can be seen on microscopic examination.
Anorectal Fissure	
Hard stools; pain, itching, bleeding.	Fissure most often in the posterior midline; spastic internal sphincter.
Anorectal Fistula	
Chills, fever, nausea, vomiting, and malaise.	Elevated, red, granular tissue at external opening, possibly with serosanguineous or purulent drainage on compression of the area; palpable indurated tract.
Hemorrhoids	
Itching and bleeding; discomfort.	May or may not be visible; may be palpable as soft swellings. Thrombosed hemorrhoids appear as blue, shiny masses at anus.
Rectal Carcinoma	
Bleeding; may be asymptomatic.	Sessile polypoid mass with nodular raised edges and areas of ulceration; consistency often stony with irregular contour.

SUBJECTIVE DATA	OBJECTIVE DATA
Prostatic Carcinoma	
Early carcinoma asymptomatic; symptoms of urinary obstruction as carcinoma advances.	Hard, irregular nodule may be palpable on prostate examination; prostate asymmetric, median sulcus may be obliterated; biopsy required for diagnosis.
Prostatitis	
Acute: Pain, urination problems, sexual dysfunction, fever, chills, shakes. *Chronic:* Asymptomatic, frequent bladder infections, frequent urination, persistent pain in the lower abdomen or back.	*Acute:* Prostate enlarged, acutely tender, and often asymmetric. May have urethral discharge and fever; bacteria in the urine. *Chronic:* Prostate boggy, enlarged, and tender or have palpable areas of fibrosis.
Benign Prostatic Hypertrophy	
Symptoms of urinary obstruction: hesitancy, decreased force and caliber of stream, dribbling, incomplete emptying of the bladder, frequency, urgency, nocturia, and dysuria.	Prostate smooth, rubbery, symmetric, and enlarged; median sulcus may or may not be obliterated.

Prostate Enlargement

Prostate enlargement is classified by the amount of protrusion into the rectum

Grade I: 1–2 cm
Grade II: 2–3 cm
Grade III: 3–4 cm
Grade IV: >1 cm

PEDIATRIC VARIATIONS

EXAMINATION

TECHNIQUE	FINDINGS
Examine the patency of the anus and its position in all newborn infants. To determine patency, insert a lubricated catheter no more than 1 cm into the rectum.	**EXPECTED:** Catheter inserts; patency confirmed by passage of meconium. **UNEXPECTED:** Not able to insert catheter; no evidence of stool.
Inspect perianal area.	**UNEXPECTED:** Parental concerns about infant's or child's irritability at night or evidence that child has itching in perianal area may indicate presence of parasites such as roundworms or pinworms. Specimen collection and microscopic examination are necessary to confirm findings. Shrunken buttocks suggest a chronic debilitating disease. Asymmetric creases occur with congenital dislocation of the hips. Perirectal redness and irritation are suggestive of pinworms, *Candida*, or other irritants of the diaper area. Rectal prolapse results from constipation, diarrhea, or sometimes severe coughing or straining. Hemorrhoids are rare in children, and their presence suggests a serious underlying problem such as portal hypertension. Small, flat flaps of skin around the rectum (condylomata) may be syphilitic in origin. Sinuses, tufts of hair, and dimpling in the pilonidal area may indicate lower spinal deformities.

CHAPTER

19 Musculoskeletal System

Equipment

- Goniometer
- Skin-marking pencil
- Reflex hammer
- Tape measure

EXAMINATION

Begin examination by observing gait and posture as patient enters room. During examination, note ease of movement when patient walks, sits, rises, takes off garments, and responds to directions.

TECHNIQUE	FINDINGS
Posture and General Guidelines	
Inspect skeleton and extremities, comparing sides	
Inspect anterior, posterior, lateral aspects of posture; ability to stand erect; extremities.	
• *Size, alignment, contour, symmetry* Measure extremities when lack of symmetry is noted in length or circumference.	**EXPECTED:** Bilateral symmetry of length, circumference, alignment, position, and number of skinfolds; aligned extremities. **UNEXPECTED:** Gross deformity, lordosis, kyphosis, scoliosis, bony enlargement.
Inspect skin and subcutaneous tissues over muscles, cartilage, bones, joints	**UNEXPECTED:** Discoloration, swelling, or masses.
Inspect muscles and compare sides	
• *Size and symmetry*	**EXPECTED:** Approximately symmetric bilateral muscle size. **UNEXPECTED:** Gross hypertrophy or atrophy, fasciculations, or spasms.

TECHNIQUE	FINDINGS
Palpate all bones, joints, surrounding muscles (palpate inflamed joints last)	
• *Muscle tone*	**EXPECTED:** Firm. **UNEXPECTED:** Hard or doughy, spasticity.
• *Characteristics*	**UNEXPECTED:** Heat, tenderness, swelling, fluctuation of a joint, synovial thickening, crepitus, resistance to pressure, or discomfort to pressure on bones and joints.
Test each major joint and related muscle groups for active and passive range of motion, and compare sides	
Ask patient to move each joint through range of motion (see instructions for specific joints and muscles in individual sections that follow), then ask patient to relax as you passively move same joints until end of range is felt. 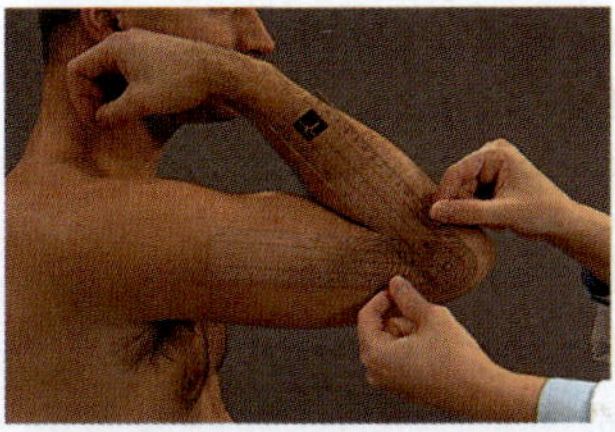 *Goniometer.*	**EXPECTED:** Passive range of motion often exceeds active range of motion by 5 degrees. Range of motion with passive and active maneuvers should be equal between contralateral joints. **UNEXPECTED:** Pain, limitation of motion, spastic movement, joint instability, deformity, contracture, discrepancies greater than 5 degrees between active and passive range of motion. When increase or limitation in range of motion is found, measure angles of greatest flexion and extension with goniometer, as shown in the accompanying figure, and compare with values as described for specific joints in individual extremities.
Test major muscle groups for strength, and compare contralateral sides	
For each muscle group, ask patient to contract a muscle by flexing or extending a joint and to resist as you apply opposing force. Compare bilaterally.	**EXPECTED:** Bilaterally symmetric strength with full resistance to opposition. **UNEXPECTED:** Inability to produce full resistance. Grade muscular strength according to the following table.

Muscle Strength Assessment

MUSCLE FUNCTION LEVEL	GRADE
No muscle activation	0
Trace muscle activation (twitch)	1
Muscle activation with gravity eliminated, full range of motion*	2
Muscle activation with full range of motion against gravity but not against resistance	3
Muscle activation with full range of motion against gravity and some weak resistance	4
Muscle activation with full range of motion against full resistance	5

*Passive movement.
https://www.ncbi.nlm.nih.gov/books/NBK436008/.

TECHNIQUE	FINDINGS

Hands and Wrists

Inspect dorsum and palm of each hand

- *Characteristics and contour*

  EXPECTED: Palmar and phalangeal creases, palmar surfaces with central depression with prominent, rounded mound on thumb side (thenar eminence), and less prominent hypothenar eminence on little-finger side.

- *Position*

  EXPECTED: Fingers able to fully extend and align with forearm when in close approximation to each other.

  UNEXPECTED: Deviation of fingers to ulnar side or inability to fully extend fingers; swan neck or boutonnière deformities.

- *Shape*

  EXPECTED: Lateral finger surfaces gradually tapered from proximal to distal aspects.

  UNEXPECTED: Spindle-shaped fingers, bony overgrowths, or synovial swelling at phalangeal joints.

TECHNIQUE	FINDINGS
Palpate each joint in hand and wrist	
Palpate interphalangeal joints as shown in figure below, panel A; metacarpophalangeal joints with both thumbs, panel B; and wrist and radiocarpal groove with thumbs on dorsal surface and fingers on palmar aspect of wrist, panel C.	**EXPECTED:** Joint surfaces smooth. **UNEXPECTED:** Nodules, swelling, bogginess, tenderness, or ganglion.

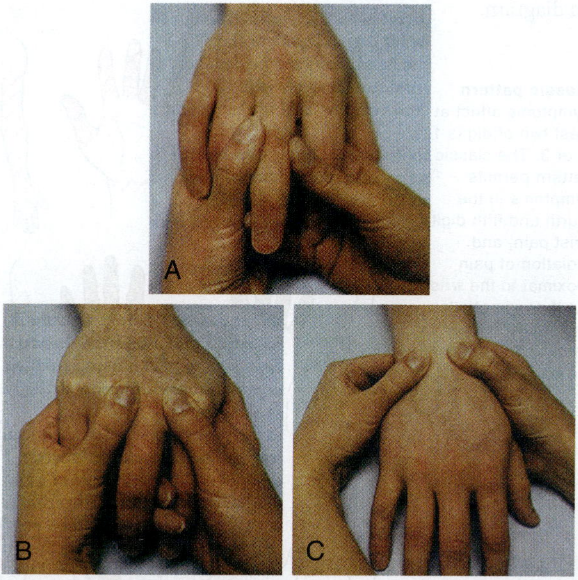

(A) Palpating the interphalangeal joints. (B) Palpating metacarpophalangeal joints with both thumbs. (C) Palpating radiocarpal groove with thumbs on dorsal surface and fingers on palmar aspect of wrist.

TECHNIQUE	FINDINGS
Assess integrity of median nerve	
• *Tinel sign* Strike median nerve where it passes through carpal tunnel with index or middle finger.	**UNEXPECTED:** Tingling sensation radiating from wrist to hand along pathway of median nerve.
• *Thumb abduction test* Apply downward pressure on thumb as patient holds thumb perpendicular to hand, palm side up.	**EXPECTED:** Full resistance to pressure. **UNEXPECTED:** Inability to produce full resistance.

TECHNIQUE	FINDINGS
• *Phalen test* Have patient hold both wrists in fully palmar-flexed position with dorsal surfaces pressed together for 1 minute.	**UNEXPECTED:** Numbness, paresthesia in distribution of median nerve.
• *Katz hand diagram* Have patient mark specific locations of pain, numbness, tingling in hands and arms on diagram.	**UNEXPECTED:** Pain, numbness, tingling in pattern shown in the following figure.

Classic pattern
Symptoms affect at least two of digits 1, 2, or 3. The classic pattern permits symptoms in the fourth and fifth digits, wrist pain, and radiation of pain proximal to the wrist, but it does not allow symptoms on the palm or dorsum of the hand.

Probable pattern
Same symptom pattern as classic except palmar symptoms are allowed unless confined solely to the ulnar aspect.
In the **possible pattern,** not shown, symptoms involve only one of digits 1, 2, or 3.

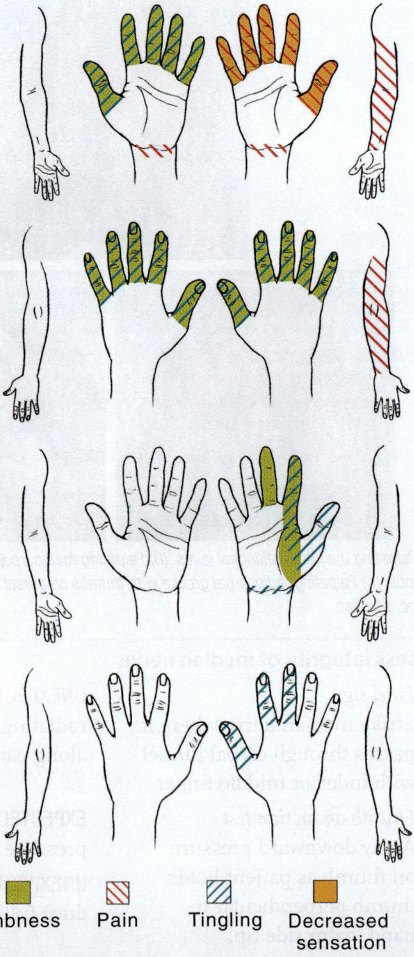

TECHNIQUE	FINDINGS
Test range of motion	
Ask patient to perform the following movements:	
• *Metacarpophalangeal flexion and hyperextension* Bend fingers forward at metacarpophalangeal joint, then stretch fingers up and back at knuckle.	EXPECTED: 90-degree metacarpophalangeal flexion and as much as 30-degree hyperextension.
• *Thumb opposition* Touch thumb to each fingertip and to base of little finger, then make a fist.	EXPECTED: Able to perform all movements.
• *Finger abduction and adduction* Spread fingers apart and then touch them together.	EXPECTED: Both movements possible.
• *Wrist extension and hyperextension* Bend hand at wrist up and down.	EXPECTED: 90-degree flexion and 70-degree hyperextension.
• *Radial and ulnar motion* With palm side down, turn each hand to right and left.	EXPECTED: 20-degree radial motion and 55-degree ulnar motion.
Test muscle strength	
Ask patient to perform the following movements:	
• *Wrist extension and hyperextension* Maintain wrist flexion while you apply opposing force.	EXPECTED: Bilaterally symmetric with full resistance to opposition. UNEXPECTED: Inability to produce full resistance.
• *Hand strength* Grip two of your fingers tightly.	EXPECTED: Firm, sustained grip. UNEXPECTED: Weakness or pain.

TECHNIQUE	FINDINGS
Elbows	
Inspect elbows in flexed and extended positions	
• *Contour*	**UNEXPECTED:** Subcutaneous nodules along pressure points of extensor surface of ulna.
• *Carrying angle* Inspect with arms at sides passively extended, palms facing forward.	**EXPECTED:** Usually 5–15 degrees laterally. **UNEXPECTED:** Lateral angle exceeding 15 degrees (cubitus valgus) or a medial carrying angle (cubitus varus).
Palpate extensor surface of ulna, olecranon process, medial and lateral epicondyles of humerus, groove on each side of olecranon process	
Palpate with patient's elbow flexed at 70 degrees.	**UNEXPECTED:** Boggy, soft, tenderness at lateral epicondyle or along grooves of olecranon process and epicondyles.
Test range of motion	
Ask patient to perform the following movements:	
• *Flexion and extension* Bend and straighten elbow.	**EXPECTED:** 160-degree flexion from full extension at 0 degree.
• *Pronation and supination* With elbow flexed at right angle, rotate hand from palm side down to palm side up.	**EXPECTED:** 90-degree pronation and 90-degree supination. **UNEXPECTED:** Increased pain with pronation and supination of elbow.
Test muscle strength	
Ask patient to maintain flexion and extension, as well as pronation and supination, while you apply opposing force.	**EXPECTED:** Bilaterally symmetric with full resistance to opposition. **UNEXPECTED:** Inability to produce full resistance.

TECHNIQUE	FINDINGS
Shoulders	
Inspect shoulders, shoulder girdle, clavicles and scapulae, area muscles	
• *Size and contour*	**EXPECTED:** All shoulder structures symmetric in size and contour. **UNEXPECTED:** Asymmetry, hollows in rounding contour, or winged scapula.
Palpate sternoclavicular and acromioclavicular joints, clavicle, scapulae, coracoid process, greater trochanter of humerus, biceps groove, area muscles	
Palpate the biceps groove by rotating the arm and forearm externally. Follow the biceps muscle and tendon along the anterior aspect of the humerus into the biceps groove.	**EXPECTED:** No tenderness or masses, bilateral symmetry.
Palpate the muscle insertion for the supraspinatus, infraspinatus, and teres minor near the greater tuberosity of the humerus by lifting the elbow posteriorly to extend the shoulder.	**UNEXPECTED:** Pain, tenderness, mass.
Test range of motion	
Ask patient to perform the following movements:	
• *Shoulder shrug*	**EXPECTED:** Symmetric rising.
• *Forward flexion* Raise both arms forward and straight up over head.	**EXPECTED:** 180-degree forward flexion.
• *Hyperextension* Extend and stretch both arms behind back.	**EXPECTED:** 50-degree hyperextension.
• *Abduction* Lift both arms laterally and straight up over head.	**EXPECTED:** 180-degree abduction.

TECHNIQUE	FINDINGS
• *Adduction* Swing each arm across front of body.	**EXPECTED:** 50-degree adduction.
• *Internal rotation* Place both arms behind hips, elbows out.	**EXPECTED:** 90-degree internal rotation.
• *External rotation* Place both arms behind head, elbows out.	**EXPECTED:** 90-degree external rotation.

Test shoulder girdle muscle strength

Ask patient to maintain the following positions while you apply opposing force:

TECHNIQUE	FINDINGS
• *Shrugged shoulders* (This also tests cranial nerve XI.)	**EXPECTED:** Bilaterally symmetric with full resistance to opposition. **UNEXPECTED:** Inability to produce full resistance.

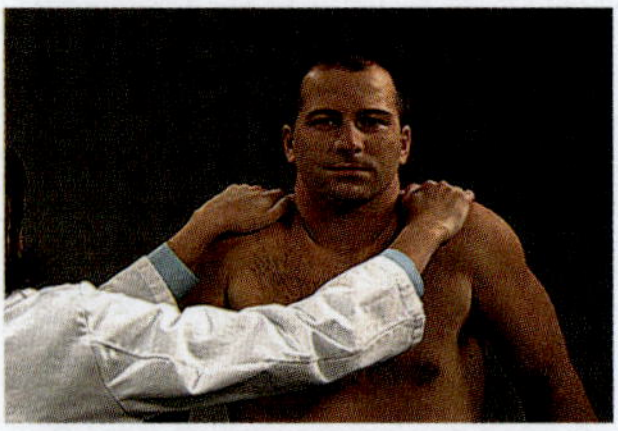

Shrugged shoulders.

TECHNIQUE	FINDINGS
• *Forward flexion*	**EXPECTED:** Bilaterally symmetric with full resistance to opposition. **UNEXPECTED:** Inability to produce full resistance.
• *Abduction*	**EXPECTED:** Bilaterally symmetric with full resistance to opposition. **UNEXPECTED:** Inability to produce full resistance.

TECHNIQUE	FINDINGS
Assess rotator cuff muscles	
Abduct the arm 90 degrees and flex the shoulders forward 30 degrees to test the supraspinatus muscle. Apply downward pressure on the distal humerus when the arm is rotated so that thumb points down or up.	UNEXPECTED: Pain and weakness with opposing force.
Flex the elbow 90 degrees and rotate the forearm medially against resistance to test the subscapularis muscle.	UNEXPECTED: Pain and weakness with opposing force.
With the arm at the side and elbow flexed 90 degrees, rotate the arm laterally against resistance to test the infraspinatus and teres minor muscles.	UNEXPECTED: Pain and weakness with opposing force.
Evaluate the rotator cuff for impingement or a tear	
• *Neer test* Have the patient internally rotate and forward flex the arm at the shoulder, pressing the supraspinatus muscle against the anterior inferior acromion.	UNEXPECTED: Increased shoulder pain.
• *Hawkins-Kennedy test* Abduct the shoulder to 90 degrees, flexing the elbow to 90 degrees and then internally rotating the arm to its limit.	UNEXPECTED: Increased shoulder pain.

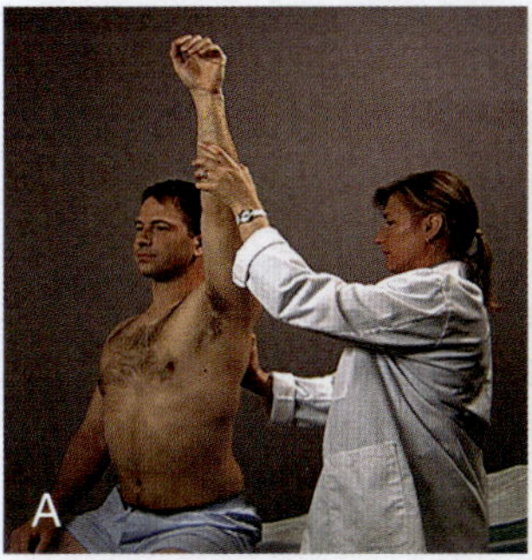

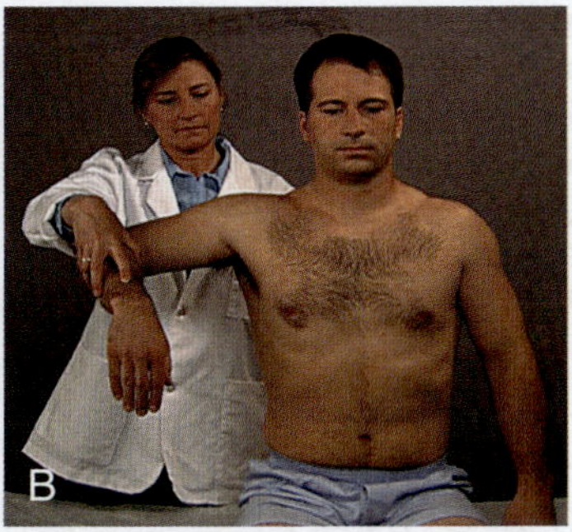

*Assessment for rotator cuff inflammation or tear: **(A)** Neer test and **(B)** Hawkins-Kennedy test.*

TECHNIQUE	FINDINGS

Temporomandibular Joint

Palpate joint space for clicking, popping, pain

Locate temporomandibular joints with fingertips placed just anterior to tragus of each ear, as shown in figure at right. Ask patient to open mouth and allow fingertips to slip into joint space. Gently palpate.

EXPECTED: Audible or palpable snapping or clicking may be noted.

UNEXPECTED: Pain, crepitus, locking, or popping.

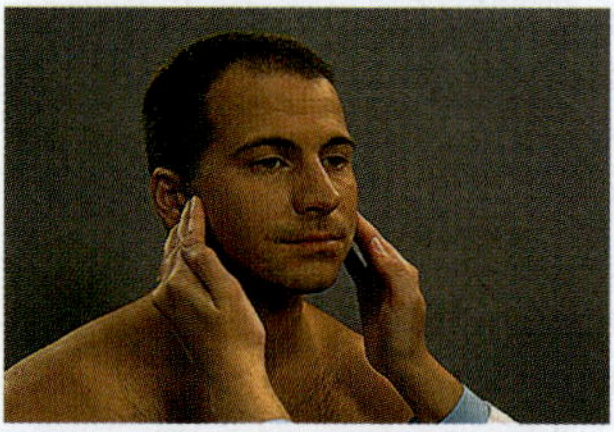

Palpating temporomandibular joint.

Test range of motion

Ask patient to:

- *Open and close mouth* — **EXPECTED:** Opens 3–6 cm between upper and lower teeth.
- *Move jaw laterally to each side* — **EXPECTED:** Mandible moves 1–2 cm in each direction.
- *Protrude and retract jaw* — **EXPECTED:** Both protrusion and retraction possible.

Test strength of temporalis and masseter muscles with patient's teeth clenched

Ask patient to clench teeth while you palpate contracted muscles and apply opposing force. (This also tests cranial nerve V motor function.)

EXPECTED: Bilaterally symmetric with full resistance to opposition.

UNEXPECTED: Inability to produce full resistance.

Cervical Spine

Inspect neck from anterior and posterior positions

- *Alignment* — **EXPECTED:** Cervical spine straight with head erect and in approximate alignment.
- *Symmetry of skinfolds* — **UNEXPECTED:** Asymmetric skinfolds, webbed neck.

TECHNIQUE	FINDINGS
Palpate posterior neck, cervical spine, and paravertebral, trapezius, and sternocleidomastoid muscles	
	EXPECTED: Good muscle tone, symmetry in size. **UNEXPECTED:** Palpable tenderness or muscle spasm.
Test range of motion	
• *Forward flexion* Bend head forward, chin to chest.	**EXPECTED:** 45-degree flexion.
• *Hyperextension* Bend head backward, chin toward ceiling.	**EXPECTED:** 45-degree hyperextension.
• *Lateral bending* Bend head to each side, ear to each shoulder.	**EXPECTED:** 40-degree lateral bending.
• *Rotation* Turn head to each side, chin to shoulder.	**EXPECTED:** 70-degree rotation.
Test strength of sternocleidomastoid and trapezius muscles	
Ask patient to maintain each of the previous positions while you apply opposing force. (Cranial nerve XI is also tested with rotation.)	**EXPECTED:** Bilaterally symmetric strength with full resistance to opposition. **UNEXPECTED:** Inability to produce full resistance.

Thoracic and Lumbar Spine

Inspect spine for alignment

TECHNIQUE	FINDINGS
Note major landmarks of back—each spinal process of vertebrae (C7 and T1 usually most prominent), scapulae, iliac crests, paravertebral muscles.	**EXPECTED:** Head positioned directly over gluteal cleft, vertebrae straight (as indicated by symmetric shoulder, scapular, and iliac crest heights), curves of cervical and lumbar spines concave, curve of thoracic spine convex, and knees and feet aligned with trunk and pointing directly forward. **UNEXPECTED:** Lordosis, kyphosis, scoliosis, or sharp angular deformity (gibbus).

TECHNIQUE	FINDINGS
Palpate spinal processes and paravertebral muscles	
Ask patient to stand erect.	**UNEXPECTED:** Muscle spasm or spinal tenderness.
Percuss for spinal tenderness	
Patient is still standing erect. First, tap each spinal process with one finger, then more firmly tap each side of spine along paravertebral muscles with ulnar aspect of fist.	**UNEXPECTED:** Muscle spasm or spinal tenderness.
Test range of motion and curvature	
Ask patient to perform the following movements (mark each spinal process with skin pencil if unexpected curvature suspected):	
• *Forward flexion* Bend forward at waist and try to touch toes. Observe patient from behind to check curvature.	**EXPECTED:** 75–90-degree flexion; back remains symmetrically flat as concave curve of lumbar spine becomes convex with forward flexion. **UNEXPECTED:** Lateral curvature or rib hump.
• *Hyperextension* Bend back at waist as far as possible.	**EXPECTED:** 30-degree hyperextension with reversal of lumbar curve.
• *Lateral bending* Bend to each side as far as possible.	**EXPECTED:** 35-degree lateral bending on each side.
• *Rotation* Swing upper trunk from waist in circular motion, front to side to back to side, while you stabilize pelvis.	**EXPECTED:** 30-degree rotation forward and backward.

TECHNIQUE	FINDINGS
Test for lumbar nerve root irritation or disk herniation at L4, L5, or S1 levels (patient supine with neck slightly flexed)	
• *Straight-leg raising test* Ask patient to raise leg with knee extended. Repeat with other leg.	**EXPECTED:** No pain below knee with leg raising. **UNEXPECTED:** Unable to raise leg more than 30 degrees without pain. Pain below knee in dermatome pattern. Flexion of knee often eliminates pain with leg raising. Crossover pain in affected leg.
• *Bragard stretch test* Hold patient's lower leg with knee extended and raise it slowly until pain is felt. Lower leg slightly, briskly dorsiflex foot, and internally rotate hip.	**UNEXPECTED:** Pain when leg is raised less than 70 degrees; aggravated by dorsiflexion and internal rotation of hip.

Hips

TECHNIQUE	FINDINGS
Inspect hips for symmetry and level of gluteal folds	
With patient standing, inspect anteriorly and posteriorly using major landmarks of iliac crest and greater trochanter of femur.	**UNEXPECTED:** Asymmetry in iliac crest height, size of buttocks, or number and level of gluteal folds.
Test range of motion	
While in position indicated, patient should perform the following movements:	
• *Flexion, knee extended* With patient supine, raise leg over body.	**EXPECTED:** Up to 90-degree flexion.
• *Hyperextension* While standing or prone, swing straightened leg behind body without arching the back.	**EXPECTED:** Up to 30-degree hyperextension.

TECHNIQUE	FINDINGS
• *Flexion, knee flexed* While supine, raise one knee to chest while keeping other leg straight.	**EXPECTED:** 120-degree flexion.
• *Abduction and adduction* While supine, swing leg laterally and medially with knee straight. During adduction movement, lift patient's opposite leg to permit examined leg full movement.	**EXPECTED:** Some degree of both abduction and adduction.
• *Internal rotation* While supine, flex knee and rotate leg inward toward other leg.	**EXPECTED:** 40-degree internal rotation.
• *External rotation* While supine, place lateral aspect of foot on knee of other leg. Move flexed leg toward table.	**EXPECTED:** 45-degree external rotation.

Test hip muscle strength

TECHNIQUE	FINDINGS
• *Knee in flexion and extension* Ask patient to maintain flexion of hip with knee in flexion and then extension while applying opposing force.	**EXPECTED:** Bilaterally symmetric with full resistance to opposition.
• *Resistance to uncrossing legs while seated*	**UNEXPECTED:** Inability to produce full resistance. **EXPECTED:** Bilaterally symmetric with full resistance to opposition.

TECHNIQUE	FINDINGS

Perform Trendelenburg test to inspect for weak hip abductor muscles

Ask patient to stand and balance, first on one foot, then on other. Observe from behind.

UNEXPECTED: Asymmetry or change in level of iliac crests.

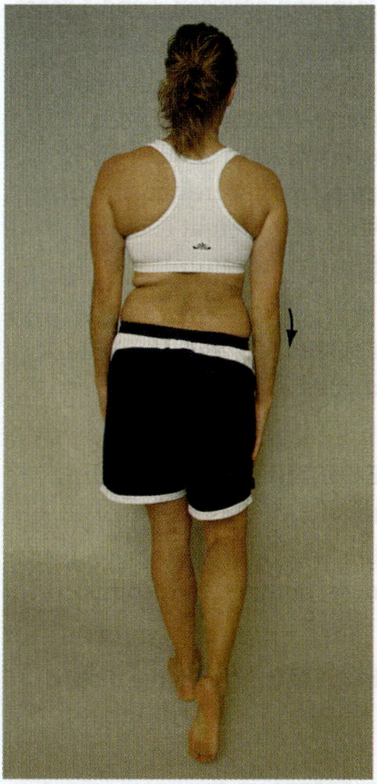

Legs and Knees

Inspect knees and popliteal spaces, flexed and extended

Note major landmarks—tibial tuberosity, medial and lateral tibial condyles, medial and lateral epicondyles of femur, adductor tubercle of femur, patella.

EXPECTED: Natural concavities on anterior aspect, on each side, above patella.

UNEXPECTED: Convex rather than usual concave indentation above patella.

TECHNIQUE	FINDINGS
Observe lower leg alignment	
	EXPECTED: Angle between femur and tibia less than 15 degrees. Bowlegs common until 18 months of age; knock-knees common between 2 and 4 years of age. **UNEXPECTED:** Knock-knees (genu valgum) or bowlegs (genu varum) at other ages, excessive hyperextension of knee with weight bearing (genu recurvatum).
Palpate popliteal space	
	UNEXPECTED: Swelling or tenderness.
Palpate tibiofemoral joint space	
Identify patella, suprapatellar pouch, infrapatellar fat pad.	**EXPECTED:** Smooth and firm joint. **UNEXPECTED:** Tenderness, bogginess, nodules, or crepitus.
Test range of motion	
• *Flexion* Ask patient to bend each knee.	**EXPECTED:** 130-degree flexion.
• *Extension* Ask patient to straighten leg and stretch it.	**EXPECTED:** Full extension and up to 15-degree hyperextension.
Test muscle strength	
• *Flexion and extension* Ask patient to maintain flexion and extension while you apply opposing force.	**EXPECTED:** Bilaterally symmetric with full resistance to opposition. **UNEXPECTED:** Inability to produce full resistance.

TECHNIQUE | FINDINGS

Additional Techniques for Knees

Perform ballottement procedure to determine presence of excess fluid or effusion in knee

With knee extended, apply downward pressure on suprapatellar pouch with thumb and finger of one hand, then push patella sharply downward against femur with fingers of other hand, as shown in figure at right. Abruptly release pressure on patella while keeping fingers lightly on knee.

UNEXPECTED: A tapping or clicking is sensed when patella is pushed against femur. Patella then floats out as if a fluid wave were pushing it.

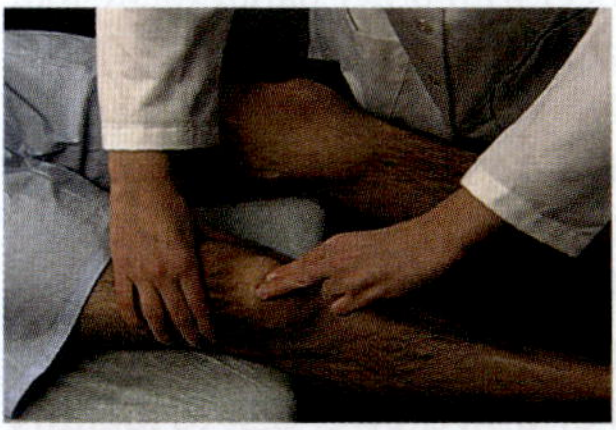

Ballottement.

Test for bulge sign to determine presence of excess fluid in knee

With knee extended, milk medial aspect of knee upward two or three times, as shown in the following figure, panel A, then tap lateral side of patella, as shown in the following figure, panel B.

UNEXPECTED: Bulge of returning fluid to hollow area medial to patella.

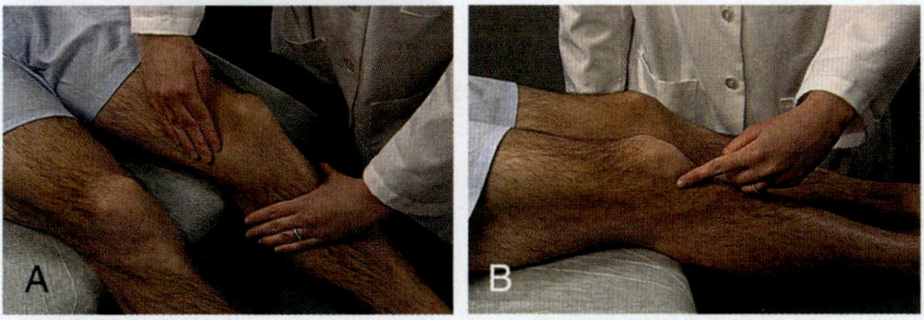

Bulge sign. ***(A)*** *Milking the medial aspect of the knee two or three times.* ***(B)*** *Tap the lateral side of the patella.*

TECHNIQUE	FINDINGS

Perform McMurray test to detect torn medial or lateral meniscus

Ask patient to lie supine and flex one knee completely with foot flat on table near buttocks. Maintain that flexion with your thumb and index finger on either side of the joint space while stabilizing knee. Hold heel with other hand; rotate foot and lower leg to lateral position. Extend knee to 90-degree angle. Return knee to full flexion, then repeat procedure rotating foot and lower leg to medial position.

UNEXPECTED: Palpable or audible click or limited extension of knee with either lateral or medial movements.

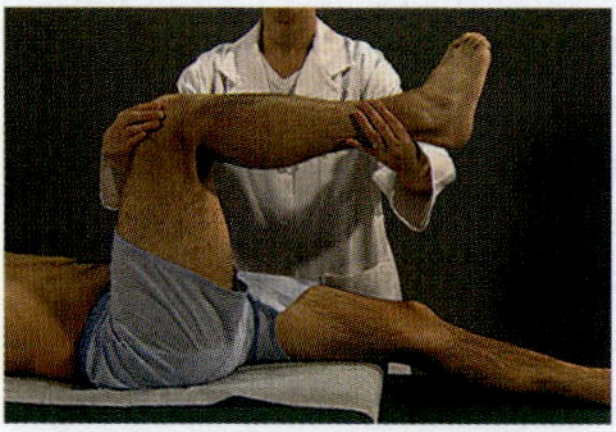

Procedure for examination of the knee with the McMurray test. Knee is flexed after lower leg was rotated to medial position.

Perform drawer test to identify instability of anterior and posterior cruciate ligaments

Ask patient, while supine, to flex knee 45–90 degrees, placing foot flat on table. Place both hands on lower leg with thumbs on ridge of anterior tibia near tibial tuberosity. Pull tibia, sliding it forward of femur. Then push tibia backward.

UNEXPECTED: Anterior or posterior movement greater than 5 mm.

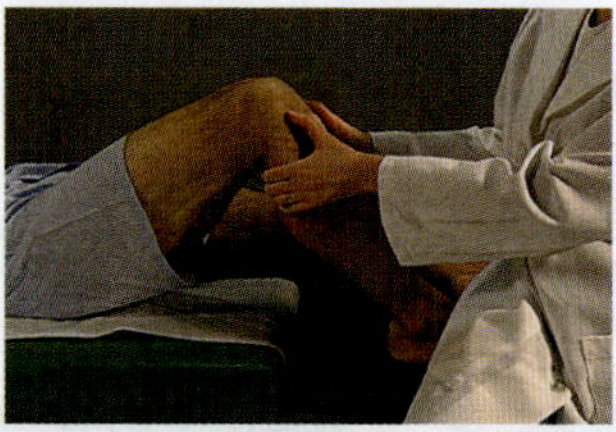

Drawer test.

Perform varus and valgus stress test to identify mediolateral collateral ligament instability

Ask patient to lie supine and extend knee. While you stabilize femur with one hand and hold ankle with other, apply varus force against the ankle (toward midline) and internal rotation.

UNEXPECTED: Excessive laxity felt as joint opening, medial or lateral movement.

TECHNIQUE	FINDINGS
Then apply valgus force against the ankle (away from midline) and external rotation. Repeat with knee flexed to 30 degrees.	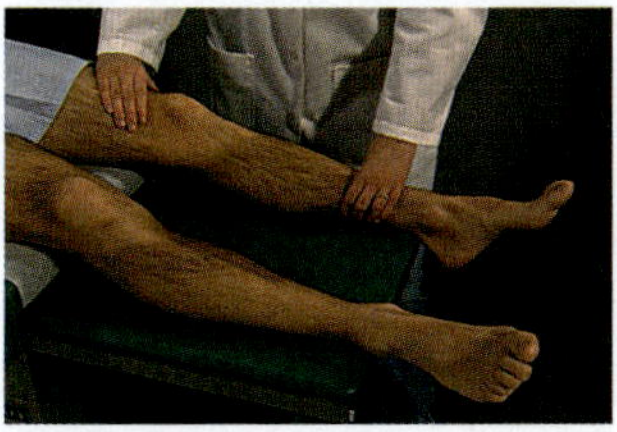 Varus and valgus stress test.

Feet and Ankles

Inspect during weight bearing (standing and walking) and nonweight bearing

Note major landmarks—medial malleolus, lateral malleolus, Achilles tendon.

TECHNIQUE	FINDINGS
• *Characteristics*	**EXPECTED:** Smooth and rounded malleolar prominence, prominent heels, prominent metatarsophalangeal joints. **UNEXPECTED:** Calluses and corns.
• *Alignment*	**EXPECTED:** Feet aligned with tibias and weight bearing on foot midline. **UNEXPECTED:** In-toeing (pes varus), out-toeing (pes valgus), deviations in forefoot alignment (metatarsus varus or metatarsus valgus), heel pronation, or pain.
• *Contour*	**EXPECTED:** Longitudinal arch that may flatten with weight bearing. Foot flat when not bearing weight (pes planus) and high instep (pes cavus) are common variations. **UNEXPECTED:** Pain with pes planus.

TECHNIQUE	FINDINGS
• *Toes*	**EXPECTED:** Toes on each foot straight forward, flat, in alignment. **UNEXPECTED:** Hammertoe; claw toe; mallet toe; hallux valgus; bunions; or heat, redness, swelling, tenderness of metatarsophalangeal joint of great toe (possibly with draining tophus).

Palpate Achilles tendon and each metatarsal joint

Using thumb and fingers of both hands, compress forefoot, palpating each metatarsophalangeal joint.	**EXPECTED:** No tenderness or masses, bilateral symmetry. **UNEXPECTED:** Pain, masses, thickened Achilles tendon.

Test range of motion

Ask patient to sit, then perform the following movements:	
• *Dorsiflexion* Point foot toward ceiling.	**EXPECTED:** 20-degree dorsiflexion.
• *Plantar flexion* Point foot toward floor.	**EXPECTED:** 45-degree plantar flexion.
• *Inversion and eversion* Bend foot at ankle, then turn sole of foot toward and away from other foot.	**EXPECTED:** 30-degree inversion and 20-degree eversion.
• *Abduction and adduction* Rotate ankle, turning away from and then toward other foot (while you stabilize leg).	**EXPECTED:** 10-degree abduction and 20-degree adduction.
• *Flexion and extension* Bend and straighten toes.	**EXPECTED:** Some flexion and extension, especially of great toes.

TECHNIQUE	FINDINGS
Test strength of ankle muscles	
Ask patient to maintain dorsiflexion and plantar flexion while you apply opposing force.	**EXPECTED:** Bilaterally symmetric with full resistance to opposition. **UNEXPECTED:** Inability to produce full resistance.

AIDS TO DIFFERENTIAL DIAGNOSIS

SUBJECTIVE DATA	OBJECTIVE DATA
Ankylosing Spondylitis	
Develops predominantly in male individuals between 20 and 40 years of age. Begins insidiously with low back pain, also involving hips and shoulders. Pain can fluctuate from one side to the other and progress to reduced spinal mobility.	Restriction in the lumbar flexion of the patient. The shoulders, hips, and knees may be affected later, developing limited range of motion. Uveitis may be present.
Carpal Tunnel Syndrome	
Numbness, burning, and tingling in the hands often occur at night. Can also be elicited by rotational movements of the wrist. Pain may radiate to the arms.	Weakness of the hand and flattening of the thenar eminence of the palm may result.
Gout	
Sudden onset of a hot, swollen joint; exquisite pain; limited range of motion. Primarily affects men older than 40 years and women of postmenopausal age. Classically affects the proximal phalanx of the great toe, although the wrists, hands, ankles, and knees may be involved.	The skin over the swollen joint may be shiny and red or purple. Uric acid crystals may form as tophi under the skin with chronic gout.

SUBJECTIVE DATA	OBJECTIVE DATA
Lumbar Disk Herniation	
Can be associated with lifting heavy objects. Common symptoms include low back pain with radiation to the buttocks and posterior thigh or down the leg in the distribution of the dermatome of the nerve root. Pain relief is often achieved by lying down.	Spasm and tenderness over the paraspinal musculature may also be present. Patient may have difficulty with heel walking (L4 and L5) or toe walking (S1). Numbness, tingling, or weakness may occur in the involved extremity.
Bursitis	
Common sites include the shoulder, elbow, hip, and knee with pain and stiffness surrounding the joint around the inflamed bursa. The pain is usually worse during activity.	Limitation of motion caused by swelling; pain on movement; point tenderness; and an erythematous, warm site. Soreness may radiate to tendons at the site.
Osteoarthritis	
See table on pp. 228–229.	
Rheumatoid Arthritis	
See table on pp. 228–229.	
Sprain	
Often associated with improper exercise warm-up, fatigue, or previous injury. Severity ranges from a mild intrafibrinous tear to a total rupture of a single muscle.	Temporary muscle weakness, spasm, pain, and contusion.
Fracture	
Usually occurs in the setting of acute trauma. Can occur more easily in patients with bone disorders (e.g., osteogenesis imperfecta, osteoporosis, bone metastasis).	Deformity, edema, pain, loss of function, color changes, and paresthesia.

SUBJECTIVE DATA	OBJECTIVE DATA
Tenosynovitis (Tendinitis)	
Pain with movement of common sites such as the shoulder, knee, heel, and wrist.	Point tenderness over the involved tendon. Pain with active movement and some limitation of movement in the affected joint.
Rotator Cuff Tear	
May be pain in the shoulder and deltoid area that can awaken the patient at night.	May be an inability to maintain a lateral raised arm against resistance. Tenderness over the acromioclavicular joint. Grating sound on movement, crepitus, and weakness in external shoulder rotation.

Differential Diagnosis of Arthritis

SIGNS AND SYMPTOMS	OSTEOARTHRITIS	RHEUMATOID ARTHRITIS
Onset	Insidious	Gradual or sudden (24–48 hours)
Duration of stiffness	Few minutes, localized, but short "gelling" after prolonged rest	Often hours, most pronounced after rest
Pain	On motion, with prolonged activity, relieved by rest	Even at rest, may disturb sleep
Weakness	Usually localized and not severe	Often pronounced, out of proportion with muscle atrophy
Fatigue	Unusual	Often severe, with onset 4–5 hours after rising
Emotional depression and lability	Unusual	Common, coincides with fatigue and disease activity, often relieved if in remission

Continued

Differential Diagnosis of Arthritis—cont'd

SIGNS AND SYMPTOMS	OSTEOARTHRITIS	RHEUMATOID ARTHRITIS
Tenderness over localized afflicted joint	Common	Almost always; most sensitive indicator of inflammation
Swelling	Effusion common, little synovial reaction, swelling rare	Fusiform soft tissue enlargement, effusion common, synovial proliferation and thickening
Heat, erythema	Unusual	Sometimes present
Crepitus, crackling	Coarse to medium on motion	Medium to fine
Joint enlargement	Mild with firm consistency	Moderate to severe

PEDIATRIC VARIATIONS

EXAMINATION

Musculoskeletal findings and motor development in infants, children, and adolescents change as they grow.

Sports Participation Screening Examination for Children and Adolescents

- Observe posture and general muscle contour bilaterally.
- Observe gait.
- Ask patient to walk on tiptoes and heels.
- Observe patient hop on each foot.
- Ask patient to duck-walk four steps with knees completely bent.
- Inspect spine for curvature and lumbar extension, fingers touching toes with knees straight.
- Palpate shoulder and clavicle for dislocation.
- Check the following for range of motion—neck, shoulder, elbow, forearm, hands, fingers, hips.
- Test knee ligaments for drawer sign.

CHAPTER 20

Neurologic System

Equipment

- Penlight
- Tongue blades (one intact and one broken with pointed and rounded edges)
- Tuning forks (200–400 Hz and 500–1000 Hz)
- Familiar objects (coins, keys, paper clip)
- Cotton wisp
- 5.07 monofilament
- Sterile needles
- Cup of water
- Reflex hammer
- Additional items for a comprehensive diagnostic neurologic examination, typically performed by a specialist:
- Test tubes of hot and cold water for temperature sensation testing
- Vials of aromatic substances (coffee, orange, peppermint extract, oil of cloves)
- Vials of solutions (glucose, salt, lemon or vinegar, and quinine—with applicators for taste testing)
- Test tubes of hot and cold water for temperature sensation testing

EXAMINATION

Assess the neurologic system during the entire encounter. When history and examination findings have not revealed a potential neurologic problem, perform a neurologic screening examination (as shown in the box) rather than a full neurologic examination. See Chapter 19 for evaluation of muscle tone and strength, because these findings are important for interpreting neurologic system examination findings. The mental status portion of the neurologic system examination can be found in Chapter 4.

Neurologic Screening Examination

This shorter screening examination is commonly used for health visits when no known neurologic problem is apparent.

Cranial Nerves

Cranial nerves (CNs) II through XII are routinely tested; however, taste and smell are not tested unless some aberration is found.

Proprioception and Cerebellar Function

One test is administered for each of the following: rapid rhythmic alternating movements, accuracy of movements, balance (Romberg test), gait, and heel-toe walking.

Sensory Function

Superficial pain and touch at a distal point in each extremity are tested; vibration and position senses are assessed by testing the great toe.

Deep Tendon Reflexes

All deep tendon reflexes are tested. Exclude the plantar reflex and the test for clonus.

Cranial Nerves I to XII

The following table summarizes the CN examination, and details of examination follow. When a sensory or motor loss is suspected, be thoughtful about determining and documenting the extent of loss when testing the relevant CN.

Procedures for Cranial Nerve (CN) Examination

CN	PROCEDURE
CN I (olfactory)	When a concern exists, test ability to identify familiar aromatic odors, one naris at a time, with eyes closed.
CN II (optic)	Test distance and near vision. Perform an ophthalmoscopic examination. Test visual fields by confrontation and extinction of vision.

Procedures for Cranial Nerve (CN) Examination—cont'd

CN	PROCEDURE
CN III (oculomotor), CN IV (trochlear), CN VI (abducens)	Test extraocular movement. Inspect eyelids for drooping. Inspect pupils for size equality and direct and consensual response to light and accommodation.
CN V (trigeminal)	Inspect face for muscle atrophy and tremors. Palpate jaw muscles for tone and strength when patient clenches teeth. Test superficial pain and touch sensation in each nerve branch. (Test temperature sensation if findings to pain and touch sensation are unexpected.) Test corneal reflex.
CN VII (facial)	Inspect symmetry of facial features with various expressions (e.g., smile, frown, puffed cheeks, wrinkled forehead). Test ability to identify sweet and salty tastes on each side of tongue.
CN VIII (acoustic)	Test hearing with whisper screening tests or by audiometry. Compare bone and air conduction of sound. Test for lateralization of sound. Test balance with Romberg maneuver.
CN IX (glossopharyngeal) and CN X (vagus)	When a concern exists, test ability to identify sour and bitter tastes on each side of the tongue. Test gag reflex and ability to swallow. Inspect palate and uvula for symmetry with speech sounds and gag reflex. Observe for swallowing difficulty. Evaluate quality of guttural speech sounds (presence of nasal or hoarse quality to voice).

Continued

Procedures for Cranial Nerve (CN) Examination—cont'd

CN	PROCEDURE
CN XI (spinal accessory)	Test trapezius muscle strength (shrug shoulders against resistance). Test sternocleidomastoid muscle strength (turn head to each side against resistance).
CN XII (hypoglossal)	Inspect tongue in mouth and while protruded for symmetry, tremors, atrophy. Inspect tongue movement toward nose and chin. Test tongue strength with index finger when tongue is pressed against cheek. Evaluate quality of lingual speech sounds (**l, t, d, n**).

TECHNIQUE	FINDINGS
Assess olfactory nerve (CN I)	
Ask patient to close eyes. Occlude one naris, hold vial (using least irritating aromatic substances first [e.g., orange or peppermint extract]) under nose, and ask patient to breathe deeply and identify odor. Allow patient to breathe comfortably, then occlude other naris and repeat with different odor. Continue, alternating two or three odors.	**EXPECTED:** Able to perceive and usually identify odor on each side. **UNEXPECTED:** Anosmia, loss of smell, or inability to discriminate odors.
Assess optic nerve (CN II)	
See tests for near and distance visual acuity and visual fields in Chapter 9.	**EXPECTED:** Vision 20/20 without or with lenses each eye; full visual fields.

TECHNIQUE	FINDINGS
Assess oculomotor, trochlear, abducens nerves (CN III, CN IV, CN VI)	
See tests for six cardinal points of gaze, pupil size, shape, response to light and accommodation, and opening of upper eyelids in Chapter 9.	**EXPECTED:** Equal pupil size, equal and consensual response to light and accommodation, symmetric eye movements in all six cardinal points of gaze. **UNEXPECTED:** Absence of lateral gaze. Absence of any expected finding, ptosis.
Assess trigeminal nerve (CN V)	
• *Facial muscle tone* Inspect face for symmetry or muscle twitching. Ask patient to clench teeth tightly as you palpate muscles over jaw.	**EXPECTED:** Symmetric tone. **UNEXPECTED:** Muscle atrophy, deviation of jaw to one side, or fasciculation.
• *Sensation* Ask patient to close eyes and report if sensation to touch is sharp or dull as you touch each side of face at scalp, cheek, and chin areas, alternately using sharp and rounded edges of tongue blade or paper clip in an unpredictable pattern. Ask patient to report when the stimulus is felt as you stroke the same six areas with cotton wisp or brush. Finally, test sensation over buccal mucosa inside the mouth with wooden applicator.	**EXPECTED:** Symmetric discrimination of sensations in each location to all stimuli. **UNEXPECTED:** Impaired sensation with identified distribution. If impaired, use test tubes of hot and cold water to evaluate temperature sensation. 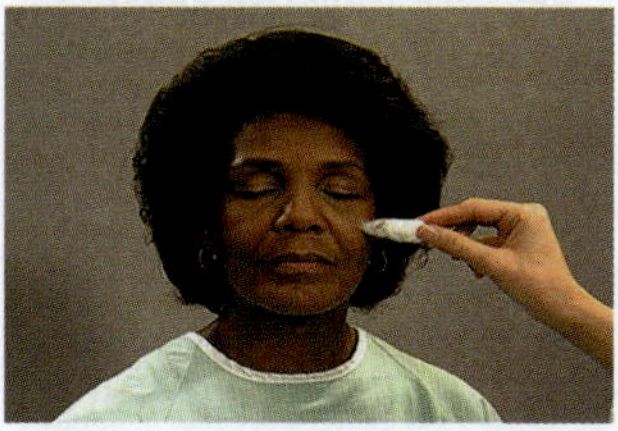 *Testing sensation over distribution of cranial nerve V.*
• *Corneal reflex* See test for corneal sensitivity in Chapter 9.	**EXPECTED:** Symmetric blink reflex. May be diminished or absent if patient wears contact lenses.

TECHNIQUE	FINDINGS
Assess facial nerve (CN VII)	
• *Expressions* Assess motor function by asking patient to make the following facial expressions: • *Raise eyebrows and wrinkle forehead* • *Smile* • *Frown* • *Puff out cheeks* • *Purse lips and blow out* • *Show teeth* • *Squeeze eyes shut against resistance*	**EXPECTED:** Facial symmetry. 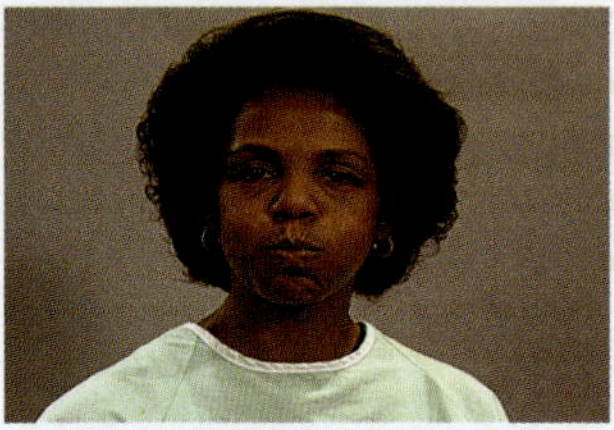 *Assessing motor function of cranial nerve VII.* **UNEXPECTED:** Tics, unusual facial movements, or asymmetry of expression (flattened nasolabial fold, lower eyelid sagging, side of mouth drooping).
• *Speech* Listen to articulation and clarity of speech.	**UNEXPECTED:** Difficulty with enunciation of *b*, *m*, and *p* (labial sounds).
• *Taste (CN VII and CN IX)* Hold card listing tastes in patient's view. Ask patient to extend tongue. Apply one of four solutions to lateral side of tongue in appropriate taste bud region. Ask patient to point to the taste perceived. Offer patient a sip of water, then repeat with different solution and applicator, testing each side of tongue with each solution.	**EXPECTED:** Able to identify sweet, salty, sour, bitter taste bilaterally when placed in appropriate taste bud region.

TECHNIQUE	FINDINGS

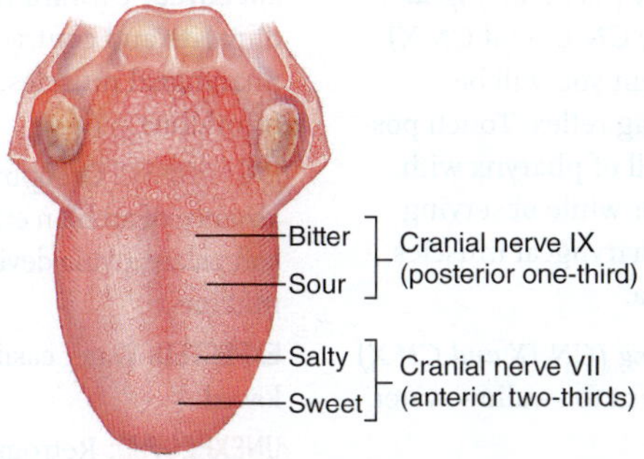

Sites for taste assessment.

Assess acoustic nerve (CN VIII)

TECHNIQUE	FINDINGS
• *Hearing* Perform screening tests as described in Chapter 10 or use an audiometer to test hearing.	**EXPECTED:** Adequate hearing bilaterally.
• *Balance* See Romberg test on p. 239.	

Assess glossopharyngeal nerve (CN IX)

- *Taste*
  See CN VII.
- *Gag reflex (nasopharyngeal sensation)*
  See CN X.

Assess vagus nerve (CN X)

TECHNIQUE	FINDINGS
• *Motor function* Ask patient to say "aah" while observing movement of palate and uvula.	**EXPECTED:** Soft palate rises with uvula remaining in midline. **UNEXPECTED:** Failure of soft palate to rise or uvula deviates from midline.

TECHNIQUE	FINDINGS
• *Gag reflex (nasopharyngeal sensation; CN IX and CN X)* Tell patient you will be testing gag reflex. Touch posterior wall of pharynx with applicator while observing palate, pharyngeal muscles, and uvula.	**EXPECTED:** Upward movement of palate and contraction of pharyngeal muscles, with uvula in midline. **UNEXPECTED:** Drooping or absence of arch on either side of soft palate; uvula deviates from midline.
• *Swallowing (CN IX and CN X)* Ask patient to swallow water.	**EXPECTED:** Water easily swallowed. **UNEXPECTED:** Retrograde passage of water through nose.
• *Speech*	**UNEXPECTED:** Hoarseness, nasal quality, or difficulty with guttural sounds.

Assess spinal accessory nerve (CN XI)

See Chapters 8 and 19 for evaluations of size, shape, strength of trapezius and sternocleidomastoid muscles of the neck.	**EXPECTED:** Symmetric size, shape, and strength.

Assess hypoglossal nerve (CN XII)

• *Tongue resting and protruded* Inspect while at rest on floor of mouth and while protruded.	**EXPECTED:** Tongue midline, symmetric size. **UNEXPECTED:** Fasciculation, asymmetry, atrophy, or deviation from midline.

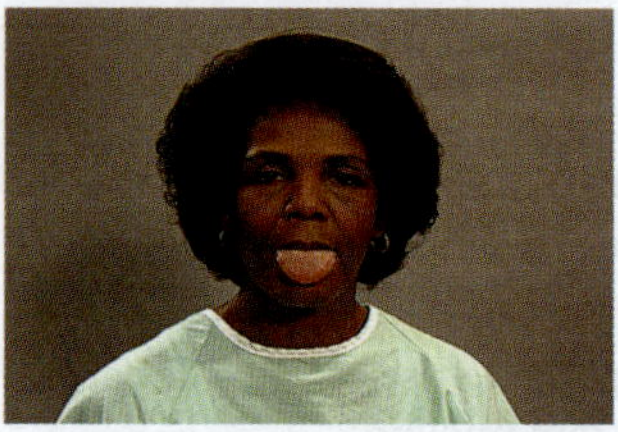

Assessing motor function of cranial nerve XII.

• *Tongue movement* Ask patient to move tongue in and out, side to side, curled up toward nose, curled down toward chin.	**EXPECTED:** Able to perform most tongue movements.

TECHNIQUE	FINDINGS
• *Tongue strength* Ask patient to push tongue against cheek while you apply resistance with index finger.	**EXPECTED:** Steady, firm pressure.
• *Speech*	**UNEXPECTED:** Problems with *l, t, d,* or *n* (lingual sounds).

Proprioception and Cerebellar Function

Evaluate Coordination and Fine Motor Skills

Have patient sit.

TECHNIQUE	FINDINGS
• *Rapid, rhythmic, alternating movements* Ask patient to pat knees with both hands, alternately turning up and down the palmar surfaces of the hands and increasing the speed gradually; or, ask the patient to touch the thumb to each finger of the same hand, sequentially from index finger to little finger and back, one hand at a time.	**EXPECTED:** Smooth execution, maintaining rhythm with increasing speed. **UNEXPECTED:** Stiff, slowed, nonrhythmic, or jerky clonic movements.
• *Accuracy of movement: Finger-to-nose test* Position your index finger about 18 in from patient. Ask patient to touch their nose and your index finger with the index finger of one hand, as shown below. Move your index finger several times encouraging the patient to reach full arm extension. Repeat with patient's other hand. Alternatively, ask the patient to close both eyes and touch their nose with index finger of each hand, alternating hands and gradually increasing speed.	**EXPECTED:** Movements rapid, smooth, and accurate. **UNEXPECTED:** Consistent past pointing (missing examiner's index finger).

TECHNIQUE	FINDINGS

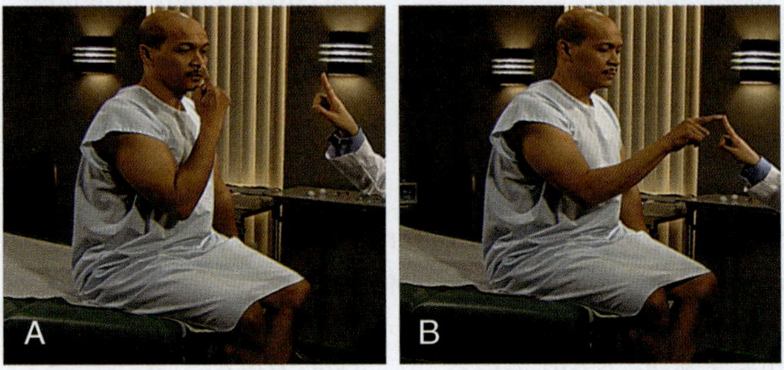

Assess the patient's accuracy of moving a finger between (A) the patient's nose and (B) the examiner's finger.

TECHNIQUE	FINDINGS
• *Accuracy of movement: Heel-to-shin test (can be performed sitting, standing, or supine)* Ask patient to run heel of one foot along shin of opposite leg from knee to ankle. Repeat with other heel.	**EXPECTED:** Able to move heel up and down shin in straight line. **UNEXPECTED:** Irregular deviations to side of leg.

Evaluate balance

TECHNIQUE	FINDINGS
• *Balance: Romberg test* Ask patient to stand with feet together and arms at sides, with eyes first open, then closed. **Stand close by in case patient starts to fall.**	**EXPECTED:** Slight swaying movement, no danger of falling. **UNEXPECTED:** Staggering, losing balance, or swaying to the extent of falling.
• *Balance: Recovery* After explaining test to patient, ask patient to spread feet slightly, then push shoulders with enough effort to throw patient off balance. **Be prepared to catch patient.**	**EXPECTED:** Quick recovery of balance. **UNEXPECTED:** Must catch patient to prevent a fall.

TECHNIQUE	FINDINGS
• *Balance: Standing and hopping* Have patient (with eyes closed) stand in place on one foot, then the other. Then have patient (with eyes open) hop on each foot.	**EXPECTED:** Able to stand and hop on each foot for 5 seconds without losing balance. **UNEXPECTED:** Instability, need to continually touch floor with opposite foot, or tendency to fall.
• *Gait: Walking* Ask patient to walk without shoes around room or down hallway, with eyes open, then closed.	**EXPECTED:** Smooth, regular gait, rhythm, and symmetric stride length; upright trunk posture swaying with gait phase; and arm swing smooth and symmetric. **UNEXPECTED:** Shuffling, widely placed feet, toe walking, foot flop, leg lag, scissoring, loss of arm swing, staggering, lurching, or waddling motion.
• *Gait: Heel-toe walking* Ask patient (with arms at side and eyes open) to walk forward in a straight line, touching toes of one foot with heel of other foot. Then repeat, walking backward.	**EXPECTED:** Consistent contact between toe and heel, slight swaying. **UNEXPECTED:** Extension of arms for balance, instability, tendency to fall, or lateral staggering and reeling.
• *Timed Up and Go Test* Time how long it takes the patient to stand up from a chair without using the chair arms, walk 10 ft (3 m) to mark on floor, turn around, walk 10 ft (3 m) back to the chair, and sit down without using chair arms (CDC, 2017).	**EXPECTED:** This simple screening test of balance, strength, and cerebellar function is completed in less than 12 seconds. **UNEXPECTED:** Taking 12 seconds or longer to complete indicates a higher risk for falls.

TECHNIQUE	FINDINGS
Sensory Function	
Test primary sensory functions	
Ask patient to close eyes for all tests. Use minimal stimulation initially, then increase gradually until patient becomes aware. Test contralateral areas, asking patient to compare perceived sensations side to side.	**EXPECTED:** For all tests, minimal differences side to side, correct interpretation of sensations (e.g., sharp, dull), identifies side of body tested and location of sensation (e.g., proximal or distal to previous stimulus). **UNEXPECTED:** For all tests, map gait, and heel-toe walking by distribution of major peripheral nerves or dermatomes.

TECHNIQUE FINDINGS

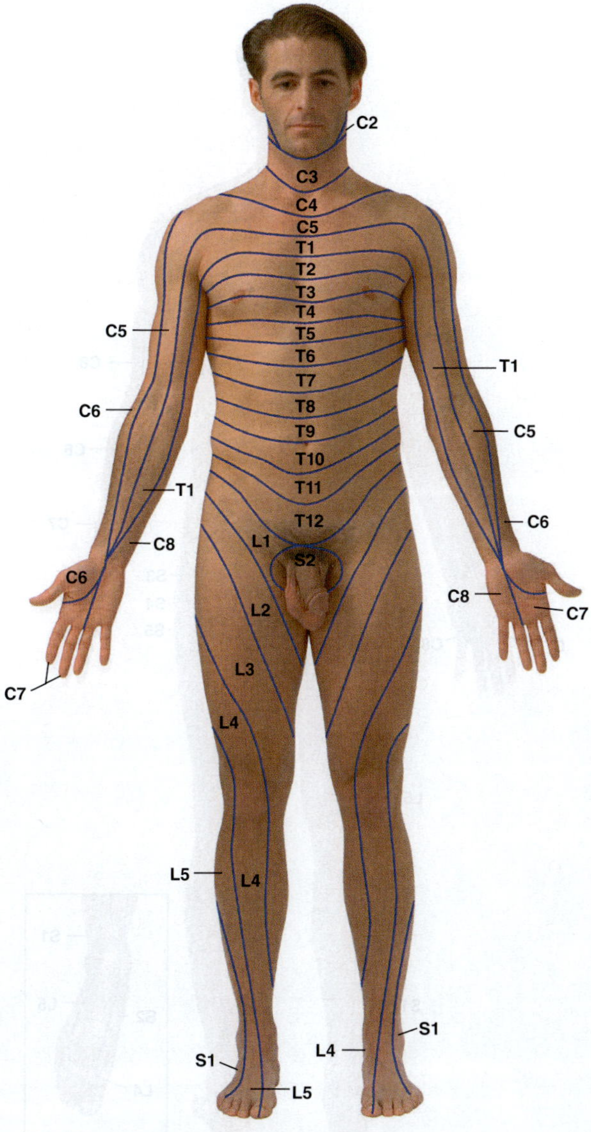

Dermatomes of the body, anterior view.

TECHNIQUE FINDINGS

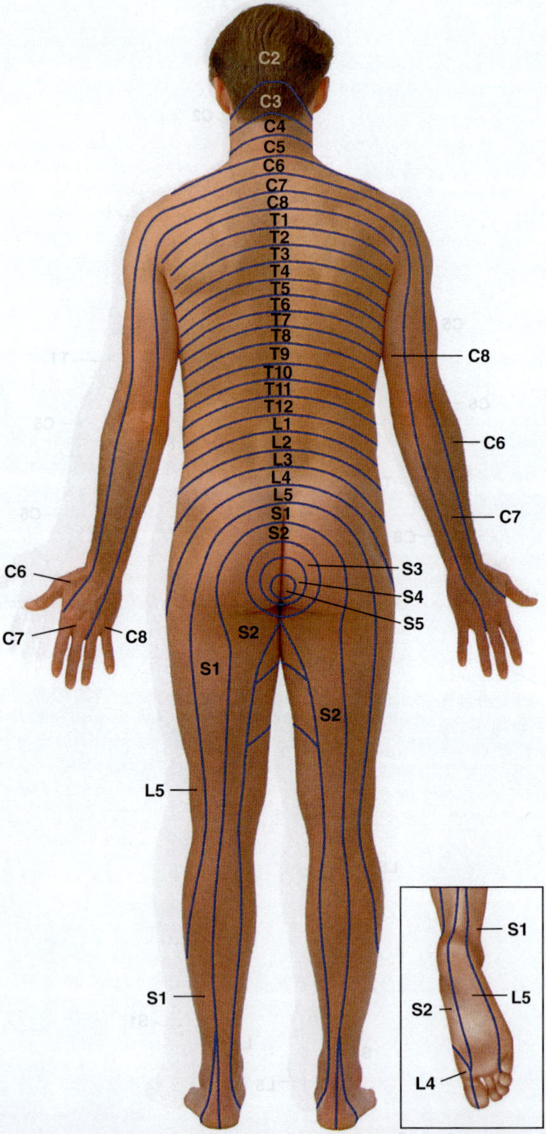

Dermatomes of the body, posterior view.

TECHNIQUE	FINDINGS
• *Superficial touch* Lightly touch skin with cotton wisp or your fingertips, as shown at right. Ask patient to point to area touched or indicate when and where the sensation is felt.	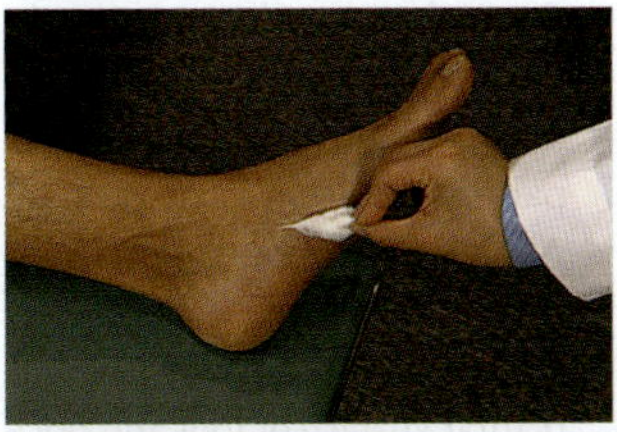 *Superficial touch assessment.*
• *Superficial pain* Alternate the sharp and smooth edges of broken tongue blade or round end and point of a paper clip, touching the skin in an unpredictable pattern. Allow 2 seconds between sensations. Ask patient to identify sensation (sharp or dull) and where it is felt.	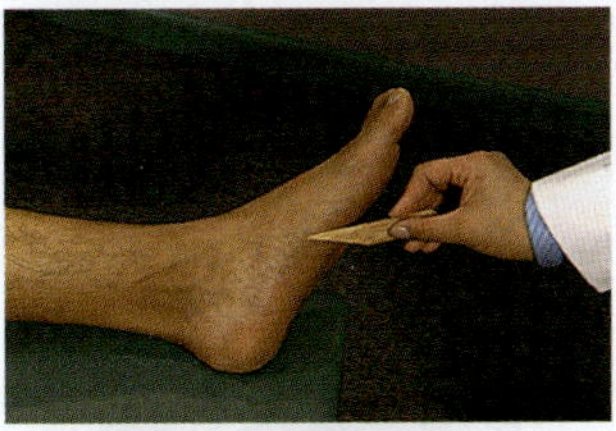 *Superficial pain assessment.*
• *Temperature and deep pressure* Perform test only if superficial pain sensation is not intact.	
• *Temperature* Alternately roll test tubes of hot and cold water against skin in an unpredictable pattern. Ask patient to indicate hot or cold and where it is felt.	**EXPECTED:** Distinguishes between hot and cold and location of sensation.
• *Deep pressure* Squeeze trapezius, calf, or biceps muscle.	**EXPECTED:** Discomfort with deep pressure.

TECHNIQUE	FINDINGS
• *Protective sensation* Perform test only if patient has diabetes mellitus or impaired sensation is suspected. Apply 5.07 monofilament until filament bends. Use a random pattern to test several sites on plantar surface of foot and once on dorsal surface. Avoid calloused areas and broken skin.	**EXPECTED:** Sensation felt at all sites touched. **UNEXPECTED:** Loss of sensation at any site.

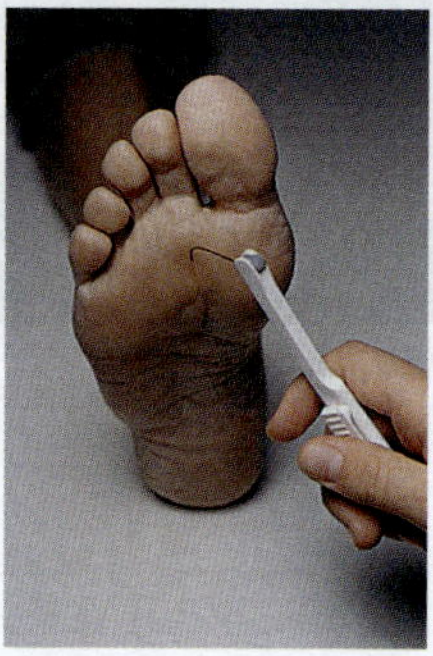

Monofilament testing of superficial touch.

TECHNIQUE	FINDINGS
• *Vibration* Place stem of vibrating tuning fork against several bony prominences (e.g., toes, ankle, shin, finger joints, wrist, elbow, shoulder, sternum), beginning distally. Ask patient when and where sensation is felt and how it feels. Occasionally dampen tines to see if patient notices the difference.	**EXPECTED:** Buzzing or tingling sensation, correct location of stimulus. **UNEXPECTED:** Does not distinguish between vibrating and nonvibrating tuning fork.

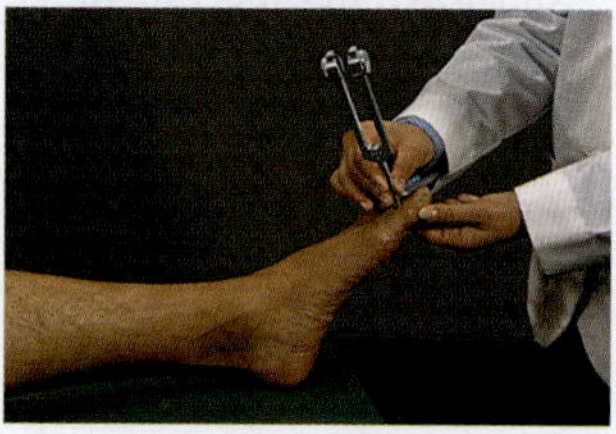

Assessment of vibration sensation.

TECHNIQUE	FINDINGS

- *Position of joints*
  Hold joint to be tested (great toe or finger) by lateral aspects in neutral position, then raise or lower the digit. Ask the patient which way the joint was moved. Return the digit to neutral before moving it another direction. Repeat and test a joint in both feet and both hands.

EXPECTED: Patient correctly identifies position of joint.

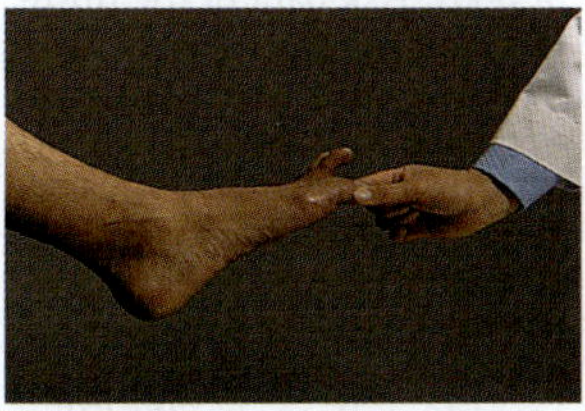

Position sense assessment.

Test cortical sensory functions

Ask patient to close eyes for all tests.

- *Stereognosis*
  Hand patient familiar objects (e.g., key, coin) and ask them to identify object by touch.

UNEXPECTED: Inability to recognize objects (tactile agnosia).

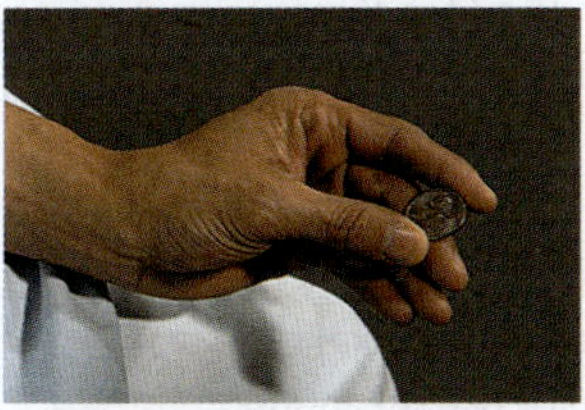

Stereognosis.

- *Two-point discrimination*
  Using two paper clip ends or sharp edges of a broken tongue blade, alternately touch patient's skin with one or both points simultaneously at various locations. Find distance at which patient can no longer distinguish two points.

EXPECTED: Correctly identifies one or two points used. On the fingertips and toes, points are commonly felt when 2–8 mm apart. Discrimination of two points varies on other body parts, such as the back (40–70 mm) or chest and forearms (40 mm).

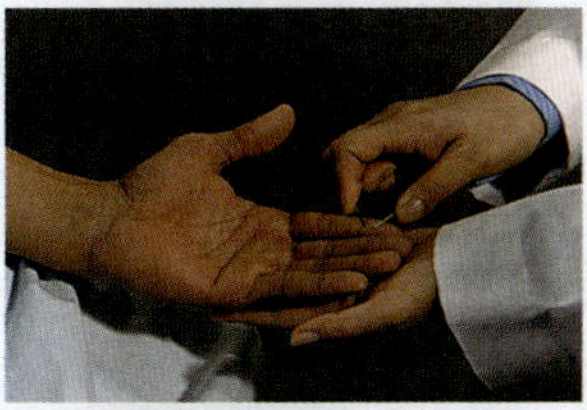

Two-point discrimination.

TECHNIQUE | **FINDINGS**

- *Extinction phenomenon*
  Use sharp points of a broken tongue blade to simultaneously touch cheek and hand, or two other areas on each side of body. Ask patient the number of stimuli and locations.

EXPECTED: Correct number and location of both sensations identified bilaterally.

- *Graphesthesia*
  With blunt pen or applicator stick, draw letter, number, or shape on palm of patient's hand, then ask patient to identify it. Repeat with different figure on other hand.

EXPECTED: Letter, number, or figure readily recognized.

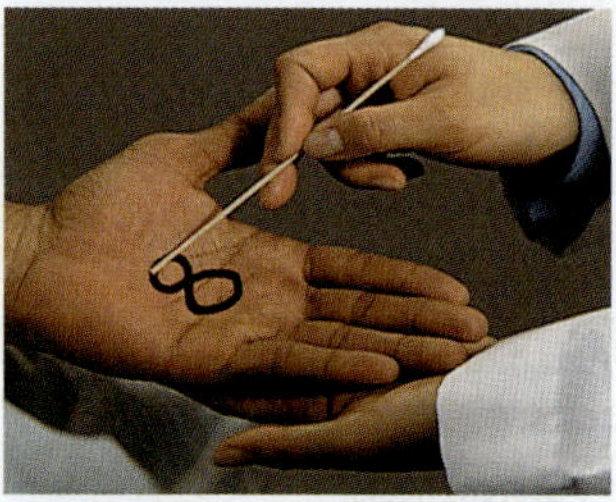

Graphesthesia.

- *Point location*
  Touch area on patient's skin and withdraw stimulus. Ask patient to point to area touched.

EXPECTED: Able to locate stimulus.

Reflexes

Test superficial reflexes

Have patient supine

- *Plantar reflex*
  Using pointed object, stroke lateral side of foot from heel to ball and then across ball of foot to medial side.

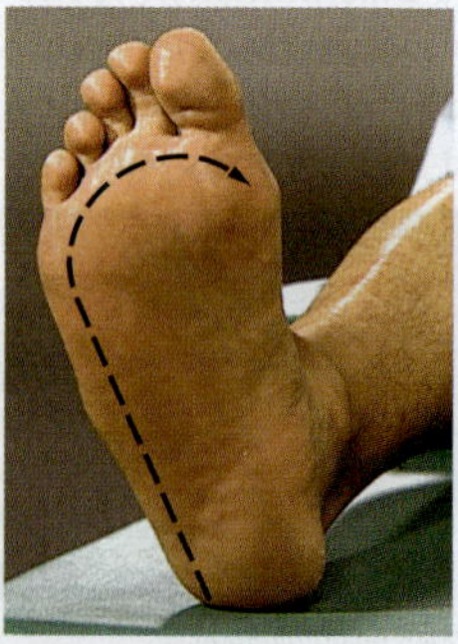

Plantar reflex assessment.

EXPECTED: Plantar flexion of all toes. Dorsiflexion of great toe and fanning of other toes in children younger than 2 years.

UNEXPECTED: Fanning of toes or dorsiflexion of great toe with or without fanning of other toes (Babinski sign positive) in all patients older than 2 years.

TECHNIQUE	FINDINGS
• *Abdominal* Stroke each quadrant of abdomen from umbilicus outward with end of reflex hammer or with tongue blade edge.	**UNEXPECTED:** Slight, bilaterally equal movements of umbilicus toward each area of stimulation. May have diminished response in obese patient or when abdominal muscles stretched by pregnancy.

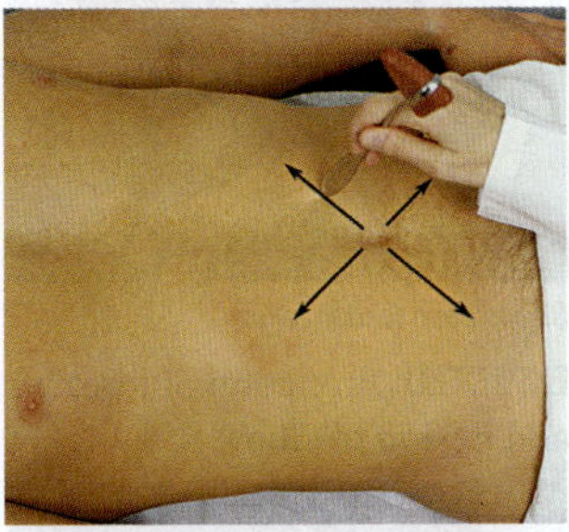

Abdominal reflex assessment.

TECHNIQUE	FINDINGS
• *Cremasteric (male patients)* Stroke inner thigh, proximal to distal.	**EXPECTED:** Testicle and scrotum rise on stroked side.

Test deep tendon reflexes

TECHNIQUE	FINDINGS
Patient is relaxed and either sitting or lying for most procedures. Test each reflex, comparing responses side to side. Score deep tendon reflexes on scale shown in table below.	**EXPECTED:** Symmetric visible or palpable responses. **UNEXPECTED:** Absent or diminished responses (0 or 1+), or hyperactive reflexes (3+ or 4+).

Scoring Deep Tendon Reflexes

GRADE	DEEP TENDON REFLEX RESPONSE
0	No response
1+	Sluggish or diminished
2+	Active or expected response
3+	More brisk than expected, slightly hyperactive
4+	Brisk, hyperactive, with intermittent or transient clonus

TECHNIQUE	FINDINGS
• *Biceps* Flex arm 45 degrees at elbow, then palpate biceps tendon in antecubital fossa. Place thumb over tendon and fingers under elbow. Strike your thumb with reflex hammer.	**EXPECTED:** Visible or palpable flexion of elbow, contraction of biceps muscle.

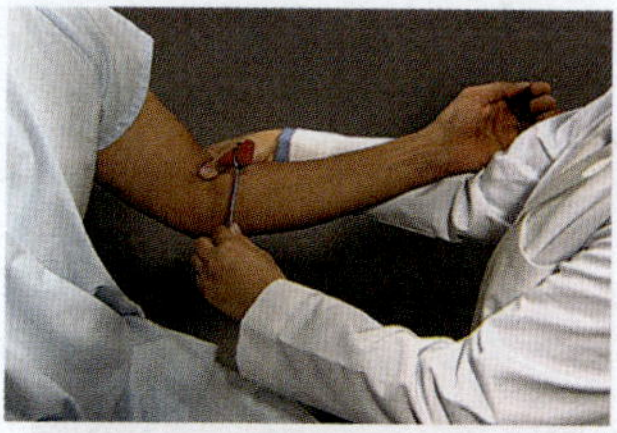

Biceps deep tendon reflex.

TECHNIQUE	FINDINGS
• *Brachioradial* Flex patient's arm up to 45 degrees while resting patient's forearm on your arm, with hand slightly pronated. Strike brachioradial tendon directly.	**EXPECTED:** Pronation of forearm and flexion of elbow.

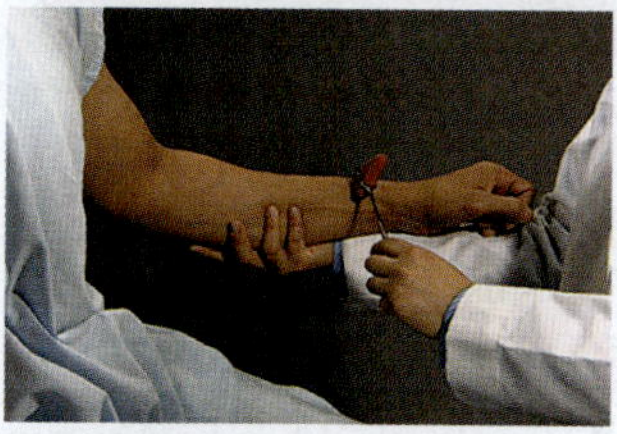

Brachioradialis deep tendon reflex.

TECHNIQUE	FINDINGS
• *Triceps* Flex patient's arm at elbow up to 90 degrees while supporting the patient's forearm on your arm. Palpate triceps tendon and strike directly with reflex hammer just above elbow.	**EXPECTED:** Visible or palpable extension of elbow, contraction of triceps muscle.

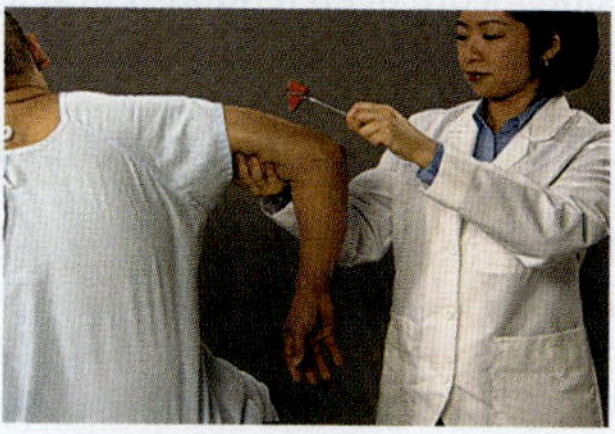

Triceps deep tendon reflex.

TECHNIQUE	FINDINGS
• *Patellar* Flex patient's knee up to 90 degrees, allowing lower leg to hang loosely. Support upper leg so it does not rest against edge of examining table, then strike patellar tendon just below patella.	**EXPECTED:** Extension of lower leg, contraction of quadriceps muscle. 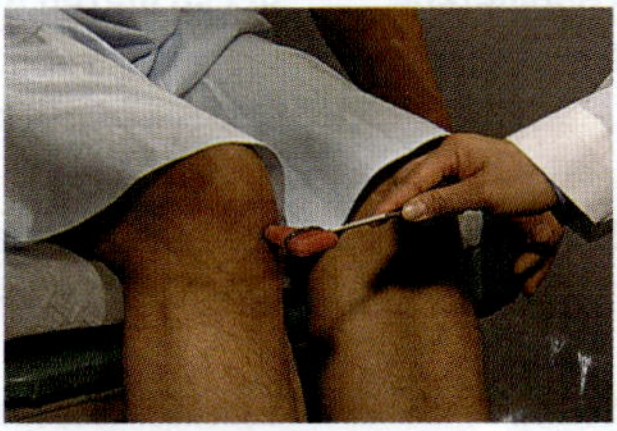 *Patellar deep tendon reflex.*
• *Achilles* With patient sitting, flex a knee and dorsiflex the ankle up to 90 degrees, holding heel of foot. Strike Achilles tendon at level of ankle malleoli.	**EXPECTED:** Plantar flexion, contraction of gastrocnemius muscle. 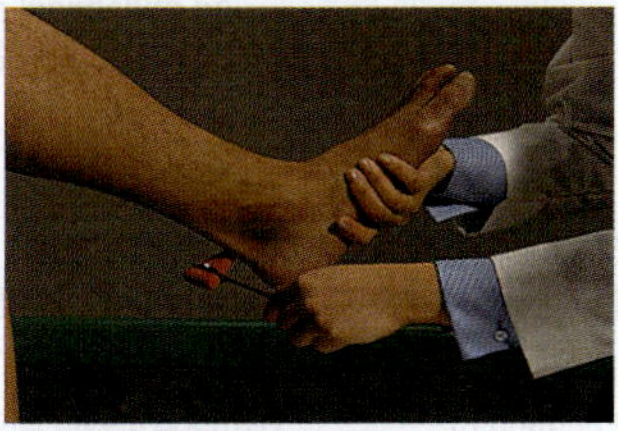 *Achilles deep tendon reflex.*
• *Clonus* Support patient's knee in partially flexed position and briskly dorsiflex foot with other hand, maintaining foot in flexion.	**EXPECTED:** No rhythmic oscillating movements. **UNEXPECTED:** Sustained clonus, rhythmic oscillating movements between dorsiflexion and plantar flexion palpated. 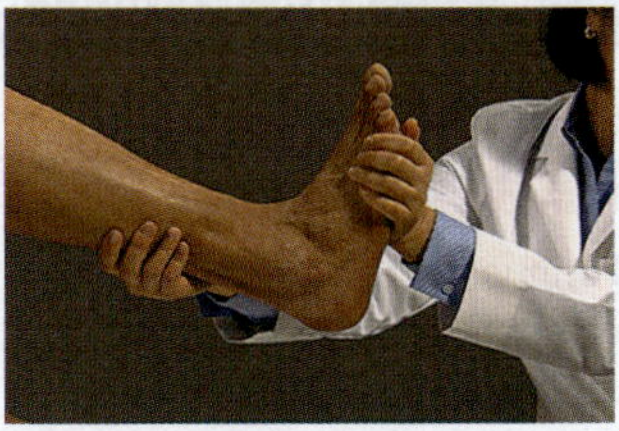 *Clonus assessment.*

Differential Diagnosis of Upper and Lower Motor Neuron Disorders

ASSESSMENT PARAMETERS	UPPER MOTOR NEURON	LOWER MOTOR NEURON
Muscle tone	Increased tone, muscle spasticity, risk for contractures	Decreased tone, muscle flaccidity
Muscle atrophy	Little or no muscle atrophy, but decreased strength	Loss of muscle strength; muscle atrophy or wasting
Sensation	Sensation loss may affect entire limb	Sensory loss that follows the distribution of dermatomes or peripheral nerves
Reflexes	Hyperactive deep tendon and abdominal reflexes; positive Babinski sign	Weak or absent deep tendon, plantar, and abdominal reflexes, negative plantar reflex, no pathologic reflexes
Fasciculation	No fasciculation	Fasciculation
Motor effect	Paralysis of voluntary movements	Paralysis of muscles
Location of insult	Damage above level of brainstem will affect opposite side of body, damage below the brainstem will affect the same side of the body	Damage affects muscle on same side of body

AIDS TO DIFFERENTIAL DIAGNOSIS

SUBJECTIVE DATA	OBJECTIVE DATA
Multiple Sclerosis	
Fatigue; vertigo, weakness, numbness; blurred vision, diplopia, vision loss; urinary frequency, urgency, hesitancy; sexual dysfunction; emotional changes	Muscle weakness, ataxia; hyperactive deep tendon reflexes; paresthesia, sensory loss; intention tremor; optic neuritis; cognitive changes

SUBJECTIVE DATA	OBJECTIVE DATA
Generalized Seizure Disorder	
Premonition or aura, stiff body followed by rhythmic jerking movements, eyes rolled upward, drooling; loss of bladder and bowel control	Tonic phase (brief flexion then extension for 10–15 minutes, eyes deviated upward, dilated pupils), clonic phase (alternating muscle contraction and relaxation), postictal (coma followed by confusion and lethargy)
Meningitis	
Fever, chills, headache, stiff neck, lethargy, malaise, vomiting, irritability, seizures	Altered mental status, confusion, nuchal rigidity, may see positive Brudzinski and Kernig signs
Encephalitis	
Recovery from mild viral illness with fever, then onset of lethargy, restlessness, mental confusion	Altered mental status, confusion, stupor, coma, photophobia, stiff neck, muscle weakness, paralysis, ataxia
Intracranial Tumor	
Headaches, may awaken from sleep; nausea and vomiting; memory loss and confusion; unsteady gait, impaired coordination; behavioral or personality changes	Signs vary by location of lesion; altered consciousness, confusion, papilledema, CN impairment, aphasia, vision loss, gait disturbance, ataxia
Stroke (Cerebrovascular Accident or Brain Attack)	
Sudden onset of numbness or weakness (often unilateral); sudden confusion, difficulty speaking or understanding speech; sudden trouble seeing in one or both eyes; sudden trouble walking, loss of balance, or loss of coordination; sudden severe headache with no known cause	Signs vary by part of brain affected. Altered consciousness, elevated blood pressure, difficulty managing secretions, weakness or paralysis of extremities or facial muscles on one or both sides of body, aphasia (receptive or expressive), articulation impairment, impaired horizontal gaze, or hemianopia

SUBJECTIVE DATA	OBJECTIVE DATA
Parkinson Disease	
Tremors at rest and with fatigue that disappear with intended movement and sleep; slowing of voluntary movement; bilateral pill rolling of fingers; may have numbness, aching, tingling, and muscle soreness; difficulty swallowing, drooling	Tremors; muscle rigidity, cogwheel rigidity with jerks; stooped posture; balance instability; short steps, shuffling, freezing gait; voice softening, slowed, slurred, monotonous speech; impaired cognition, dementia
Peripheral Neuropathy	
Gradual onset of numbness, tingling, burning in hands and feet; strange sensation when walking on cotton or floors; inability of fingers to feel difference between coins; night pain in feet	Reduced protective sensation (to pain and touch) in foot and may progress up lower leg; distal pulses diminished, diminished deep tendon reflexes in ankles and knees, loss of vibratory sensation below knee, distal muscle weakness, cannot stand on toes or heels
Trigeminal Neuralgia	
Sharp pain episodes on one side of face potentially caused by chewing, swallowing, talking, brushing teeth, or cold exposure	May have slight sensory impairment in regions of pain; may have normal neurologic findings
Bell's Palsy	
Rapid (2–3 days) progression of muscle weakness on one side of face, feeling of facial numbness	Unilateral disappearance of facial creases and nasolabial fold, eyelid does not close and lower lid sags. Facial sensation is intact

SUBJECTIVE DATA	OBJECTIVE DATA
Cerebral Palsy	
Delays in gross motor development, activity limitation; stiff joints and positioning; may have hearing, speech, or language disorders, feeding difficulties	Increased or decreased muscle tone, tremors, scissor gait or wide-based gait, toe walking, ataxia, exaggerated posturing, cognitive disability or learning disabilities, persistent primitive reflexes

PEDIATRIC VARIATIONS

EXAMINATION

Neurologic findings in the infant and child change as the child matures. (See Chapter 23 for a complete description of expected developmental findings by age.)

TECHNIQUE	FINDINGS
Indirectly evaluate CNs in newborns and infants	
• *Optical blink reflex (CN II, CN III, CN IV, CN VI)* Shine a light at infant's open eyes. Observe quick closure of eyes and dorsal flexion of head.	**EXPECTED:** Gazes intensely at close object or face. Focuses on and tracks an object with both eyes. **UNEXPECTED:** No response may indicate poor light perception.
• *Rooting reflex (CN V)* Touch one corner of infant's mouth.	**EXPECTED:** Infant opens mouth and turns head in direction of stimulation. Minimal or no response expected if infant was recently fed.
• *Sucking reflex (CN V)* Place your finger in infant's mouth, feeling sucking action. Note pressure, strength, pattern of sucking.	**EXPECTED:** Tongue should push up against your finger with decent strength.

TECHNIQUE	FINDINGS
• *Infant's facial expression (CN VII)* Note symmetry of facial expression and wrinkling of forehead when crying.	**EXPECTED:** Facial symmetry with all expressions.
• *Acoustic blink reflex (CN VIII)* Loudly clap your hands about 30 cm from infant's head; avoid producing an air current.	**EXPECTED:** Blink and movement of eyes in response to sound. Infant will habituate to repeated testing. Freezes position with high-pitched sound. **UNEXPECTED:** No response after 2–3 days of age.
• *Doll's eye maneuver (CN VIII)* Hold infant under axilla in upright position, head held steady, facing you. Rotate infant first in one direction and then in other.	**EXPECTED:** Infant's eyes turn in direction of rotation and then in opposite direction when rotation stops. **UNEXPECTED:** Eyes do not move in expected direction.
• *Swallowing and gag reflex (CN IX and CN X)*	**EXPECTED:** Coordinated sucking and swallowing ability.
• *Sucking and swallowing (CN XII)* Pinch infant's nose.	**EXPECTED:** Mouth will open, and tip of tongue will rise in midline position.
Evaluate common newborn reflexes in infant	
• *Palmar grasp (present at birth)* Making sure infant's head is in midline, touch palm of infant's hand from ulnar side (opposite thumb).	**EXPECTED:** Strong grasp of your finger. Sucking facilitates grasp. Grasp should be strongest between 1 and 2 months of age and disappear by 3 months.
• *Plantar grasp (present at birth)* Touch plantar surface of infant's feet at the base of toes.	**EXPECTED:** Toes should curl downward. Reflex should be strong up to 8 months of age.

TECHNIQUE	FINDINGS
• *Moro reflex (present at birth)* With infant supported in semisitting position, allow head and trunk to drop back to a 30-degree angle.	**EXPECTED:** Symmetric abduction and extension of arms. Fingers fan out, and thumb and index finger form a C. Arms then adduct in an embracing motion followed by relaxed flexion. Reflex diminishes in strength by 3–4 months and disappears by 6 months.
• *Placing (at 4 days of age)* Hold infant upright under axilla next to a table or chair. Touch dorsal side of foot to table or chair edge.	**EXPECTED:** Flexion of hip and knee, lifting of foot as if stepping up on table. Age of disappearance varies.
• *Stepping (between birth and 8 weeks)* Hold infant upright under axilla and allow soles of feet to touch surface of table.	**EXPECTED:** Alternate flexion and extension of legs, simulating walking. Disappears before voluntary walking.
• *Asymmetric tonic neck or "fencing" (by 2–3 months)* With infant lying supine and relaxed or sleeping, turn the head to one side so jaw is over shoulder. Then turn infant's head to other side.	**EXPECTED:** Extension of arm and leg on side to which head is turned, and flexion of opposite arm and leg. Reversal of extremities' positions with head turned opposite way. Reflex diminishes by 3–4 months of age and disappears by 6 months. **UNEXPECTED:** Be concerned if infant never exhibits reflex or seems locked in fencing position.

CHAPTER

21 Head-to-Toe Examination: Adult

Components of the Examination

The physical examination can be sequenced several ways. You are encouraged to consider and then to adapt the following suggested approach, minimizing the number of position changes, as appropriate for the unique needs of the patient's condition and abilities.

GENERAL INSPECTION

Start the examination the moment the patient is within your view. As you first observe the patient, take note of the following characteristics:

- Signs of distress or disease
- Habitus
- Manner of sitting
- Degree of facial relaxation

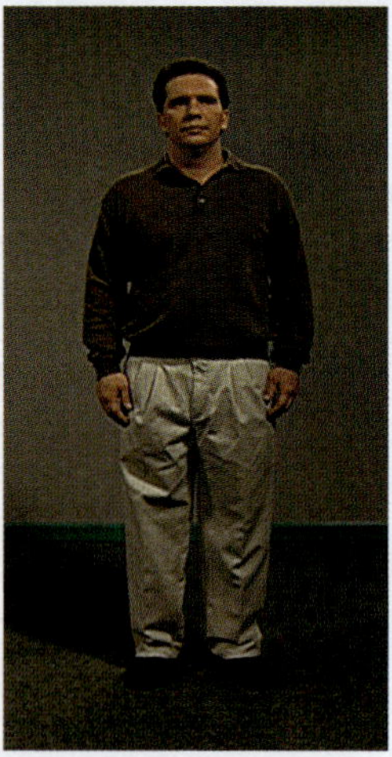

- Relationship with others in room
- Degree of interest in what is happening in room

- Manner with which you are met
- Moistness of palm when you shake hands
- Facial expression
- Eyes (luster and expression of emotion)
- Eye contact with you
- Skin color
- Mobility:
    - Use of assistive devices
    - Gait
    - Sitting, rising from chair
    - Taking off coat
- Stature, build
- Musculoskeletal deformities
- Dress, posture
- Speech pattern, disorders, foreign language
- Difficulty hearing, assistive devices
- Vision problems, assistive devices
- Orientation, mental alertness
- Nutritional state
- Respiratory problems
- Significant others accompanying patient

PATIENT INSTRUCTIONS (PLAN EACH STEP TO MINIMIZE THE PATIENT'S EFFORT AND TO CONSERVE ENERGY)

- Empty bladder.
- Remove as much clothing as necessary (always respecting modesty).
- Put on a gown.

MEASUREMENTS

- Measure weight and height.
- Calculate body mass index.
- Assess distance vision using Snellen chart.
- Document vital signs—temperature, pulse, respiration, blood pressure in both arms, oxygen saturation, and pain assessment.

PATIENT SEATED, WEARING GOWN

Stand in front of patient as they are seated on examining table.

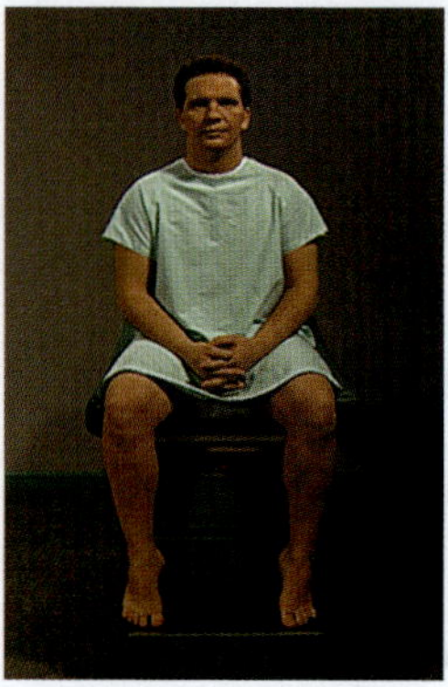

Head and Face

- Inspect skin characteristics.
- Inspect symmetry and external characteristics of eyes and ears.
- Inspect configuration of skull.
- Inspect and palpate scalp and hair for texture, distribution, and quantity of hair.
- Palpate facial bones.
- Palpate temporomandibular joint while patient opens and closes mouth.
- Palpate and percuss sinus regions.
- Inspect ability to clench teeth, squeeze eyes tightly shut, wrinkle forehead, smile, stick out tongue, and puff out cheeks (cranial nerve [CN] V, VII).
- Test sensation using light touch on forehead, cheeks, chin (CN V).

Eyes

- External examination:
  - Inspect eyelids, eyelashes, palpebral folds.
  - Determine alignment of eyebrows.
  - Inspect sclerae, conjunctivae, irides.
  - Palpate lacrimal apparatus.
  - Test near-vision—Rosenbaum chart (CN II).
- Eye function:
  - Test pupillary response to light and accommodation.
  - Perform cover–uncover test and corneal light reflex.
  - Test extraocular eye movements (CN III, IV, VI).

- Assess visual fields (CN II).
- Test corneal reflexes (CN V).
- Ophthalmoscopic examination:
  - Test red reflex.
  - Inspect lens.
  - Inspect disc, cup margins, vessels, retinal surface.

Ears

- Inspect alignment and placement.
- Inspect surface characteristics.
- Palpate auricle.
- Assess hearing with whisper test or ticking watch (CN VIII).
- Perform otoscopic examination:
  - Inspect canals.
  - Inspect tympanic membranes for landmarks, deformities, inflammation.
- Perform Rinne and Weber tests.

Nose

- Note structure, position of septum.
- Determine patency of each nostril.
- Inspect mucosa, septum, turbinates with nasal speculum.
- Assess sense of smell when clinically necessary (CN I).

Mouth and Pharynx

- Inspect lips, buccal mucosa, gums, hard and soft palates, floor of mouth for color and surface characteristics.
- Inspect oropharynx: note anteroposterior pillars, uvula, tonsils, posterior pharynx, mouth odor.
- Inspect teeth for color, number, surface characteristics.
- Inspect tongue for color, characteristics, symmetry, movement (CN XII).
- Test gag reflex and observe rising soft palate with patient saying "aah" (CN IX, X).
- Test sense of taste when clinically indicated (CN VII, IX).

Neck

- Inspect for symmetry and smoothness of neck and thyroid.
- Inspect for jugular venous distention (also when patient is supine).
- Perform active and passive range of motion; test resistance against examiner's hand.

- Test strength of shoulder shrug (CN IX).
- Palpate carotid pulses, one side at a time (also when patient is supine).
- Palpate tracheal position.
- Palpate thyroid.
- Palpate lymph nodes—preauricular and postauricular, tonsillar, submaxillary, submental, submandibular, superficial cervical chain, posterior cervical, deep cervical, supraclavicular, infraclavicular.
- Auscultate carotid arteries and thyroid.

Upper Extremities

- Inspect skin and nail characteristics.
- Inspect symmetry of muscle mass.
- Inspect and palpate hands, arms, shoulders, including epitrochlear nodes; note musculoskeletal deformities.
- Assess joint range-of-motion and muscle strength in fingers, wrists, elbows, and shoulders.
- Assess pulses—radial, brachial.

PATIENT SEATED, BACK EXPOSED

Stand behind patient seated on examining table. Have male patients pull gown down to the waist so entire chest and back are exposed. Have females expose back, keeping breasts covered.

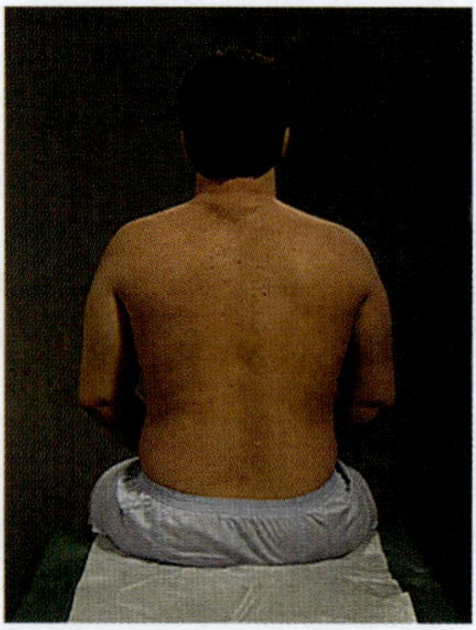

Back and Posterior Chest

- Inspect skin and thoracic configuration.
- Inspect symmetry of shoulders, musculoskeletal development.

- Inspect and palpate scapulae and spine.
- Palpate and percuss costovertebral angle.

Lungs

- Inspect chest movement with respiration—excursion, depth, rhythm, pattern.
- Palpate for expansion and tactile fremitus.
- Palpate scapular and subscapular nodes.
- Percuss posterior chest and lateral walls systematically for resonance.
- Percuss for diaphragmatic excursion.
- Auscultate systematically for breath sounds. Note characteristics and adventitious sounds.

PATIENT SEATED, CHEST EXPOSED

Move around to front of patient. Have female patients lower gown to expose anterior chest.

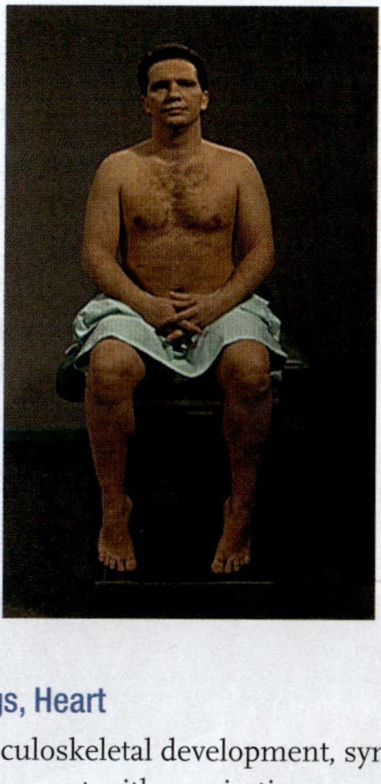

Anterior Chest, Lungs, Heart

- Inspect skin, musculoskeletal development, symmetry.
- Inspect chest movement with respirations—patient posture, respiratory effort.
- Inspect for pulsations or heaving.
- Palpate chest wall for stability, crepitation, tenderness.

- Palpate precordium for thrills, heaves, pulsations, and location of apical impulse.
- Palpate for tactile fremitus.
- Palpate axillary nodes.
- Percuss systematically for resonance.
- Auscultate systematically for breath sounds.
- Auscultate systematically for heart sounds in aortic, pulmonic, second pulmonic, tricuspid, and mitral areas.

Female Breasts

- Inspect in these positions—patient's arms hanging loosely at the sides, extended over head or flexed behind the neck, pushing hands on hips, patient leaning forward from waist.
- Perform chest wall sweep from clavicles to nipples.
- Perform bimanual digital palpation of each breast.
- Palpate for axillary, supraclavicular, and infraclavicular lymph nodes (if not already performed).

Male Breasts

- Inspect breasts and nipples for symmetry, enlargement, surface characteristics.
- Palpate breast tissue.
- Palpate for axillary, supraclavicular, and infraclavicular lymph nodes.

PATIENT RECLINING 45 DEGREES

Assist patient to a reclining position at a 45-degree angle. Stand to side of patient that allows greatest comfort and approach for examination.

- Inspect chest in recumbent position.
- Inspect jugular venous pulsations; measure right jugular venous pressure.

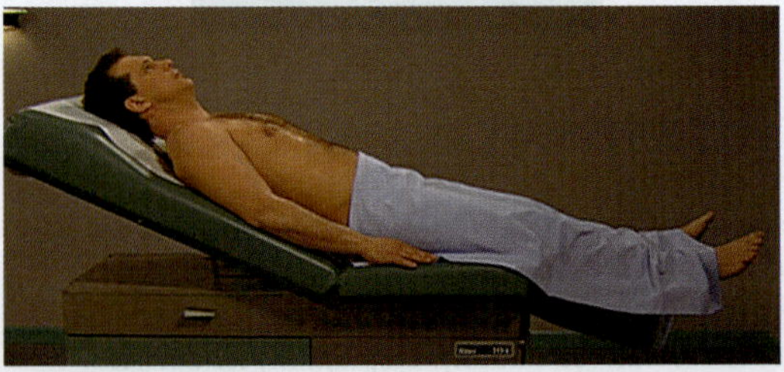

PATIENT SUPINE, CHEST EXPOSED

Assist patient into supine position. If patient cannot tolerate lying flat, maintain head elevation at 30-degree angle. Uncover chest while keeping abdomen and lower extremities draped.

Female Breasts

- Palpate all areas of breast tissue systematically using light, medium, and deep palpation with the patient's arm (on same side as breast being examined) over their head.
- Depress nipple into well behind the areola.

Heart

- Palpate chest wall for thrills, heaves, pulsations.
- Auscultate systematically; turn patient slightly to left side and repeat auscultation.

PATIENT SUPINE, ABDOMEN EXPOSED

Have patient remain supine. Cover chest with patient's gown. Arrange draping to expose abdomen from pubis to epigastrium.

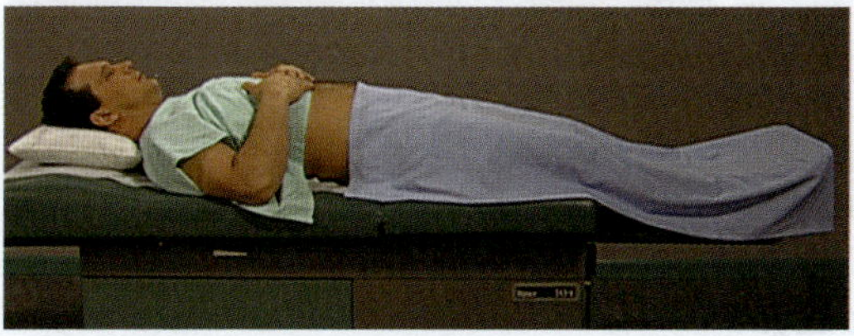

Abdomen

- Inspect skin characteristics, contour, pulsations, movement.
- Auscultate all quadrants for bowel sounds.
- Auscultate aorta and renal, iliac, and femoral arteries for bruits or venous hums.
- Percuss all quadrants for tone.
- Percuss liver borders and estimate span.
- Percuss left midaxillary line for splenic dullness.
- Lightly palpate all quadrants.
- Deeply palpate all quadrants:
  - Palpate right costal margin for liver border.
  - Palpate left costal margin for spleen.

  - Palpate at the flanks for right and left kidneys.
  - Palpate midline for aortic pulsation.
  - Test abdominal reflexes.
- Have patient raise head as you inspect abdominal muscles.

Inguinal Area

- Palpate for lymph nodes, femoral pulses, hernias.

External Genitalia, Males

- Inspect penis, urethral meatus, scrotum, pubic hair.
- Palpate scrotal contents.
- Test cremasteric reflex.

PATIENT SUPINE, LEGS EXPOSED

Have patient remain supine. Arrange drapes to cover abdomen and pubis, and to expose lower extremities.

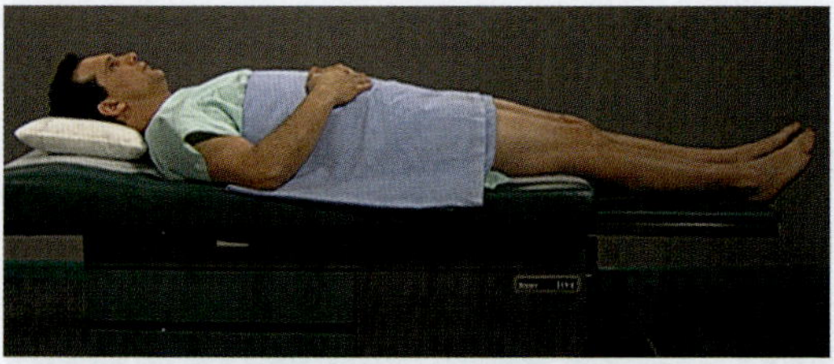

Feet and Legs

- Inspect for skin characteristics, hair distribution, muscle mass, musculoskeletal configuration.
- Palpate for temperature, texture, edema, pulses (dorsalis pedis, posterior tibial, popliteal).
- Test range of motion and strength of toes, feet, ankles, knees.

Hips

- Palpate hips for stability.
- Test range of motion and strength of hips.

PATIENT SITTING, LAP DRAPED

Assist patient into a sitting position. Have patient wear gown with a drape across lap.

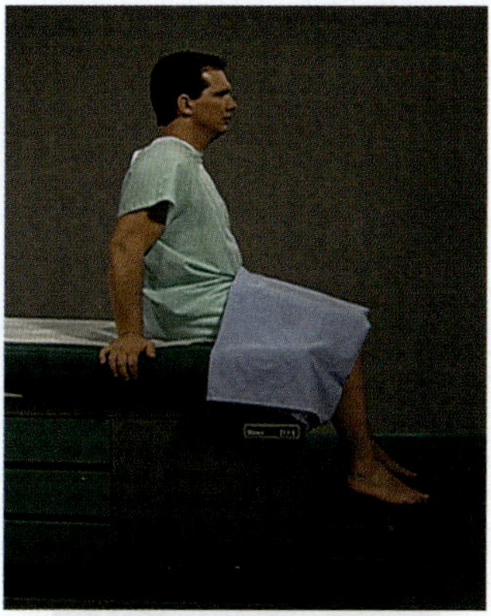

Musculoskeletal

- Observe patient moving from lying to sitting position.
- Note coordination, use of muscles, ease of movement.

Neurologic

- Test sensory function—dull and sharp sensation of forehead, cheeks, chin, lower arms, hands, lower legs, feet.
- Test position sense and vibratory sensation of wrists, ankles.
- Test two-point discrimination of palms, thighs, back.
- Test stereognosis, graphesthesia.
- Test fine motor function and coordination of upper extremities, asking patient to do the following:
  - Touch nose with alternating index fingers.
  - Rapidly alternate touching fingers to thumb.
  - Rapidly move index finger between own nose and examiner's finger.
- Test fine motor function and coordination of lower extremities, asking patient to do the following:
  - Run heel down tibia of opposite leg.
- Test deep tendon reflexes and compare bilaterally—biceps, triceps, brachioradial, patellar, Achilles.
- Test plantar reflex bilaterally.

PATIENT STANDING

Assist patient to standing position. Stand next to patient.

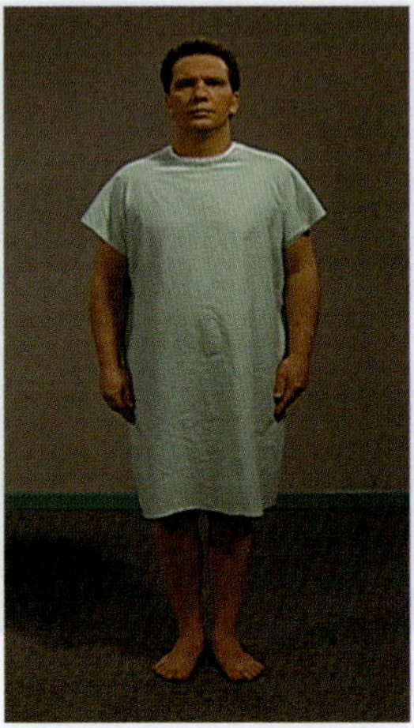

Spine

- Inspect and palpate spine as patient bends over at waist.
- Test range of motion—hyperextension, lateral bending, rotation of upper trunk.

Neurologic

- Observe gait.
- Test proprioception and cerebellar function:
  - Perform Romberg test.
  - Ask patient to walk heel to toe.
  - Ask patient to stand on one foot, then the other, with eyes closed.
  - Ask patient to hop in place on one foot, then the other, with eyes open.

Abdominal/Genital

- Test for inguinal and femoral hernias.

FEMALE PATIENT, LITHOTOMY POSITION

Assist female patient into lithotomy position and drape appropriately. Examiner is seated.

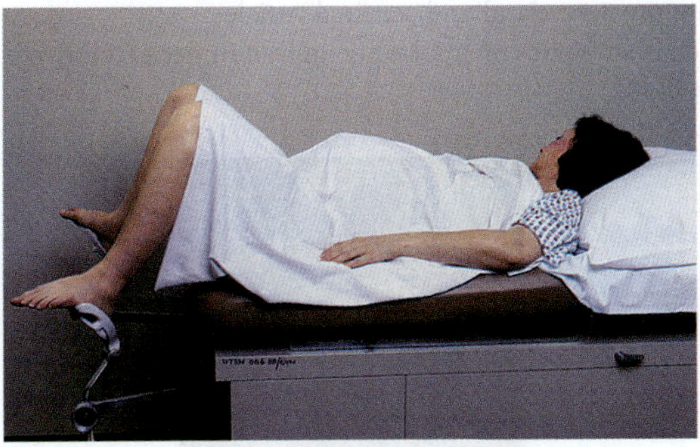

External Genitalia

- Inspect pubic hair, labia, clitoris, urethral opening, vaginal opening, perineal and perianal area, anus.
- Palpate labia and Bartholin glands; milk skene glands.

Internal Genitalia

- Perform speculum examination:
  - Inspect vagina and cervix.
  - Collect Pap smear/human papillomavirus and other necessary specimens.
- Perform bimanual palpation to assess for characteristics of vagina, cervix, uterus, adnexa (examiner standing).
- Perform rectovaginal examination to assess rectovaginal septum, broad ligaments.
- Perform rectal examination:
  - Assess anal sphincter tone and surface characteristics; palpate circumferentially for rectal mass.
  - Obtain rectal culture if needed.
  - Note characteristics of stool when gloved finger is removed. Test for occult blood.

MALE PATIENT, BENDING FORWARD

- Assist male patient to lean over examining table (or into knee–chest or lateral decubitus position). Stand behind patient.
- Inspect sacrococcygeal and perianal areas.
- Perform rectal examination:
  - Palpate sphincter tone and surface characteristics; palpate circumferentially for rectal mass.
  - Obtain rectal culture if needed.

- Palpate prostate gland and seminal vesicles.
- Note characteristics of stool when gloved finger is removed. Test for occult blood.

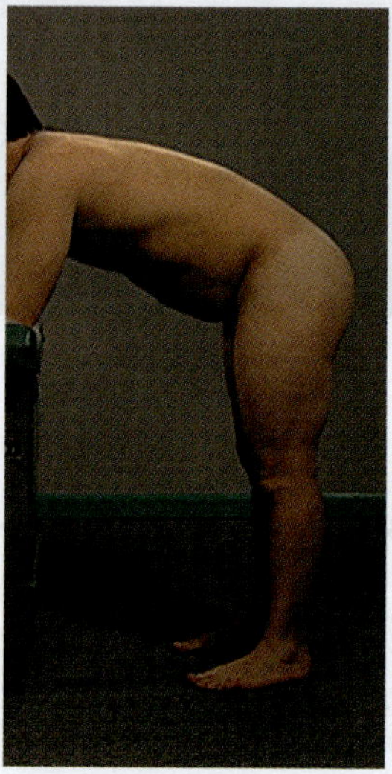

CONCLUSION

- Allow patient to dress in private.
- Take time to organize your thoughts regarding the history, physical examination, and a proposed plan of care.
- Share findings and interpretations with patient.
- Answer the patient's additional questions.
- Confirm that the patient has a clear understanding of all aspects of the situation.
- If patient is examined in a hospital bed:
  - Put everything back in order when finished.
  - Make sure patient is comfortably settled in an appropriate manner.
  - Put bedside rails up if clinical condition warrants it.
  - Make sure buttons and buzzers are easily within reach.

CHAPTER 22

Preventive Health Evaluation: Adults

The following are items to consider for inclusion as part of a routine periodic health examination or wellness visit. This is not intended as an all-inclusive list. Some items may vary depending on the patient's age, identified gender, health status, and particular risk factors. Medical history and review of systems may also be indicated. Age, gender, and risk status guidelines for preventive services are available from a variety of sources and authorities*.

Special care considerations for transgender and gender-diverse patients are addressed in Chapter 26.

History

INTERVAL HISTORY

- All patients
  - Age
  - Gender assignment at birth/gender identity (see Chapter 26)
  - Sexual history and functioning
  - Contraceptive measures and history
  - Urinary symptoms
  - Abdominal or pelvic pain or bloating
  - Rectal bleeding
  - Organ inventory (natal/acquired/absent: breasts, vagina, cervix, uterus, ovaries, penis, testes, and prostate)
  - New medical conditions, new surgeries
- As applicable
  - Last normal menstrual period
  - Menopause—age achieved, symptoms
  - Obstetric history—number of pregnancies (gravity), term pregnancies, preterm pregnancies, abortions/miscarriages, living children (GTPAL)

*Authorities that produce guidelines include American Academy of Family Physicians, American Cancer Society, American College of Obstetricians and Gynecologists, American College of Physicians, American Geriatrics Society, Canadian Task Force on the Periodic Health Examination, Centers for Disease Control and Prevention, National Cancer Institute, and US Preventive Services Task Force.

- Breast lumps, discharge, pain, and skin changes
- Unusual vaginal bleeding or discharge
- Penile discharge
- Testicular pain, lumps

RISK ASSESSMENT

- Cardiovascular—smoking, hypertension, diet, body mass index (BMI), exercise, and family history
- Cancer—personal/family history of breast, ovarian, colon, or prostate cancer; history of sun exposure and smoking
- Infection—exposure to: sexually transmitted infection (STI); HIV; tuberculosis (TB); hepatitis; and viral disease
- Immunizations:
  - Influenza
  - Respiratory syncytial virus
  - Tetanus, diphtheria, and pertussis
  - Measles, mumps, and rubella
  - Varicella
  - Herpes zoster (shingles)
  - Human papillomavirus (HPV)
  - Pneumococcal pneumonia
  - Hepatitis A
  - Hepatitis B
  - Meningococcal
  - *Haemophilus influenzae* type b
  - Mpox
  - Inactivated poliovirus
  - COVID-19 or other immunizations
- Metabolic—calcium supplement, family/personal history of osteoporosis; exercise; personal/family history of diabetes mellitus; hearing impairment in older adults; dental health; obstructive sleep apnea; visual acuity
- Injury—alcohol, seat belts, guns, falls, work-related, family/partner violence
- Mental health—depression; anxiety; vegetative symptoms (eating, sleeping, concentration, energy, social interaction)

HEALTH HABITS

- Breast/genital self-awareness
- Pap smear/date, results; any abnormal, treatment
- HPV test—date, result; any abnormal, treatment

- Mammogram—date and result
- Prostate Specific Antigen (PSA) test—date and result
- Colon cancer screening test—date, type, result
- Diet—proportion of fat, protein, carbohydrate; calcium, vitamin D
- Exercise—amount, frequency
- Smoking/tobacco use—type, amount, frequency
- Alcohol/drug use—type, amount, frequency
- Sun exposure

Physical Examination

ALL PATIENTS

- Vital signs: blood pressure
- Height and weight; BMI
- Skin—lesions, moles
- Respiratory—rate, pattern, additional sounds
- Cardiovascular—rate, rhythm, regularity, additional sounds
- Peripheral vascular—pulses, edema, clubbing
- Lymph—regional lymphadenopathy (infraclavicular and supraclavicular, axillary, inguinal)
- Abdomen—bowel sounds, masses, organ enlargement, hernias
- Rectal—hemorrhoids, masses, lesions

FOR PATIENTS WITH INDICATED ORGANS

- Breasts—contour, masses, nipple discharge, skin changes
- Pelvis—lesions, discharge; lymph nodes, Bartholin glands, urethra, Skene glands; vagina, cervix, adnexa, uterus; rectovaginal septum, perineal area, anus, rectum
- Penis and testicles—lesions, lumps, discharge; urinary meatus, penile shaft, scrotum, epididymis, lymph nodes, hernias
- Prostate—nodules, masses, hardness, softness; prostate lobes, sulcus; perianal area, anus, rectum

Screening Recommendations

This list includes the most common screening recommendations. It is not all-inclusive, and not all authorities agree on all recommendations.

CARDIOVASCULAR

- Blood pressure—begin at age 18
- Lipid profile—begin at age 45

- One-time screening for abdominal aortic aneurysm with ultrasonography in men aged 65, 70, and 75 who have ever smoked

CANCER

- Cervical: Pap smear/HPV testing:
  - Under age 25: No screening.
  - Ages 25–65 years: HPV test every 5 years, or Pap test plus an HPV test every 5 years, or Pap test alone every 3 years.
  - Testing is not recommended in patients older than 65 years who are at average risk and have had regular cervical cancer testing with normal results. Once testing is stopped, it should not be started again. Patients with a history of a serious cervical precancer (cervical intraepithelial neoplasia grade 2 or 3) should continue with routine testing for at least 25 years after diagnosis, even if testing continues past age 65.
  - Patients who have had uterus and cervix removed for reasons unrelated to cervical cancer, and who have no history of cervical cancer or serious precancer, should not be tested.
  - Patients vaccinated against HPV should follow the screening recommendations for their age group.
- Breast
  - Clinical breast examination—younger than 40 years: every 3 years; older than 40 years: annually
  - Screening mammogram—annually beginning at age 40 years; earlier if at increased risk; frequency depends on personal history, family history, and past results
- Colorectal—average risk: begin at age 45 years. Options are:
  - Tests that detect adenomatous polyps and cancer (visual examination of colon and rectum):
    - Colonoscopy every 10 years
    - Computed tomography colography (virtual colonoscopy) every 5 years
    - Flexible sigmoidoscopy every 5 years or flexible sigmoidoscopy with annual fecal immunochemical test (FIT) testing every 10 years
  - Tests that primarily detect cancer (stool-based tests):
    - Multitargeted stool DNA (every 1–3 years)
    - Highly sensitive FIT (gFBOT) every year
    - Highly sensitive FIT every year
- Prostate: Persons with a prostate
  - Begin age 50 for those at average risk; begin age 45 for those at

high risk (African American or first degree relative diagnosed before age 65); begin age 40 for those at higher risk (more than one first-degree relative diagnosed before age 65)

- Prostate examination; PSA: only after discussion of risks and benefits, and based on individual decision

- Lung
  - Ages 50–80 years: Annual screening with low-dose computed tomography in those who have a 20-pack-per-year smoking history and currently smoke or have quit within the past 15 years. Screening should be discontinued once a person has not smoked for 15 years or develops a health problem that substantially limits life expectancy or the ability or willingness to have curative lung surgery.

INFECTION

- STI testing—depending on exposure status; chlamydia screening—all sexually active women age 25 years or younger and women older than age 25 years with risk factors (e.g., women with a new or more than one sex partner); gonorrhea and syphilis screening—all sexually active women at increased risk
- HIV—adolescents and adults ages 15–65 years; antigen/antibody immunoassay
- Hepatitis B—adolescents and adults at increased risk; HBsAg tests approved by the US Food and Drug Administration, followed by a confirmatory test for initially reactive results
- Hepatitis C—ages 18–79 years; anti-HCV antibody testing followed by polymerase chain reaction testing for HCV RNA; most adults need screening only once. Those at increased risk should be screened periodically
- TB testing—depending on risk status

METABOLIC

- BMI: Obesity
- Fasting plasma glucose for those ages 40–70 years who are overweight or obese
- Bone density—women ≥65 years; begin earlier in women at increased risk for osteoporosis as determined by a formal clinical risk assessment tool

SPECIAL SENSES

- Hearing impairment—older adults
- Impaired visual acuity and glaucoma screening

INJURY

- Intimate partner violence (see Appendix A: Quick Reference to Special Histories)

MENTAL HEALTH

- Alcohol and substance abuse (see Appendix A: Quick Reference to Special Histories)
- Depression
- Anxiety

CHAPTER 23

Preventive Health Evaluation: Infants, Children, and Adolescents

Examination Guidelines

A pediatric physical examination should be developmentally and age appropriate. Not every observation and examination maneuver must be made on every pediatric patient at every visit. What you do depends on the individual circumstance and your clinical judgment, with each step being dependent on the patient's age, physical condition, and emotional state. The order of the examination can and should be modified according to individual need. There is no one correct sequence. The safety of the infant and child on the examining table must be ensured. During most of infancy and into the toddler years, an adult's lap is a more secure surface for most and often all of the examination.

- Observe child's behavior and interactions with parent (or caregiver) and with you.
- Offer toys, a book, or paper and crayons to entertain child (if age appropriate) to develop rapport and to assist you in assessing child's development and neurologic status. Attempt to gain child's cooperation and build rapport, even if it takes more time; future visits will be more pleasant for you, the child, and their caregiver.
- For young children, perform the funduscopic, otoscopic, and oral examinations at the end of the visit with the child seated on the parent's lap; with the child's back to the parent's chest their legs can be placed between the adult's legs, and the parent can then hold the child's arms with one arm and control the child's head with the other. If the parent hold is not effective and the child is unable to cooperate, be prepared to move the child to the examining table and have another person assist with holding.
- Lessen fear of these examinations by permitting child to handle instruments, blow out light, or use them on a parent, or yourself.
- Review weight, length, or height; review temperature, heart rate, and blood pressure (record extremity or extremities used, method used, and size of cuff).
- Use WHO growth charts to review percentiles for all measurements, including body mass index (BMI) for children 2 years and older.

- If clinical issues require it, include arm span, lower segment measurement (symphysis pubis to floor), upper segment measurement (subtract lower body segment from total height), upper/lower segment ratio, and chest circumference.
- Review parent-completed developmental screening tool to assess language, motor abilities, social skills, and parental concerns.
- Review other screening tools (e.g., social needs, behavioral health, sports preparticipation history form).
- Assess child's developmental skills and mental status during interactions with you and with parent.

CHILD PLAYING

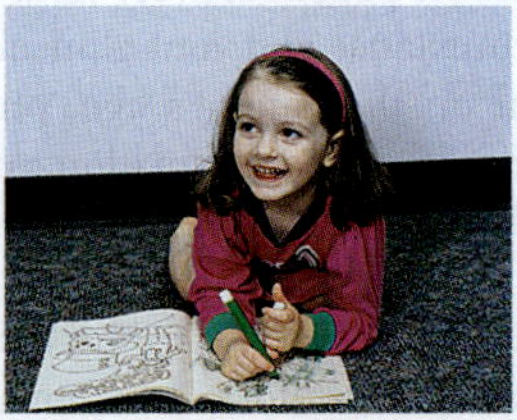

- As child plays, evaluate musculoskeletal and neurologic system while developing rapport with child.
- Observe child's spontaneous activities.
- Ask child to demonstrate skills (e.g., turning pages in a book, building block towers, drawing geometric figures, and coloring).
- Evaluate gait, jumping, hopping, and the range of motion.
- Observe child climbing on parent's lap, stooping, and recovering.

CHILD ON PARENT'S LAP

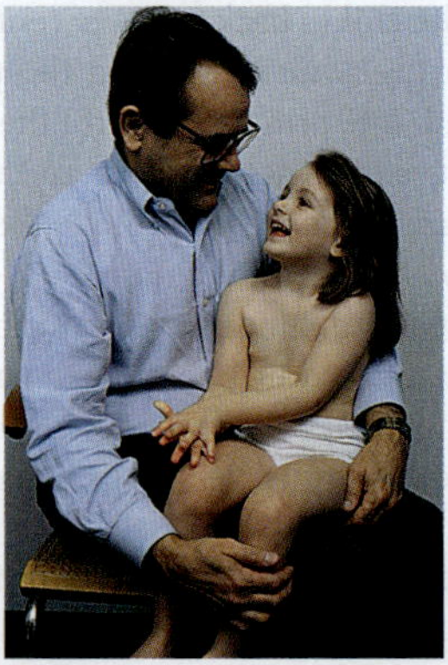

- As noted, perform examination of young children on parent's lap; the adult and the patient generally enjoy the experience more this way. You will also likely find it easier to meet the child's eye level when sitting on a stool as opposed to sitting the child on the examining table.
- Begin with child sitting and undressed except for diaper or underpants.

Upper Extremities

- Inspect arms for movement, size, shape, and skin lesions; observe use of hands; inspect hands for number and configuration of fingers and palmar creases.
- Palpate radial pulses.
- Elicit biceps and triceps reflexes.
- Check blood pressure if not previously taken or if initial measurement was abnormal.

Lower Extremities

- Child may stand for much or part of examination.
- Inspect legs for movement, size, shape, alignment, and lesions.
- Inspect feet for alignment, longitudinal arch, and the number of toes.
- Palpate femoral and dorsalis pedis pulses.
- Elicit plantar, Achilles, and patellar reflexes.

Head and Neck

- Inspect head.
- Inspect shape, alignment with neck, hairline, eyelids, palpebral folds, conjunctivae, sclerae, irides, and the position of auricles.
- Palpate anterior fontanel for size (age appropriate); head for sutures and depressions; hair for texture.
- Measure head circumference (up to age 36 months).
- Inspect neck for webbing and voluntary movement.
- Palpate neck: thyroid, muscle tone, lymph nodes, position of trachea.

Chest, Heart, and Lungs

- Inspect chest for respiratory movement, size, shape, precordial movement, deformity, and nipple and breast development.
- Palpate anterior chest, locate point of maximal impulse.
- Auscultate anterior, lateral, and posterior chest for breath sounds; count respirations.
- Auscultate all cardiac listening areas for S1 and S2, splitting and murmurs; count apical pulse.

CHILD RELATIVELY SUPINE, STILL ON LAP, DIAPER LOOSENED

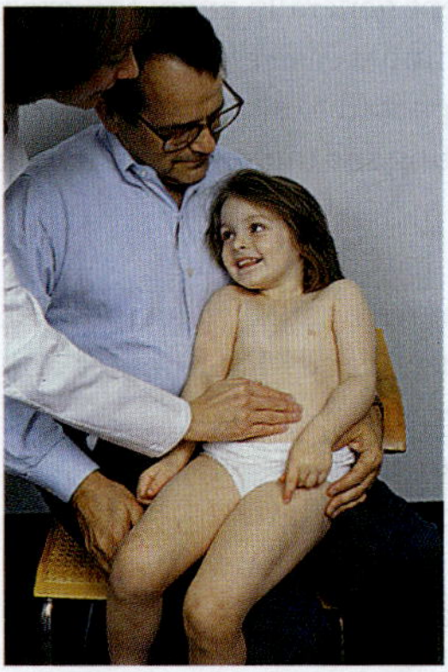

- Inspect abdomen.
- Auscultate for bowel sounds.
- Palpate: Identify size of liver and any other palpable organs or masses.
- Percuss.
- Palpate femoral pulses; compare with radial pulses.
- Palpate for inguinal lymph nodes.
- Inspect external genitalia.
- Males: Inspect penile glans and meatus, and palpate scrotum for descent of testes and other masses (see Chapter 17).
- Females: Inspect clitoris, urethral meatus, and vaginal opening (see Chapter 16).

CHILD STANDING

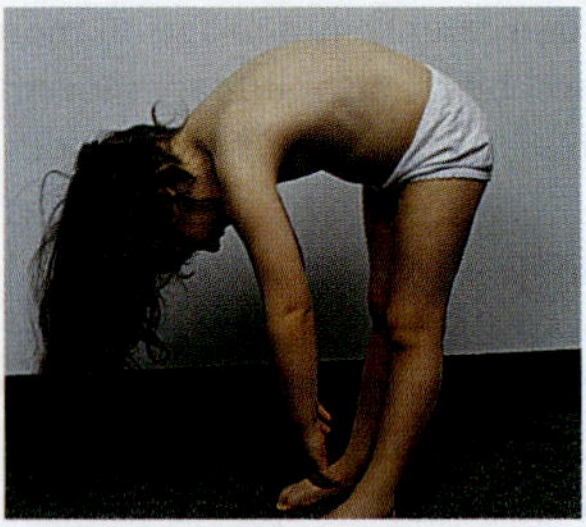

- Inspect spinal alignment as child bends slowly forward to touch toes.
- Observe posture from anterior, posterior, lateral views.
- Observe gait.

CHILD ON PARENT'S LAP

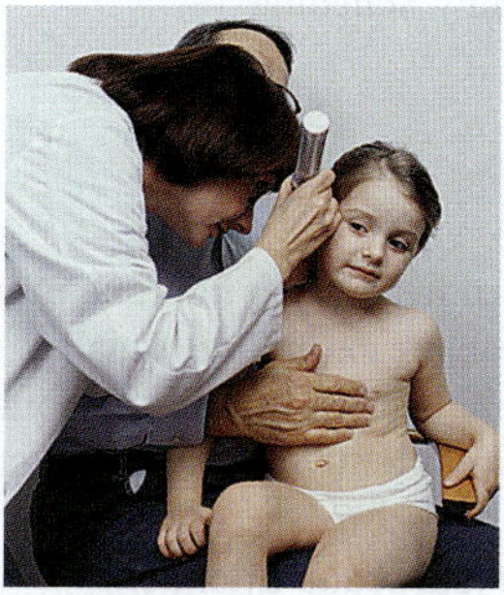

The following steps, often delayed to the end of the examination, are more easily performed with a child of appropriate age sitting on a parent's or caregiver's lap.

- Inspect eyes: Pupillary light reflex, red reflex, corneal light reflex, extraocular movements, funduscopic examination.
- Perform otoscopic examination: Note position and description of pinnae.
- Inspect nasal mucosa.
- Inspect mouth and pharynx: Note number of teeth, deciduous or permanent, and any special characteristics.

Note: By the time child is of school age, it is usually possible to use an examination sequence very similar to that for adults.

Age-Specific Recommendations

History building can be facilitated by referring to photos and videos on mobile devices, and other materials the family may have at home. This is a suggested outline, always modified by human variation, and variation exists in attainment of developmental milestones. The Centers for Disease Control and Prevention website includes resources for parents, clinicians, and trainees for assessing and tracking developmental milestones: https://www.cdc.gov/ncbddd/actearly/milestones/index.html.

BIRTH TO 2 WEEKS OF AGE

History (particular attention)

- Pertinent perinatal, maternal, and family history
- Social: Caregiver arrangements, housing, and food security
- Maternal mood and social support
- Stool pattern

- Umbilicus: Healing, discharge, granulation
- Diet: Feeding modality, schedule
- Sleep environment

Development

By this age:

- 80% will lift and turn head when in prone position.
- 40% will follow an object to midline visually.
- 35% will vocalize and become quiet in response to a voice.
- 45% will regard a face intently, diminishing activity for the moment.

Physical Examination (particular attention)

- Establish growth curves (weight, height, head circumference)
- Hips
- Femoral pulses
- Head shape
- Reflexes: Moro, root, grasp, step

Anticipatory Guidance (particular attention)

- Sleep: Emphasize supine position and safe sleep environment (alone, back, crib or bassinet, no smoking in home)
- Feeding: Breast milk or formula, use of pacifier (need to suck)
- Use of bulb syringe (nasal stuffiness)
- Safety: Falling, crib, car seats, hot water temperature for bathing
- Skin care
- Clothing
- Illness: Temperature taking
- Crying (holding the baby)

Plans and Problems

- What strengths and risks have revealed themselves as you have gotten to know the family? What are current or potential problems? Start a problem list from which to make appropriate recommendations.
- Review results of newborn metabolic screening, hearing screening, and any other notable medical or social issues requiring follow-up.
- Discuss immunization schedule based on American Academy of Pediatrics guidelines; at each visit, discuss benefits, risks, and side effects of immunizations.

2 MONTHS OF AGE

History (particular attention)

- Parental concerns
- Child's apparent temperament
- Sleep cycle
- Safe sleep positioning and environment
- Feeding patterns, frequency
- Stooling pattern, frequency, color, consistency, straining
- Social:
  Maternal well-being
  Father's involvement and other adult caregivers
  Tobacco, alcohol, and drug use in caregivers
  Living conditions, food security, housing stability
  Additional social resource needs

Development

By this age:

- Gross motor:
  80% will lift head to 45 degrees in prone position.
  45% will lift head to as much as 90 degrees in prone position.
  25% will roll over from stomach to back.
- Fine motor:
  ≥99% will follow a moving object to midline.
  85% will follow a moving object past midline.
- Language:
  Almost all will diminish activity at the sound of a voice.
  35% will spontaneously vocalize.
  Many will vocalize responsively.
- Social-emotional:
  Almost all will diminish activity when regarding a face.
  Almost all will respond to a friendly, cooing face with a social smile.
  50% may smile spontaneously or even laugh aloud.

Physical Examination (particular attention)

- Growth curves (weight, height, and head circumference)
- Hearing
- Vision
- Hips
- Skin (rashes)
- Eyes (red reflex)

Anticipatory Guidance

- Feeding and nutritional adequacy, including vitamin D
- Childcare arrangements
- Hiccups
- Straining at stool
- Visual and auditory stimulus (mirrors, rattles, singing, and talking to baby)
- Tummy time when awake
- Sibling jealousy (if there are siblings or other children in home)
- Babysitters and other caregivers (checking references, reliability)
- Safety (car seat, rolling over, smoke detectors in home); reemphasize earlier discussions
- Sleep (reemphasize safe location and supine position)
- Smoking in home and contribution to poor health

Plans and Problems

- Review immunizations and provide as appropriate.
- List problems (e.g., allergies, medications, and any areas of concern) and make appropriate plans and referrals, if necessary.

4 MONTHS OF AGE

History (particular attention)

- Parental concerns
- Infant's sleep cycle
- Safe sleep positioning and environment
- Temperament
- Feeding patterns, frequency
- Stooling pattern, frequency, color, consistency, and straining
- Social issues:
  Maternal well-being
  Father's involvement and other adult caregivers
  Review family structure, living situation, and social supports
  Tobacco, alcohol, and drug use in caregivers
  Additional social resource needs

Development

By this age:

- Gross motor:
  80%, when prone, will lift chest up with arm support.
  80% will roll over from stomach to back.

35% will have no head lag when pulled to sitting position; many will then hold head steady when kept in that position.

- Fine motor:
  60% will reach for a dangling object.
  Almost all will bring hands together.
  Almost all will follow a face or object up to 180 degrees.
- Language:
  Almost all will laugh aloud.
  20% will appear to initiate vocalization.
- Social-emotional:
  80% will smile spontaneously.
  Many will regard their own hand for several seconds.

Physical Examination (particular attention)

- Update growth curves (weight, height, and head circumference).
- Reassess hearing.
- Reassess vision.

Anticipatory Guidance

- Introduction of solid food between 4 and 6 months (iron-fortified cereal)
- Stool changes with changes in diet
- Drooling and teething
- Thumb sucking, pacifiers, bottles at bedtime
- Safety (aspiration, falls, holding baby with hot liquids, reemphasize earlier discussions [e.g., car seat, water heater temperature])
- Reemphasis on environmental stimulus and tummy time when awake
- Further discussion of babysitters and other caregivers
- Use of antipyretics (e.g., acetaminophen)

Plans and Problems

- Review immunizations and provide as appropriate.
- Maintain problem list, making appropriate plans and referrals, if necessary.

6 MONTHS OF AGE

History (Interim Details)

- Parental concerns
- Sleep patterns
- Diet

- Stooling pattern
- Reassess social needs covered in prior visits.
- If either parent has not attended visits regularly, encourage their participation and address relevant issues

Development

By this age:

- Gross motor:
  90%, when pulled to a sitting position, will have no head lag.
  60% will sit alone.
  75% will bear some weight on legs.
  Almost all will roll over.
- Fine motor:
  More than half will pass a toy from hand to hand.
  60%, in a sitting position, will look for a toy.
  40%, in a sitting position, will take two cubes.
- Language:
  60% will turn toward a voice.
  30% will initiate speech sounds (e.g., "mama," "dada") but not specifically.
- Social-emotional:
  30% may cry and turn away from strangers.
  40% may put an object in mouth to explore it, may feed self.
  60% may resist an attempt to pull away an object while holding it.

Physical Examination (Particular Attention)

- Update growth curves.
- Hearing and vision.
- Look for any new findings and recheck prior findings.

Anticipatory Guidance

- Bedtime routines (discuss putting child to bed while child is awake; waking up at night)
- Fear of strangers
- Separation anxiety
- Safety (stairgates; begin discussions about what toddlers can get into, cabinets, hot water, electrical outlets, medications and other poisons; inform about local poison control center; reemphasize earlier discussions [e.g., car seat])
- Shoes, if and when to use them

- Brushing teeth
- Teething
- Checking fluoride intake
- Offering a cup
- Addition of solid foods

Plans and Problems

- Review immunizations and provide as appropriate.
- Maintain problem list, making appropriate plans and referrals, if necessary.

9 MONTHS OF AGE

History (interim details)

- Parental concerns
- Continued attention to sleep, diet, stooling patterns
- Reassess social needs covered in prior visits

Development

By this age:

- Gross motor:
  Almost 100% will sit alone.
  80% will stand alone.
  45% will cruise.
  Some will have begun competent crawling.
- Fine motor:
  70% will have thumb-finger grasp.
  60% will bang two cubes together.
  Almost all will finger feed.
- Language:
  75% will imitate speech sounds.
  75% will use "mama" and "dada" nonspecifically.
- Social-emotional:
  Almost 100% will try to get to a toy that is out of reach.
  85% will play repetitive games (e.g., peekaboo).
  45% will be shy with strangers and may cry.

Physical Examination (particular attention)

- Update growth curves.
- Reassess earlier findings and note any new findings.

Anticipatory Guidance

- Consistent routines
- Brushing teeth
- Self-feeding
- Sleep (naps)
- Separation anxiety
- Reemphasis on checking references and reliability of babysitters and caregivers
- Safety (stair gates and toddlers, falls, window guards, poisoning, burns, aspiration, smoking in the home, etc.)
- Weaning, breast, and/or bottle feeding
- Uses of discipline

Plans and Problems

- Review immunizations and provide as appropriate.
- Perform developmental screening (using parent-administered validated tool).
- Consider need for a serum lead level, hemoglobin, or hematocrit value.
- Maintain problem list, making appropriate plans and referrals, if necessary.

12 MONTHS OF AGE

History (interim details)

- Assess parental concerns.
- Reassess social and system review.

Development

By this age:

- Gross motor:
  85% will cruise.
  70% will stand alone briefly.
  50% will walk to some extent, and more will try it with hands held.
- Fine motor:
  90% will bang two cubes together.
  70% will have a good pincer grasp.
- Language:
  80% will use “mama,” “dada” specifically.
  30% will use as many as three additional words.
  Almost all will indulge in immature jargoning.

- Psychosocial:
  Almost all will respond to parent's presence and voice.
  Almost all will wave bye-bye.
  85% will play pat-a-cake.
  50% will drink from a cup.
  About half, perhaps a bit more, will play ball with examiner.

Physical Examination (particular attention)

- Update growth curves.
- Continue reassessment.
- Evaluate gait if walking has begun.

Anticipatory Guidance

- Reduced food intake in many (this is expected)
- Weaning or eliminating bottle use (especially at night)
- Increased use of table food
- Toothbrushing
- Toilet training (expectations, attitudes)
- Discipline (e.g., limit setting)
- Limiting screen time
- Safety (childproofing house, car seat, pets, neighborhood, etc.)

Plans and Problems

- Review immunizations and provide as appropriate.
- Consider need for a serum lead level, hemoglobin or hematocrit value, tuberculosis testing.
- Maintain problem list, making appropriate plans and referrals, if necessary.

15 MONTHS OF AGE

History (Interim Details)

- Assess parental concerns.
- Reassess social and system review.

Development

By this age:

- Gross motor:
  Almost all will walk well.
  Almost all will stoop to recover an object.
  35% will walk up steps with help.

- Fine motor:
  Almost all will drink from a cup.
  Almost all will have a neat pincer grasp.
  70% will scribble with crayon.
  60% will make a tower with two cubes.
- Language:
  Almost all will use "mama" and "dada" specifically.
  75% will use as many as three additional words.
  30% will put two words together.
- Social-emotional:
  Many more than 50% will play ball with examiner.
  50% will try to use a spoon.
  45% will try to remove clothing.

Physical Examination (particular attention)

- Update growth curves.
- Continue reassessment.
- Evaluate gait.
- Teeth.

Anticipatory Guidance

- Dental health (visit to a dentist)
- Toilet training
- Weaning
- Discipline (e.g., need for consistency)
- Reading daily with child
- Consistent sleep routines
- Handling temper tantrums (distraction, praise for positive behaviors)
- Safety (all issues, repetitively)

Plans and Problems

- Review immunizations and provide as appropriate.
- Consider need for a serum lead level, hemoglobin or hematocrit value, tuberculosis testing.
- Maintain problem list, making appropriate plans and referrals, if necessary.

18 MONTHS OF AGE

History (Interim Details)

- Assess parental concerns.
- Reassess social and system review.

Development

By this age:

- Gross motor:
  55% will have begun to walk upstairs without much help.
  70% will have started to walk backward.
  More than that will have tried running with at least some success.
  45% will have tried with some success to kick a ball forward, given the opportunity.
- Fine motor:
  80% will scribble if given a crayon.
  80% will make a tower with two cubes.
  About half of those will attempt, with some success, a tower of as many as four cubes.
- Language:
  Almost all will have mature jargoning.
  85% will have at least three words in addition to "mama" and "dada."
  Many of those will put two words together.
  More than half will respond to a one-step command (e.g., when asked to point to a body part).
- Social-emotional:
  Well more than half will assist with taking off their clothes.
  75% will use a spoon successfully, albeit with some spillage.

Physical Examination (particular attention)

- Update growth curves.
- Continue reassessment; search for new findings.
- Continue to evaluate gait.

Anticipatory Guidance

- Sleep (location, naps, nightmares)
- Diet (mealtime battles)
- Dental health (toothbrushing, dentist)
- Toilet training
- Discipline (methods and, again, consistency)
- Safety (never enough discussion [e.g., car seat, guns in home, child-proofing home])
- Self-comforting (masturbation, thumb sucking, favorite blankets, and toys)
- Read, talk, and sing with child
- Childcare settings if one is necessary

Plans and Problems

- Review immunizations and provide as appropriate.
- Perform developmental and autism screening (using parent-administered validated tools).
- Consider need for serum lead level, hemoglobin or hematocrit value, tuberculosis testing.
- Maintain problem list, making appropriate plans and referrals, if necessary.

2 YEARS OF AGE

History (Interim Details)

- Assess parental concerns.
- Reassess social and system review.

Development

By this age:

- Gross motor:
  All should run well.
  All should walk up steps of reasonable height without holding on.
  90% will kick a ball forward.
  80% will throw a ball overhand.
  60% will do a little jump.
  40% may balance on one foot for 1–2 seconds.
- Fine motor:
  Almost all should scribble with a pencil.
  90% will make a tower of four cubes.
  70% will copy a vertical line.
- Language:
  All should point to and name parts of body.
  85% will readily combine two different words.
  80% will understand "on" and "under."
  75% will name a picture.
- Social-emotional:
  85% will give a toy to mother or other significant person.
  60% will put on some clothing alone and, often, also remove a garment.
  50% will play games with others.

Physical Examination (Particular Attention)

- Update growth curves.
- Calculate and plot BMI.

- Continue reassessment; note new findings.
- Examine mouth and count number of teeth.

Anticipatory Guidance

- Independence (limit setting, temper tantrums)
- Peer interaction
- Safety (over-the-counter and prescription medications, water temperature, car seat use)
- Toilet training
- Limit TV viewing to 1–2 hours per day
- Nightmares
- Use of a cup for drinking (as much as possible)

Plans and Problems

- Review immunizations and provide as appropriate.
- Perform developmental screening (using parent-administered validated tool).
- Consider need for serum lead level, hemoglobin or hematocrit value, dental referral, tuberculosis testing.
- Maintain problem list, making appropriate plans and referrals, if necessary.

3 YEARS OF AGE

History (Interim Details)

- Assess parental concerns.
- Reassess social and system review.

Development

By this age:

- Gross motor:
  75% will balance on one foot for at least 1 second.
  75% will negotiate a successful broad jump.
  40% will balance on one foot for as long as 5 seconds.
- Fine motor:
  80% will copy a circle in addition to a vertical line.
  80% will build a tower of as many as eight cubes.
- Language:
  Speech is becoming more clearly understood in more than half.
  80% will use plurals appropriately.
  Almost half will give their first and last names appropriately.

- Social-emotional:
  90% will put on clothing alone.
  75% will play interactive games.
  50% will separate from mother or other significant person without too much stress.
  Many will have begun to wash and dry hands.

Physical Examination (particular attention)

- Update growth curves.
- Measure blood pressure.
- Continue reassessment; note new findings.
- Assess whether teeth are coming in appropriately.

Anticipatory Guidance

- Degrees of independence (limit setting and encouragement, a fine balance), other aspects of discipline
- Safety (car seat, guns in the home, strangers, supervised play)
- Limit TV viewing
- Personal hygiene (handwashing, toothbrushing, and proper use of toilet tissue)
- Childcare, encourage play with peers
- Reading with child

Plans and Problems

- Review immunizations and provide as appropriate.
- Perform developmental screening (using parent-administered validated tool).
- Conduct formal vision screening.
- Consider need for serum lead level, hemoglobin or hematocrit value, tuberculosis testing.
- Maintain problem list, making appropriate plans and referrals, if necessary.

4 YEARS OF AGE

History (interim details)

- Assess parental concerns.
- Reassess social and system review.

Development

By this age:

- Gross motor:
  75% will hop on one foot.
  75% will balance on one foot for as long as 5 seconds.
  65% will be able to imitate a heel-toe walk.
  Many will have begun to throw overhand.
- Fine motor:
  Almost all will copy a circle and a plus sign.
  80% will pick longer line of two.
  50% will begin to draw a person in three parts.
- Language:
  Speech is quite understandable in almost all.
  95% will give their first and last names.
  85% will understand "cold," "tired," and "hungry."
  80% will identify three of four colors.
- Social-emotional:
  Almost all will play games with other children.
  70% will dress without supervision.

Physical Examination (particular attention)

- Update growth curves.
- Measure blood pressure.
- Continue reassessment; note new findings.

Anticipatory Guidance

- Importance of reading to child frequently
- Booster seat in the car
- Fears and fantasies
- Separation (reliance on other adults as time goes by)
- Safety (poisoning, matches and lighters out of reach, strangers, supervision when outdoors, window guards)
- Personal hygiene (again, importance of frequent toothbrushing)

Plans and Problems

- Review immunizations and provide as appropriate.
- Conduct formal hearing and vision screening.
- Consider need for serum lead level, hemoglobin, or hematocrit value.
- Maintain problem list, making appropriate plans and referrals, if necessary.

5 YEARS OF AGE

History (interim details)

- Assess parental concerns.
- Reassess social and system review.

Development

By this age:

- Gross motor:
  Almost all will hop nicely on one foot.
  75% will balance on one foot for as long as 10 seconds.
  60% will do a heel-toe walk backward reasonably well.
- Fine motor:
  85% will draw a person in three parts.
  65% will draw a person in as many as six parts.
  60% will copy a square.
- Language:
  Almost all will identify four colors.
  Almost all will understand "on," "under," "in front of," "behind."
  More than half will define adequately five of the following eight words—ball, cake, desk, house, banana, curtain, fence, ceiling.
- Social-emotional:
  Almost all will dress without supervision.
  Almost all will brush teeth without help.
  Almost all will play board and card games.
  Almost all will be relaxed when left with a babysitter.
  More than half will prepare their own cereal.

Physical Examination (Particular Attention)

- Update growth curves.
- Measure blood pressure.
- Continue reassessment; note new findings.

Anticipatory Guidance

- Reading together
- School readiness (plays with others, endures separation from parents)
- Chores
- Discipline (consistency, praising)
- Gender identity
- Peer interaction
- Limiting TV viewing and electronic device use

- Safety (booster seat, guns in home, bike helmets, pool safety)

It is not usually possible to cover so many topics at one visit, so it is usually necessary to be selective based on your knowledge of the child and family.

Plans and Problems

- Review immunizations and provide as appropriate.
- Consider need for tuberculosis testing.
- Maintain problem list, making appropriate plans and referrals, if necessary.

ELEMENTARY SCHOOL YEARS (6–12 YEARS OF AGE)

History (Interim Details)

- Parental concerns
- Child's concerns
- Reassess social and system review
- Attention span
- Behavior at home and in school
- School accomplishments and experience
- Enuresis, encopresis, constipation, nightmares

Development

By this time, gross and fine motor problems have most often become apparent (but not always; neurologic examination should not be shortchanged). Language and social-emotional skills can be readily investigated in talks with parents and child, and in explorations of school and play experiences. Socialization and developing maturity may have different expressions at home, with peers, and in school. Talks with teachers, school reports, and various drawings and other efforts that the child brings home from school can be very helpful.

Physical Examination (particular attention)

- Update growth curves.
- Measure blood pressure.
- Continue reassessment; note new findings.
- Begin Tanner stage assessment.

Anticipatory Guidance

- Parent–child rapport
- Need for praise
- Responsibility

- Safety (booster seat and seat belt use, guns in the home, fire safety, bike helmets, pool safety)
- Allowance
- Limiting TV viewing and electronic device use
- Gender identity
- Dental care
- Adult supervision
- Discipline (limit setting)

Again, time constraints almost always make it necessary to adjust the menu for anticipatory guidance to your judgment about the family's needs.

Plans and Problems

- Review immunizations and provide as appropriate.
- Consider need for tuberculosis testing.
- Consider dyslipidemia screening.
- Maintain problem list, making appropriate plans and referrals, if necessary.

ADOLESCENTS

We have assumed a continuing relationship with the patient from birth on. If you are seeing a patient for the first time, begin with a full history and physical examination. Previsit questionnaires can be helpful and are available on the American Academy of Pediatrics Bright Futures website (https://brightfutures.aap.org/materials-and-tools/tool-and-resource-kit/Pages/adolescence-tools.aspx).

History (Interim Details)

- Patient's concerns
- Parental concerns
- Menstrual history
- Use of tobacco, alcohol, and drugs
- Diet and exercise
- Gender identity
- Sexual activity (relationships, partner violence, pregnancy, and contraceptive use)
- School experience
- Depression, anxiety, suicidal ideation; past suicide attempts
- Update knowledge of home and family structure

Adolescent patients should be given time alone to assess their personal concerns and to conduct a full social history. Confidentiality should be assured and reasons why sharing information with parents and caregivers is necessary (risk of harm to self or others). Talking alone with an adolescent does not mean that parents and caregivers should not be involved. A stable, supportive, and caring relationship is fundamental to building resilience in adolescence.

DEVELOPMENT

By this time, an adolescent's physical, neurologic, and cognitive abilities should be well understood, but their social and emotional development continue to progress. Conversation with patient, parent or caregivers, and teachers; school records; and, of course, a careful physical examination should all be helpful.

Physical Examination (particular attention)

- Update growth curves.
- Continue reassessment; note new findings.
- Tanner stage assessment.
- Assess spinal curvatures.

Anticipatory Guidance

- Puberty and related concerns; body image
- Sexuality, gender identity, sexually transmitted infections, contraception
- Diet
- Tobacco, alcohol, drugs
- Other risk-taking behaviors
- Exercise
- Safety (guns in the home, fighting, weapon carrying, seat-belt use, bike helmets)
- Family and other social relationships
- Independence and responsibility
- School and future aspirations

Time constraints almost always make it necessary to adjust anticipatory guidance topics to your judgment about the adolescent's and/or the family's needs.

Plans and Problems

- Review immunizations and provide as appropriate.
- Consider need for tuberculosis testing, HIV and sexually transmitted infection screening, hemoglobin or hematocrit determination, dyslipidemia screening.
- Maintain problem list, making appropriate plans and referrals, if necessary.

CHAPTER

24 Sports Participation Evaluation

The overall goals of the preparticipation physical evaluation (PPE) are to determine the general physical and psychological health of an athlete, ensure safe participation in appropriate physical activity, and not to restrict participation unnecessarily. Whether athletes receive the PPE in the context of an ongoing primary care relationship or as a focused preseason checkup, the following objectives of the evaluation are universal:

- To identify conditions that may interfere with a person's ability to participate in a sport
- To identify existing health conditions for a person that may increase the risk of injury or death during sports participation
- To help select an appropriate sport for a person's particular abilities and physical status

Sports and disciplined physical effort enhance fitness and coordination, increase self-esteem, and provide positive social experiences for participants, including individuals with physical and intellectual disabilities. Few children and youths have conditions that should limit participation, and most of these conditions are known before the PPE takes place. The PPE should be completed at least 6–8 weeks in advance of the planned sports activity so that any needed specialist evaluations, rehabilitation, or therapy can be completed before participation begins.

Examination Guidelines

Recommended PPE History and Physical Examination Forms, as shown on the following pages, were developed by the American Academy of Family Physicians, American Academy of Pediatrics, American College of Sports Medicine, American Medical Society for Sports Medicine, American Orthopedic Society for Sports Medicine, and the American Osteopathic Academy of Sports Medicine. The physical examination component of the PPE should center on high-yield areas, particularly those related to sports participation and issues identified by the history.

Garrick's "2-minute" 14-step orthopedic screening examination consists of observing the athlete in a variety of positions and postures that highlight asymmetries in range of motion, strength, and muscle bulk. These asymmetries serve to identify acute or old, poorly rehabilitated injuries. The steps shown in the figure help in assessing most of the following:

- Posture and general muscle contour bilaterally
- Patient's duck walk, four steps with knees completely bent
- Spine for curvature and lumbar extension, fingers touching toes with knees straight
- Shoulder and clavicle for dislocation
- Neck, shoulders, elbows, forearms, hands, fingers, and hips for range of motion
- Knee ligaments for drawer sign

You should also assess the following:

- Gait
- Patient's ability to hop on each foot
- Patient's ability to walk on tiptoes and heels

Patients with findings from the PPE may require evaluation by clinicians with appropriate knowledge and experience to assess the safety of a given sport for the athlete. This may include professionals in sports medicine, orthopedic surgery, cardiology, neurology, physical therapy, and others. If a condition is identified that may restrict a patient's participation, referral to a specialist may be necessary. When it is determined there is risk to participation, shared decision-making should occur with the athlete, their family, and an interdisciplinary team. Restricting participation may lead to psychological distress, and emotional support should be offered (McDonald et al., 2021).

1

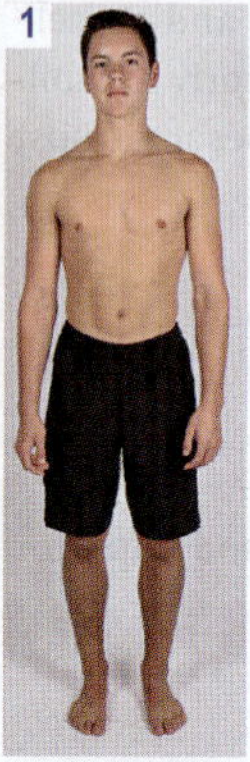

Step 1: Observe the standing athlete from the front for symmetry of trunk, shoulders, and extremities.

2

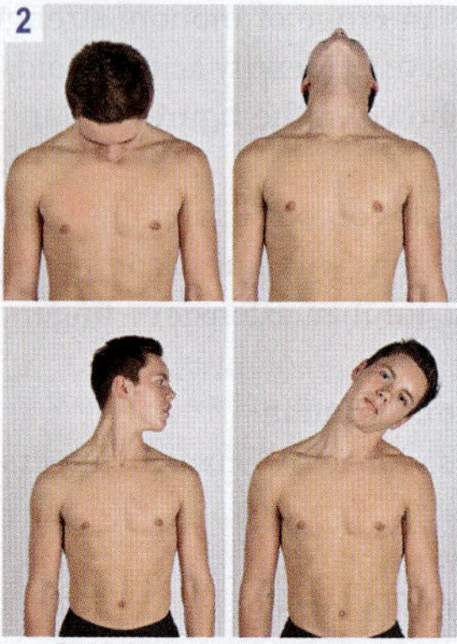

Step 2: Observe neck flexion, extension, lateral flexion on each side, and rotation to evaluate range of motion and the cervical spine.

3

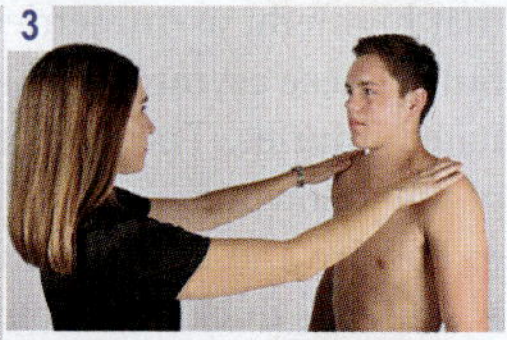

Step 3: Have the athlete shrug the shoulders against resistance from the examiner to evaluate trapezius strength.

4

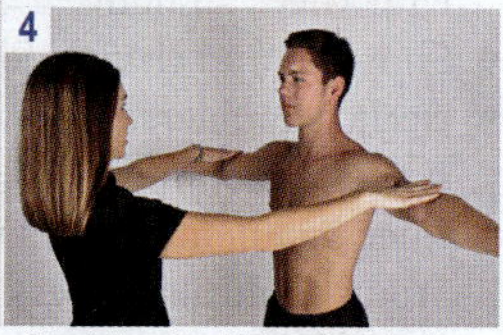

Step 4: Have the athlete perform shoulder abduction against resistance from the examiner to assess deltoid strength.

5

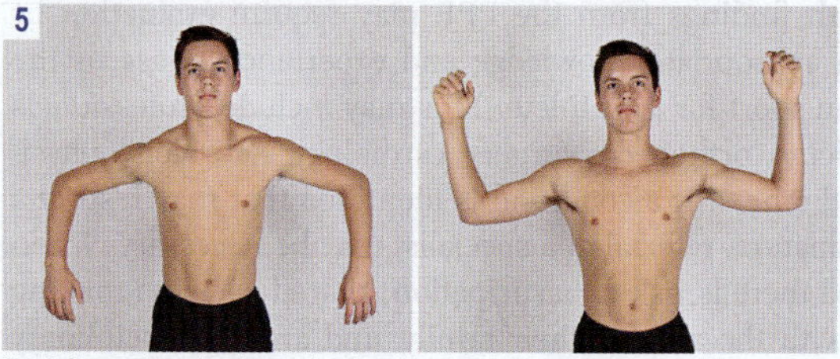

Step 5: Observe internal and external rotation of the shoulder to evaluate range of motion of the glenohumeral joint.

6

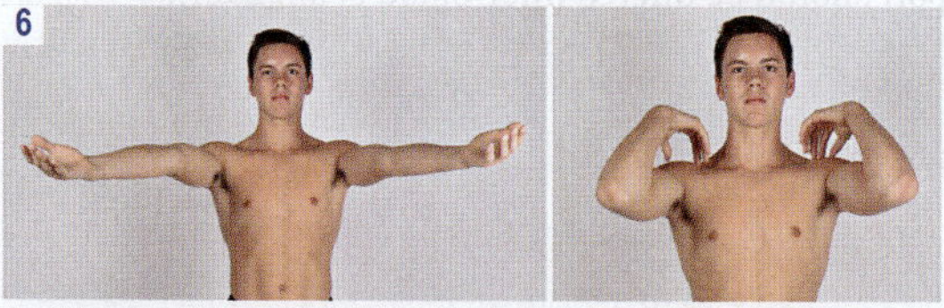

Step 6: Observe extension and flexion of the elbow to assess range of motion.

7

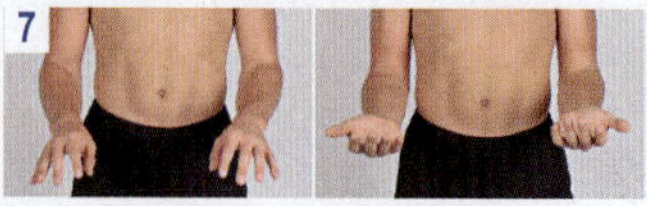

Step 7: Observe pronation and supination of the forearm to evaluate elbow and wrist range of motion.

8

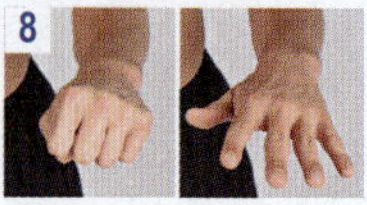

Step 8: Have the athlete clench the fist, then spread the fingers to assess range of motion in the hand and fingers.

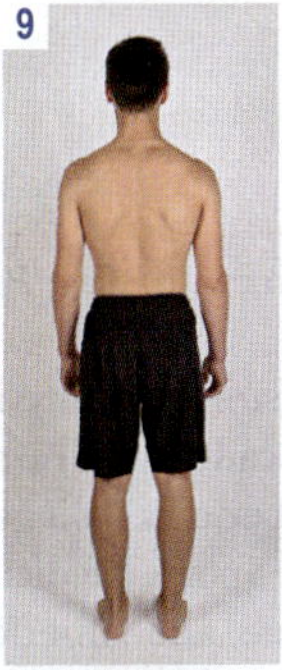

Step 9: Observe the standing athlete from the rear for symmetry of trunk, shoulders, and extremities.

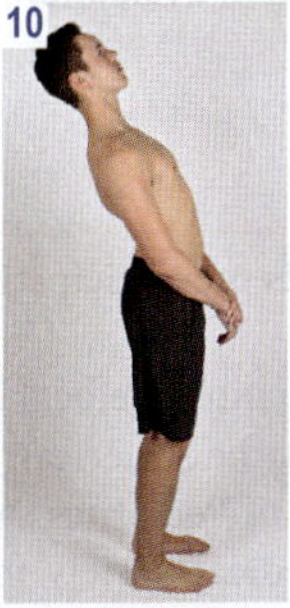

Step 10: Have the athlete stand with the knees straight and bend backward from the waist. Discomfort with extension of the lumbar spine may be associated with spondylolysis and spondylolisthesis.

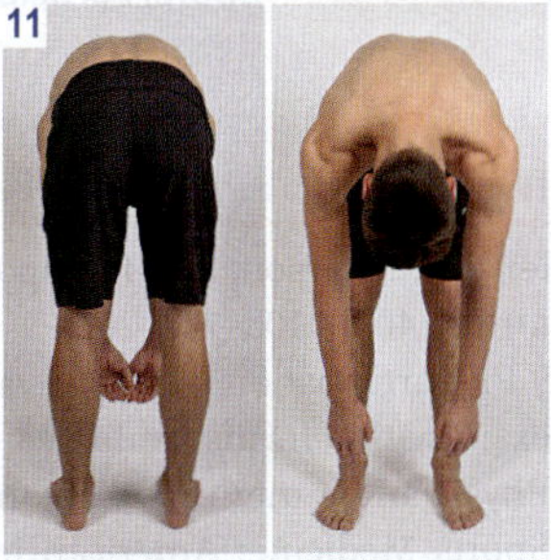

Step 11: Have the athlete stand with the knees straight and flex forward at the waist, first away from the examiner, then toward the examiner, to assess for scoliosis, spine range of motion, and hamstring flexibility.

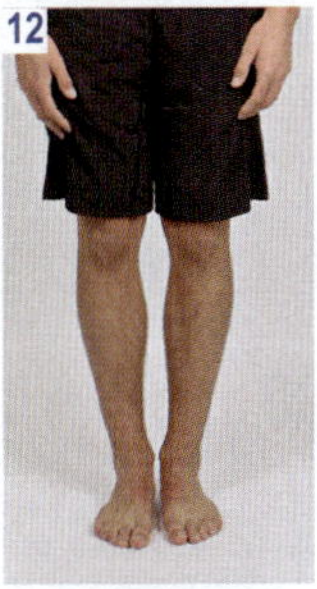

Step 12: Have the athlete stand facing the examiner with quadriceps flexed to observe symmetry of leg musculature.

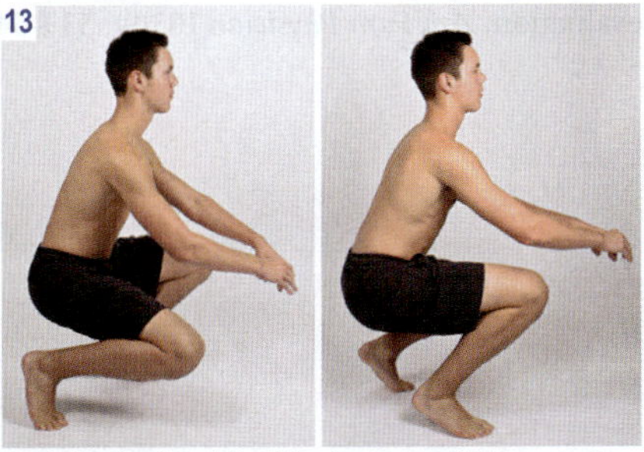

Step 13: Have the athlete duck walk four steps to assess hip, knee, and ankle range of motion, strength, and balance.

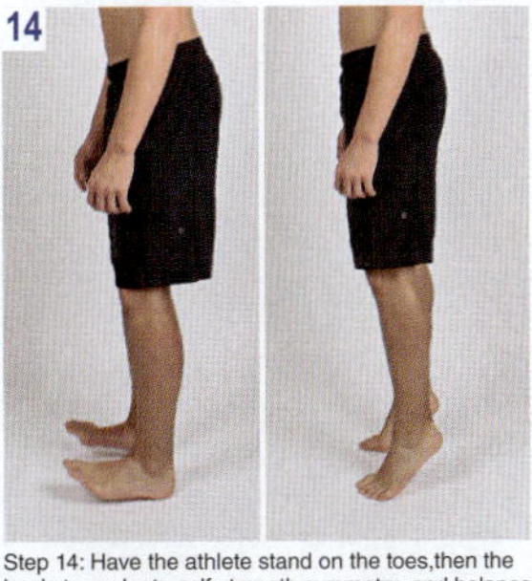

Step 14: Have the athlete stand on the toes,then the heels to evaluate calf strength,symmetry, and balance.

The 14-step screening orthopedic examination. The athlete should be dressed so that the joints and muscle groups included in the examination are easily visible; usually gym shorts for males and gym shorts and a T-shirt for females. Keep in mind that one of the most important points to look for in the orthopedic screening examination is symmetry. (From Miller SM, Peterson AR: The sports preparticipation evaluation. *Pediatrics in Review, 40(3); 108–128, 2019.)*

References

Miller, SM, Peterson, AR: The sports preparticipation evaluation. *Pediatr Rev* 40(3), 108–128, 2019.

2019 Preparticipation physical evaluation medical history and physical examination forms, endorsed by the American Academy of Family Physicians, American Academy of Pediatrics, American College of Sports Medicine, American Medical Society for Sports Medicine, American Orthopedic Society for Sports Medicine, and American Osteopathic Academy of Sports Medicine. Forms updated 2023 and publicly available at https://www.aap.org/en/patient-care/preparticipation-physical-evaluation/. (Accessed 25 November 2024).

MacDonald, J, Schaefer, M, & Stumph, J: The preparticipation physical evaluation. *Am Fam Physician* 103(9), 539–546, 2021.

CHAPTER 25

Assessment Considerations for Persons With Disabilities

Examination Guidelines

Variability among patients exists in knowledge, experience, functional status, cognitive abilities, and personality. These differences can affect your interaction. Persons with disabilities and older adults may experience some decline in their abilities, and these changes may not all occur at the same rate or may be fixed. Adaptation to patients' needs with disabling physical, intellectual, or emotional states (e.g., acute disabling illness, deafness, blindness, depression, psychosis, developmental delay, or neurologic impairment) is necessary.

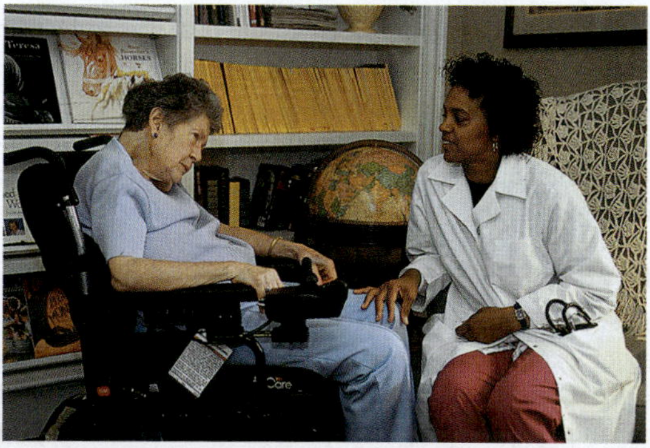

Interviewing a patient with a physical disability. Be sure the patient in a wheelchair has room to maneuver.

Some patients have sensory losses, such as hearing, that make communication more difficult. Let a hearing-, speech-, or vision-impaired patient guide you to the best communication system for your mutual purposes. For patients with hearing loss, position yourself so that the patient can see your face. Speak clearly and slowly; shouting may magnify the problem by distorting consonants and vowels. Use of a sign language interpreter is needed for patients who use sign language. Impaired vision and difficulties with light–dark adaptation are problems with written interview forms. Large print and lighting (that does not glare or reflect in the eyes) or individualized assistance is helpful.

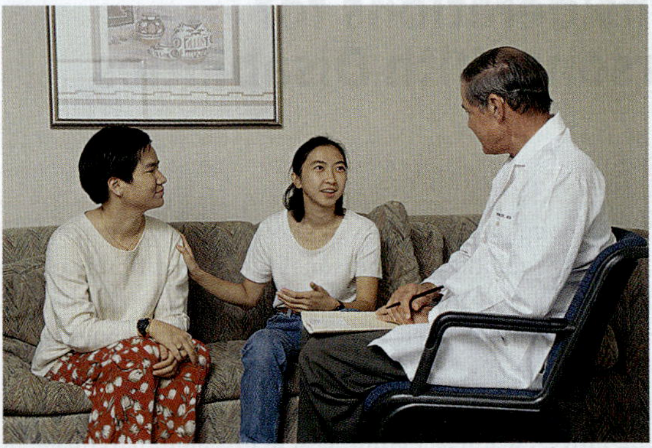

Interviewing a patient with a physical disability. Be sure the patient in a wheelchair has room to maneuver.

The patient has most often learned the best way to be transferred from a wheelchair or bed to another site or to a different position. Ask patient about this.

Bowel and bladder concerns are common to many individuals with disabilities and should be given the necessary attention during the examination process.

COGNITIVE ASSESSMENT

Some older adults or individuals with intellectual disability may be confused or experience memory loss, particularly regarding recent events. Take whatever extra time is needed. Ask short (but not leading) questions and keep language simple. Consult other family members to clarify discrepancies or to fill in the gaps. When necessary, use other healthcare professionals involved in care and the patient's record as resources for a more complete background.

Mental status is assessed continuously throughout the entire interaction with a patient by evaluating the patient's alertness, orientation, cognitive abilities, affect, and mood. Observe the patient's physical appearance, behavior, and responses to questions asked during the history. Evaluate the patient's mental status throughout the encounter (see Chapter 4).

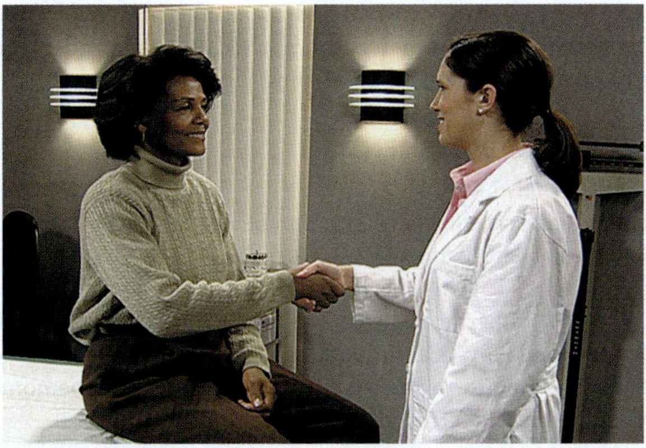

During the initial greeting, observe the patient for behavior, emotional status, grooming, and body language. Note the patient's body posture and ability to make eye contact.

TESTING MEMORY IN VISUALLY IMPAIRED PATIENTS

When a patient is visually impaired, test recent memory with unrelated words rather than observed objects. Pick four unrelated words that sound distinctly different, such as "green," "daffodil," "hero," and "sofa" or "bird," "carpet," "treasure," and "orange." Tell the patient to remember these words. After 5 minutes, ask the patient to list the four words.

Cognitive impairment that deprives ability to join in decision-making processes underscores the need for advance directives, which document the patient's wishes regarding extraordinary means of life support (e.g., ventilation assistance and feeding tubes). This document should be complemented by a surrogate (e.g., spouse, parent, child, sibling, or other person with a close relationship) who has a legally executed durable power of attorney for health care.

Many health conditions that require multiple medications increase risk for iatrogenic disorders and issues related to medication interactions or side effects. A medication history with attention to interactions of drugs, diseases, and aging is needed for prescribed and over-the-counter medications and herbal preparations. A substance use history is also relevant; people with disabilities and older patients are not immune to substance use disorders.

Aging, disability, a debilitating illness, and the onset of frailty may all increase dependency on others, concerns about tomorrow, and grieving for what has been lost. Recognize these vast concerns and the sense of loss in both the patient and the immediate caregiver. Maintaining function is a common concern of older adults. Understanding goals of care is important for developing therapeutic plans.

FUNCTIONAL ASSESSMENT

Activities of Daily Living

Functional assessment is an evaluation of a patient's ability to achieve the activities of daily living (ADLs). Questions concerning the ability to take care of one's daily needs are part of the review of systems.

The ability to perform instrumental ADLs (IADLs), or the ability to live independently, is an important assessment. Determine the patient's ability to perform ADLs and IADLs. Below is a mnemonic device to aid in remembering examples of ADLs and IADLs.

DEaTTH SHAFT (DEaTTH=ADLs, SHAFT=IADLs)

Dressing
Eating
Tabulating
Toileting
Hygiene
Shopping
Housekeeping
Accounting
Food preparation
Transportation

The personal and social history should include other dimensions of functional capacity such as social, spiritual, and economic resources; recreational activity; sleep patterns; environmental control; and the use of the healthcare system.

Functional assessment should be performed for anyone limited by disease or disability and includes:

Functional Assessment

MOBILITY	UPPER EXTREMITY FUNCTION
Difficulty walking standard distances: 1/2 mi, 2–3 blocks, 1/3 block, across a room	Difficulty grasping small objects, opening jars difficulty reaching out or up overhead (e.g., taking something off a shelf)
Difficulty climbing stairs, up and down	
Problems with balance	
Housework	**IADLs**
Heavy (vacuuming and scrubbing floors)	Bathing
Light (dusting)	Dressing
Meal preparation	Toileting
Shopping	Moving from bed to chair, chair to standing
	Eating
	Walking in home

Any limitations will affect a patient's independence and autonomy and increase reliance on other people and assistive devices.

In older patients, these limitations indicate the loss of physical reserve and the potential loss of physical function and independence, signifying the onset of frailty.

Characteristics of Frailty

Unintentional weight loss of 5% or more in past year	Weak grip strength
Unable to walk up a flight of steps	Low activity
Feeling of exhaustion	Increased number of illnesses

Frailty is an at-risk state caused by the age-associated accumulation of deficits resulting from cardiovascular and respiratory diseases and diabetes. Identification is important because of its association with functional decline, disability, and poor health outcomes (Phillips-Burkhart, 2016).

CHAPTER

26 Care of Transgender and Gender-Diverse Persons

Patients

This chapter is intended to highlight health history questions and physical examination considerations specific to Transgender and Gender Diverse (TGD) patients. The chapter is not a comprehensive guideline for care of TGD patients. Not addressed in this chapter are gender incongruence, dysphoria, and mental health issues; transition decisions, issues, and management; criteria for hormonal and/or surgical intervention; hormonal management and monitoring; surgical complications; and fertility considerations. Resources for more in-depth care guidelines and standards are included in the chapter.

History

SEXUAL ORIENTATION, GENDER IDENTITY

Sexual orientation, gender identity data are part of the requirements for the interoperability of electronic health records.

- Gender identity
  - Cisgender male
  - Cisgender female
  - Transgender man, transman, transmasculine
  - Transgender woman, transwoman, transfeminine
  - Genderqueer
  - Genderfluid
  - Other
- Sex assigned at birth: female, male
- Sexual orientation: gay, lesbian, straight/heterosexual, bisexual, queer, pansexual, asexual, other
- Preferred name
- Preferred pronouns: she/her/hers; he/him/his; they/them/theirs

MEDICAL HISTORY

- Use of hormones that may have feminizing or masculinizing effects (see Box 26.1)

Box 26.1 Gender-Affirming Hormone Therapies

Estrogen, Spironolactone, Progesterone Effects

Irreversible

- Breast tissue growth
- Decreased testicular volume
- Infertility

Reversible

- Redistribution of body fat
- Decreased muscle mass
- Softening of skin
- Decreased libido
- Decreased spontaneous erections
- Decreased terminal hair growth

Possible Risks

- Venous thromboembolic diseases
- Gallstones
- Elevated liver enzymes
- Weight gain
- Hypertriglyceridemia
- Cardiovascular disease
- Hypertension
- Hyperprolactinemia or prolactinoma
- Type 2 diabetes

Testosterone Effects

Irreversible

- Facial hair growth
- Voice deepening
- Clitoral enlargement
- Balding

Reversible

- Increased muscle mass
- Fat redistribution
- Acne and oily skin
- Increased libido
- Decreased fertility (but does not eliminate the possibility of pregnancy)

Possible Risks

- Polycythemia
- Weight gain
- Acne
- Androgenic alopecia (balding)

Continued

Box 26.1 Gender-Affirming Hormone Therapies—cont'd

- Sleep apnea
- Elevated liver enzymes
- Hyperlipidemia
- Destabilization of certain psychiatric disorders
- Cardiovascular disease
- Hypertension
- Type 2 diabetes

- Use of silicone or other soft-tissue fillers to enhance breast contour
- Adolescents: use of gonadotropin-releasing hormone agonists to suppress puberty
- Use of nonsurgical or nonhormonal methods to affirm gender identity (binding, packing, tucking, voice modulation); see Box 26.2 for description of gender affirming practices

Box 26.2 Gender-Affirming Practices

Some gender-affirming practices create special health concerns for transgender patients. These practices may or may not be relevant to the presenting health concern and should be used only if relevant.

Binding: Used by some transmasculine people, the practice involves the use of tight-fitting sports bras, shirts, ace bandages, or a specially made binder to flatten the breasts and provide a flat chest contour. Prolonged binding may result in breast pain, local skin breakdown, or fungal infection.

Packing: Used by some transmasculine people, the patient places a penile prosthesis in the underwear, creating an outward appearance of the presence of a penis.

Tucking: Used by some feminine people, the practice creates a visibly smooth crotch contour. The patient tucks the testicles (if present) into the inguinal canal and positions the penis and scrotum posteriorly in the perineal region. Tight-fitting underwear or a special undergarment known as a gaffe may be worn to maintain this alignment. Sometimes patients use adhesive or duct tape. This practice can result in urinary retention, hernias, or skin breakdown.

Voice modulation: Used by some transgender people to alter pitch, resonance, intonation, and intensity as a means to make the voice congruent with the identified gender. Patients may experience vocal fatigue. Specialty-trained speech language pathologists are best equipped to facilitate overall vocal health and efficiency.

- Other providers seen for gender-affirming treatment
- Previous cancer screenings and results

SURGICAL HISTORY

- Gender-affirming surgeries.
  - Gender-affirming surgeries may be specific to TGD people or be performed in cisgender populations. Any complications that have occurred as a result of surgery should be noted.
  - Box 26.3 summarizes gender-affirming surgeries.
- Organ inventory: To guide the assessment and management of specific health concerns and cancer screening. The inventory includes what gender-related organs (breasts, vagina, clitoris, ovaries, penis, prostate, and testes) are present and whether they are natal or surgically constructed. The inventory also includes the organs that have been surgically removed (breasts, uterus, ovaries, penis, prostate, and testes).

SOCIAL HISTORY

- Social support
- Challenges, concerns, or difficulties in relationships (e.g., family, friends, and coworkers) created by gender identity
- Concerns related to employment
- Adequacy of resources for daily needs

Box 26.3 Gender-Affirming Surgeries

Surgeries That May Be Considered by Trasnfeminine People

- Feminizing vaginoplasty
- Breast augmentation
- Orchiectomy
- Facial feminization procedures
- Reduction thyrochondroplasty (tracheal cartilage shave)
- Vocal cord surgery
- Lipo suction
- Lipo filling

Surgeries That May Be Considered by Transmansculine People

- Metaoidioplasty (clitoral release/enlargement, may include urethral lengthening)
- Masculinizing chest surgery (top surgery): mastectomy and chest contouring
- Hysterectomy or oophorectomy
- Vaginectomy
- Masculinizing phalloplasty or scrotoplasty

- Experiences of discrimination, bodily harm, or threats of bodily harm
- Thoughts about self-harm or suicide
- Tobacco use
- Alcohol or other substance use

CANCER SCREENING

- TGD patients are less likely to have undergone routine cancer screening.
- Research in the transgender population is lacking, and thus there are no established guidelines for TGD patients. Routine screening should continue based on the patient's organ inventory and existing anatomy. For example, a transmasculine person with an intact uterus still needs cervical cancer screening, and patients with breasts should have clinical breast examinations and mammograms. Prostate cancer screening should be considered in transmasculine people with a prostate, using the same guidelines as for cisgender men. Box 26.4 summarizes cancer screening recommendations for TGD patients.

Box 26.4 Cancer Screening Recommendations for TGD Patients

Transfeminine People

- Prostate cancer screening if prostate intact:
  - Prostate-specific antigen not reliable if testosterone levels are low
  - Digital rectal examination
- Breast cancer screening:
  - Mammograms after age 50 if on estrogen for more than 5 years
  - Clinical breast examination
- Colon cancer screening: The same age-appropriate screening recommendations and schedule as cisgender patients

Transmasculine People

- Breast cancer screening:
  - Mammogram: Follow guidelines until after breast surgery.
  - Clinical breast examination: Follow guidelines until after breast surgery.
- Cervical cancer screening (Pap smear and human papillomavirus testing):
  - Follow guidelines if the cervix is intact.
  - Clarify specimen is cervical.
  - Alert the pathologist to the use of testosterone.
  - No screening after hysterectomy unless there is a history of high-grade cervical lesions.
- Colon cancer screening: the same age-appropriate screening recommendations and schedule as cisgender patients

Physical Examination

- The physical examination should be relevant to the anatomy that is present in the patient regardless of gender identity or expression and should be specific to the presenting health concern. For example, the examination of the genitalia is not appropriate for a visit for headache or cough. A prostate examination in a transfeminine person and a pelvic examination in a transmasculine person would be appropriate for a relevant presenting symptom or for cancer screening.
- The physical examination should also be performed without assumptions as to anatomy or gender identity. Maintaining an organ inventory will help guide the appropriate examination. It is important to respect the patient's wishes regarding potentially sensitive examinations such as pelvic examination. It may take more than a single encounter to establish a relationship that will support the performance of such examinations.

SECONDARY SEX CHARACTERISTICS AND PHYSICAL CHANGES

- Patients using hormone therapy may present with secondary sex characteristics that fall along a continuum of development. The degree of secondary sex characteristics is somewhat dependent on the age at which hormone therapy was started, the duration of the therapy, and whether the patient went through puberty suppression therapy as an adolescent.
- Transmasculine people may have facial and body hair, clitoromegaly, increased muscle mass, masculine fat redistribution, androgenic alopecia, and acne.
- Transfeminine people may have some breast development and feminine fat redistribution. The breast tissue that develops as a result of hormone therapy should not be referred to as gynecomastia. Patients who have had silicone injections may have disfigured breasts or hard, lumpy masses. Transfeminine people who have used hormone therapy may have reduced muscle mass; thinned or absent body hair; thinned or absent facial hair; softened, thinner skin; and testicles that have decreased in size or have completely retracted. Electrolysis is commonly used by transfeminine people.
- Patients who have undergone gender-affirming surgeries may have varying physical examination findings depending on what procedures were performed, the surgical approaches used, and sequelae from complications.

PELVIC EXAMINATION WITH TRANSGENDER PATIENTS

- Pelvic examination in transfeminine people who have had vaginoplasty—the creation of a neovagina—may be appropriate to screen for lesions, granulation tissue, or stenosis, or to test for sexually transmitted infections (STIs).
- Differences between a natal vagina and a neovagina alter both the examination and the findings. The neovagina ends in a blind cuff, does not have a cervix or fornices, and may have a more posterior orientation. The neovagina does not self-lubricate and requires the use of a lubricant.
- Pelvic examination in transmasculine people who have an intact vagina and cervix may be appropriate for cancer screening or to test for STIs. Transmasculine people are less likely to be up to date on cervical cancer screenings. When sending a specimen for Pap smear or Human Papillomavirus (HPV) testing, it is essential to make clear to the laboratory that the specimen is cervical, especially if the listed gender is "male." Otherwise, the specimen may be discarded or incorrectly run as an anal Pap. The use of testosterone or presence of amenorrhea should be indicated.
- Pelvic examination in a transgender patient requires special consideration and care because the examination may induce anxiety and be perceived as traumatic. Many transgender patients have experienced violence, including sexual violence; therefore providing patients with information, choices, decision-making ability, and a sense of control is important. In testing for STIs, some transgender patients may prefer to collect their own specimens. If a patient declines speculum examination, consider offering an external or bimanual examination as a beginning step. A positive experience can establish trust and comfort and may facilitate further examination in the future.

PROSTATE EXAMINATION IN TRANSFEMININE PEOPLE

- In a transfeminine person with a prostate, prostate examination may be appropriate for cancer screening or for evaluation of prostate-specific symptoms, or both rectal and neovaginal approaches may be considered.
- In a transfeminine person who has undergone vaginoplasty, the prostate is anterior to the vaginal wall, and a digital neovaginal examination may be more effective.

Special Health Concerns

BREAST PAIN IN TRANSMASCULINE PEOPLE

- Prolonged breast binding may result in breast pain, local skin breakdown, bruising, or fungal infection. Patients may be reluctant to remove the binder for physical examination. In some patients with larger breasts, multiple garments may be used, and breathing may be restricted.
- Binding can also cause back pain. The workup for breast pain for feminine people is the same as that for cisgender patients.

PELVIC PAIN IN TRANSMASCULINE PEOPLE

- The use of testosterone creates a hypoestrogenic state that promotes tissue atrophy, increases vaginal pH, and increases the risk of vaginitis and cervicitis. As with cisgender women, the atrophic tissue is susceptible to traumatic irritation from sexual contact and can result in dyspareunia or vaginitis. The workup of pelvic pain in transmasculine people will be the same as that for cisgender patients.
- Transmasculine people may have decreased access to screening for and treatment of STIs. Genital or pelvic surgery may cause adhesions, scarring, bladder dysfunction, or nerve injury, which may cause or contribute to pain.

VAGINAL BLEEDING IN TRANSMASCULINE PEOPLE

- Cessation of menses is typically expected within 6 months of initiation of therapy in transmasculine people using testosterone. Cessation of menses driven by endometrial atrophy and testosterone-induced ovulation suppression may be incomplete. The time to cessation of menses may vary depending on dose and frequency of testosterone, presence and functioning of ovaries, and body habitus.
- Patients with intact organs not taking testosterone will continue to have menses, and the workup for abnormal bleeding will be the same as that for cisgender patients. The workup includes ruling out pregnancy in transmasculine people who have sex with sperm-producing partners.

BREAST PAIN IN TRANSFEMININE PEOPLE

- Early potential adverse effects from soft-tissue fillers include localized skin papules and inflammatory nodules that may become infected. Noninflammatory nodules may also develop and cause pain, itching, and abnormal pigmentation.

- Potential long-term adverse effects include migration of silicone with associated pain or deformity. Silicone granulomas may develop, which can produce pain, swelling, ulcerations, and lymphadenopathy.

SCROTAL PAIN IN TRANSFEMININE PEOPLE

- A common cause of scrotal pain in transfeminine people is the practice of tucking, described in Box 26.2. Many transfeminine people find this practice to be gender-affirming and may maintain positioning throughout the night while asleep. The scrotal pain may be of traumatic, mechanical, or neuropathic origin.
- Prolonged tucking may also result in urinary reflux and symptoms of epididymitis, orchitis, prostatitis, or cystitis.
- Prolonged positioning of the urethral meatus near the anus may serve as a portal of infection.

VOICE ISSUES AND VOCAL HEALTH

- Lowering of voice pitch may occur as a desired effect of hormone therapy in transmasculine people.
- Transfeminine people may use strategies to increase the tension in the vocal folds to elevate pitch. This requires continuous muscular effort, and patients may report a sensation of vocal effort or fatigue. Vocal cord surgeries have been designed to elevate pitch by altering vocal fold tension, mass, or both.
- Voice surgery undertaken by transgender people to alter the pitch of their voice can injure the delicate tissue of the vocal folds and negatively alter normal vocal quality.
- Patients may have voice-related issues not related to transition.

Guidelines and Standards for Care

The following sources provide guidelines and standards for care of transgender patients.

- Huynh V, Conroy M, Carroll EF, et al.: Contemporary considerations for breast cancer risk and screening in transgender, nonbinary, and gender-diverse populations, *Curr Breast Cancer Rep* 17(8), 2025. https://doi.org/10.1007/s12609-025-00573-6
- Green J: 13 The evolution of professional organizations and standards of care an inside-outsider's perspective. In Wolf-Gould C, Denny D, Green J, Lynch K, editors: *A history of transgender medicine in the United States: from Margins to mainstream,* Seattle, WA, 2025, SUNY Press, pp. 435–473. https://doi.org/10.1515/9798855801231-015

- Mclachlan C: Navigating gender diversity in healthcare: a guide for doctors, psychologists and social workers, *Mental Health Matters* 11(2), 2024. https://hdl.handle.net/10520/ejc-menhm_v11_n2_a1
- Taylor J, Hall R, Heathcote C, et al.: Clinical guidelines for children and adolescents experiencing gender dysphoria or incongruence: a systematic review of guideline quality (part 1), *Arch Dis Child* 109:s65–s72, 2024.

CHAPTER

27 Emergency or Life-Threatening Situations

Life-threatening emergencies occur in all settings. This assessment is intended to guide the initial response for a patient with an emergency in a health care setting.

Assessment Equipment Needed	Emergency Response Equipment Needed
Personal protective equipment	Bag valve mask
Pulse oximetry	Cervical collar
Stethoscope	Defibrillator
Sphygmomanometer	Endotracheal tube and laryngoscope
	Intravenous (IV) cannulas and fluids
	Oxygen
	Suction equipment
	Tourniquet

Primary Survey

This is a systematic assessment to rapidly identify potentially life-threatening physiologic derangements. Immediate treatment is initiated as soon as a life threat is identified. This assessment takes less than 30 seconds when the patient is stable, but it continues longer when life threats exist and must be managed. A similar assessment sequence is used for serious illnesses and injuries.

TECHNIQUE	FINDINGS
Hemorrhage	
Inspect for excessive bleeding and estimate blood loss.	**EXPECTED:** No bleeding. **UNEXPECTED:** Excessive bleeding. *Apply manual pressure to control bleeding, or apply a tourniquet if bleeding in an extremity cannot be controlled.*

Pulse—Palpate for the presence of the carotid or brachial pulse for 10 seconds.

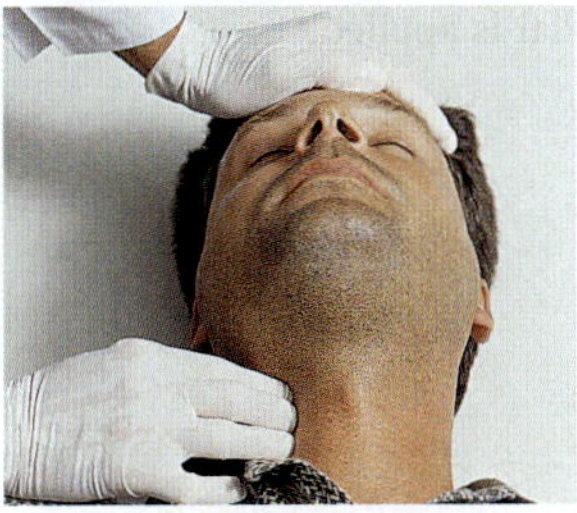

EXPECTED: Pulse is present, regular, and greater than 60 bpm in adults.

UNEXPECTED: No pulse palpated within 10 seconds. *Begin chest compressions. Call for help and a defibrillator.*

Airway and Responsiveness

Assess for a patent airway by asking the patient a question. If no response, place your ear close to patient's nose and mouth to detect air movement while looking for chest movement.

EXPECTED: Patient is able to talk, air movement through the nose is detected, and chest rise is observed.

UNEXPECTED: No air movement. *Begin rescue breathing with a bag valve mask and perform basic life support.*

If patient is supine and unresponsive, perform a chin lift or jaw thrust to open the airway.

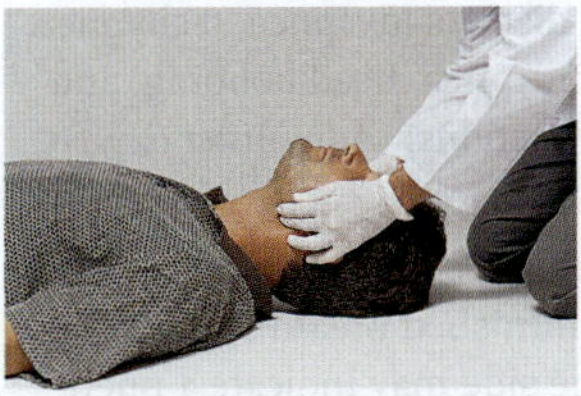

EXPECTED: Air movement is detected along with chest rise.

UNEXPECTED: No air movement.

Listen for an audible hoarse voice, stridor, drooling, barking cough, or wheezing.

UNEXPECTED: Presence of any of these sounds may be associated with an obstructed airway.

Inspect for any blood, vomitus, teeth, or foreign bodies that could obstruct the airway.

EXPECTED: No foreign bodies observed.

UNEXPECTED: Excessive secretions or a foreign body observed. *Remove the obstruction, if visible. Suction secretions.*

Cervical spine

Stabilize the head and neck in neutral position, without hyperextension, to reduce head movement when a patient has been injured.

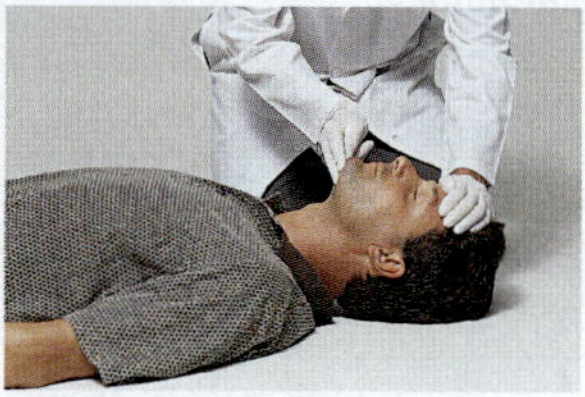

EXPECTED: Head and neck are held in position until a cervical collar is applied.

Breathing

Assess the rate and depth of respirations. Apply a pulse oximeter. Auscultate for breath sounds.

EXPECTED: Respiratory rate is 12–20 breaths per minute for adults; oxygen saturation (SpO2) is 93% or higher. Breathing is unlabored, bilateral breath sounds are auscultated, and chest rise is synchronized with breathing.
UNEXPECTED: Gasping, respiratory distress (dyspnea, tachypnea, bradypnea, head bobbing, and retractions). *Administer oxygen.*

Observe the chest for bilateral movement synchronized with breathing and signs of injury.

UNEXPECTED: Open chest wound, bruising over chest, and diminished breath sounds on one side may indicate a pneumothorax. *Cover an open chest wound immediately with your gloved hand until an occlusive dressing can be applied.*

Circulation

Assess skin color and quality, rate, and rhythm of carotid and distal pulses.

EXPECTED: Pulses present, strong, and regular rate.
UNEXPECTED: Pallor, weak distal pulses, irregular pulse rhythm.

Assess the blood pressure.	**EXPECTED:** Systolic blood pressure within expected range or slightly elevated. **UNEXPECTED:** Hypertension or hypotension. Systolic blood pressure of 90 mm Hg or lower in injured patient indicates hypovolemia from dehydration or blood loss. *IV fluid resuscitation should be initiated.*
Use capillary refill to assess tissue perfusion. Press firmly over a nail bed or bony prominence until the skin blanches, then release. Count seconds until skin color returns.	**EXPECTED:** 2 seconds or less. **UNEXPECTED:** Greater than 2 seconds.
Check dark clothing for dampness or signs of bleeding. Consider the possibility of internal bleeding in injured patients.	**EXPECTED:** No signs of bleeding. **UNEXPECTED:** Excessive bleeding and low systolic blood pressure are associated with hypovolemia/hypovolemic shock. *IV fluid resuscitation and blood products should be administered.*

Disability

Assess the Glasgow Coma Scale score to determine responsiveness. Repeat the test at regular intervals when hypoxemia, hypovolemic shock, or head injury is suspected. See Table 27.1.	**EXPECTED:** Score greater than 13. **UNEXPECTED:** Score of 13 or less indicates decreased level of consciousness. Decreasing score over time indicates worsening of condition. *Airway protection with an endotracheal tube should be provided for decreased level of consciousness.*
Shine a light at the eyes to assess pupillary size and responsiveness to light.	**EXPECTED:** Pupils are equal in size, not dilated, and respond briskly to light. **UNEXPECTED:** Pupils are unequal in size and are sluggish or nonreactive to light.

Table 27.1 Glasgow Coma Scale

ASSESSED BEHAVIOR	ADULT CRITERIA	INFANT AND YOUNG CHILD CRITERIA	SCORE
Eye opening	Spontaneous opening	Spontaneous opening	4
	To verbal stimuli	To loud noise or voice	3
	To pain	To pain	2
	No response	No response	1
Verbal response	Oriented to appropriate stimulation	Smiles, coos, cries	5
	Confused	Irritable, cries	4
	Inappropriate words	Inappropriate crying	3
	Incoherent	Grunts, moans	2
	None	No response	1
Motor response	Obeys commands	Spontaneous movement	6
	Localizes pain	Withdraws to touch	5
	Withdraws from pain	Withdraws to pain	4
	Flexion to pain (decorticate)	Abnormal flexion (decorticate)	3
	Extension to pain (decerebrate)	Abnormal extension (decerebrate)	2
	None	No response	1

Match the patient's best response in each category to the criteria for scoring. Appropriate verbal stimuli are questions eliciting the patient's level of orientation to person, place, and time. Painful stimuli are used when necessary to obtain eye opening and motor responses. Begin with less painful stimuli (e.g., pinching the skin) and progress to squeezing muscle mass or tendons if there is no response. Three scores are summed for the total Glasgow Coma Scale score. A maximum score of 15 indicates the optimal level of consciousness, and the minimal score of 3 indicates deepest coma.

Modified from Bethel (2012), James (1986), Teasdale and Jennett (1974), Teasdale et al. (2014).

Observe extremity movement and strength, and facial expression for any lateralizing signs of impairment.

EXPECTED: Extremity movement and strength, as well as facial expression, are bilaterally symmetric.

UNEXPECTED: Movement and strength are impaired on one side of the body.

Exposure and Environmental Control—Cut clothing off of the injured patient and perform a brief body search to identify any additional injuries, including on the back.

EXPECTED: Body temperature is maintained with heat lamps, warm blankets, and surface warmer.

UNEXPECTED: Additional injuries found.

Cover the patient with warmed blankets to prevent hypothermia.

Repeat the primary survey frequently during resuscitation to identify improvement or worsening of the patient's physiologic status.

Transition to the Secondary Assessment

History

Obtain an abbreviated history of the event (AMPLE):

A Allergies

M Medications or drugs of any type currently being used by the patient

P Past illnesses (e.g., diabetes, epilepsy, and hypertension); Pregnancy

L Last meal

E Events and their timing preceding the precipitating event; Environment related to the injury. Ask about the mechanism of injury to learn about energy forces transmitted and potential injury patterns that will guide treatment.

Secondary Assessment

Perform a rapid head-to-toe physical assessment to identify additional injuries or to begin developing a differential diagnosis.

Reassess the vital signs and oxygen saturation. **EXPECTED:** Vital signs and SpO2 improve and stabilize. **UNEXPECTED:** Deterioration in vital signs and SpO2.

For the patient with injuries, identify signs of severe injury in each body region. **UNEXPECTED:** See Table 27.2 and begin treatment.

For the patient with a medical condition, identify signs of serious illness. **UNEXPECTED:** See Table 27.3 and begin treatment.

Data from Perman, S.M., Elmer, J., Maciel, C.B., Uzendu, A., May, T., Mumma, B.E., Bartos, J.A., Rodriguez, A.J., Kurz, M.C., Panchal, A.R., Rittenberger, J.C., on behalf of the American Heart Association. 2023 American Heart Association Focused update on adult advanced cardiovascular life support: an update to the American Heart Association Guidelines for cardiopulmonary resuscitation and emergency cardiovascular care. doi:https://doi.org/10.1161/CIR.0000000000001194 (Published Print: 2024-01-30; Update policy: https://doi.org/10.1161/crossmarkpolicy).

Table 27.2 Signs of Serious Injury and Potential Conditions

SIGNS	POTENTIAL CONDITIONS
Raccoon eyes—ecchymosis and swelling around eyes	Basilar skull fracture or facial bone fracture
Battle sign—bruising and swelling behind the ear(s), in line with posterior auricular artery	Basilar skull fracture
Clear or amber-colored fluid from ears or nose	Basilar skull fracture
Hamman sign or crunch—precordial crunching, slicking, or knocking sound synchronous with heartbeat	Hemothorax, acute mediastinitis, pneumomediastinum, pneumothorax, or respiratory failure
Kehr sign—severe pain in subscapular area of shoulder, often on left side	Phrenic nerve irritation from splenic rupture, ectopic pregnancy, or gastrointestinal disease
Cullen sign—Bluish skin discoloration around the umbilicus, indicating bleeding in the tissues	Intraperitoneal or intraabdominal hemorrhage, ectopic pregnancy, or acute hemorrhagic pancreatitis
Grey-Turner sign—bruising and induration of the skin of the flanks, umbilicus, and costovertebral angle	Retroperitoneal hematoma or acute hemorrhagic pancreatitis
Diminished or absent breath sounds	Pneumothorax or hemothorax
Bruising over iliac wings, pubis, labia, or scrotum and pain by palpation	Pelvic fracture
Paralysis or paresthesia	Spinal cord injury, injury to peripheral nervous system

Table 27.3 Serious or Life-threatening Medical Signs and Potential Conditions

SERIOUS MEDICAL SIGNS	POTENTIAL CONDITIONS
Vomiting blood or material looking like coffee grounds, black or tarry stools	Bleeding from ulcer in stomach, duodenum, or esophageal varices
Crushing pain in middle of chest, pain radiation to left arm, neck, jaw, or shoulder	Myocardial infarction
Severe throbbing pain in and around one blood-shot eye, blurry vision, or acute loss of vision	Acute glaucoma
Flashes of light in field of vision of one eye, partial loss of vision spreading as a shadow from top or one side of eye	Retinal detachment
Sudden, severe, and progressive abdominal pain	Acute abdomen (e.g., appendicitis, intestinal obstruction)
Sudden onset of breathing difficulty that worsens rapidly	Pulmonary edema, pneumothorax, pulmonary embolism
Sudden weakness or paralysis, unsteadiness, possible loss of consciousness, speech difficulty, headache	Brain attack (stroke) or transient ischemic attack

PEDIATRIC VARIATIONS

The primary assessment sequence is the same for children as for adults, with attention to responsiveness, airway, breathing, and circulation (see Table 27.4).

Table 27.4 Assessment Findings Indicating a Sense of Urgency in Infants and Children

ASSESSMENT FOCUS	SIGNS AND SYMPTOMS OF CONCERN
Responsiveness	• Combative or inconsolable • Decreased responsiveness, lethargy • Poor muscle tone • Weak or high-pitched cry, moaning • Personality change, failure to make eye contact, glassy-eyed stare, lack of interest in play or interaction • Does not recognize parents

Continued

Table 27.4 Assessment Findings Indicating a Sense of Urgency in Infants and Children—cont'd

ASSESSMENT FOCUS	SIGNS AND SYMPTOMS OF CONCERN
Airway and Breathing	• Respiratory rate greater than 60 breaths per minute, sustained, especially with oxygen administration • Respiratory rate less than 20 breaths per minute, especially in the presence of acute illness or with injury to the chest or abdomen • Respiratory distress, nasal flaring, retractions (intercostal, supraclavicular, and sternal) • Airway sounds: Stridor, muffled speech, grunting, signs of obstruction • Head bobbing with each breath: impending respiratory failure • Position: Tripod, refusing to lie down • Asymmetric chest movements or see-saw respirations (chest rises as abdomen falls and vice versa)
Circulation	• Pale, cool skin—mottling, pallor, and peripheral cyanosis are indicators of poor tissue perfusion or respiratory distress • Pulses—absence of peripheral pulses indicates poor tissue perfusion; diminished central pulse is an ominous sign • Capillary refill time—greater than 2 seconds indicates poor tissue perfusion, hypothermia, constricted blood flow (e.g., tight cast) • Sunken fontanel, doughy skin texture, dry mucous membrane may indicate hypovolemia due to dehydration • Heart rate—greater than 160 or less than 80 per minute sustained in child under age 5 years; greater than 140 per minute sustained in child at least 5 years of age • Bradycardia—sign of impending cardiac arrest • Sustained sinus tachycardia—indicates hypovolemia, fever, or infection • Blood pressure—hypotension is a late sign of hypovolemia and indicates cardiovascular decompensation (a decrease of 10 mm Hg is significant) • Oliguria

AIDS TO DIFFERENTIAL DIAGNOSIS

SUBJECTIVE	OBJECTIVE
Increased Intracranial Pressure	
History of brain injury, seizure, and stroke. Headache, nausea, and vomiting	Change in mental status (lethargy, irritability, stupor, or coma), seizures or syncope, papilledema, cranial nerve VI palsy, Cushing triad (bradycardia, rising blood pressure, irregular respirations)
Pulmonary embolism	
History of surgery in past month, long plane trip, oral contraceptives, pregnancy; reduced mobility associated with conditions such as cancer, fractured femur Shortness of breath, stabbing chest pain that worsens with breathing or coughing, coughing up blood, palpitations, anxiety, leg pain, and swelling	Tachycardia, diaphoresis, tachypnea, pain with deep leg vein palpation, unilateral leg swelling, syncope, cough, hemoptysis
Status asthmaticus	
History of dyspnea and increasing asthma medication use over several days or sudden symptom onset Shortness of breath, wheezing, coughing, fatigue	Unable to speak or can say only a few words between breaths, tachycardia, tachypnea, hypertension, dyspnea, hypoxemia, wheezing (unless airflow is so diminished it obscures wheezing), pulsus paradoxus greater than 20 mm Hg, altered mental status

SUBJECTIVE	OBJECTIVE
Status epilepticus	
History of seizures, neurologic disorder, or injury Shaking movements, loss of consciousness, and unresponsive longer than usual with seizures	Tonic-clonic movements or unresponsiveness lasting longer than 5 minutes, or second seizure without return to baseline, despite appropriate emergency antiepileptic medications; hypotension, cardiac dysrhythmias, hypoxemia from impaired ventilation during tonic stage, hypoglycemia due to increased metabolic rate

References

Teasdale, G, Jennet, B: Assessment of coma and impaired consciousness: a practical scale, *Lancet*, 2: 81–84, 1974.

Teasdale, G, Maas, A, Lecky, F., et al.: The Glasgow Coma Scale at 40 years: standing the test of time, *Lancet Neurol*, 13: 844–854, 2014.

Maconochie, IK, Aickin, R, Hazinski, MF., et al.: Pediatric life support 2020 International Consensus on Cardiopulmonary Resuscitation and Emergency Cardiovascular Care Science With Treatment Recommendations. *Pediatrics* 147(Suppl 1): e2020038505B, 2021. doi:10.1542/peds.2020-038505B.

Slovis, JC, Bach, A, Beaulieu, F., et al.: Neuromonitoring after pediatric cardiac arrest: cerebral physiology and injury stratification. *Neurocrit Care* 40: 99–115, 2024. https://doi.org/10.1007/s12028-023-01685-6.

Perman, S.M., Elmer, J., Maciel, C. B., Uzendu, A., May, T., Mumma, B.E., Bartos, J.A., Rodriguez, A.J., Kurz, M.C., Panchal, A.R., Rittenberger, J.C., on behalf of the American Heart Association. 2023 American Heart Association Focused update on adult advanced cardiovascular life support: an update to the American Heart Association Guidelines for cardiopulmonary resuscitation and emergency cardiovascular care. doi:link: https://doi.org/10.1161/CIR.0000000000001194 (Published Print: 2024-01-30; Update policy: https://doi.org/10.1161/crossmarkpolicy)

Signs and Symptoms That Can Be Caused by Drugs

Innumerable symptoms and physical findings are caused by the drugs we commonly use in practice. An adverse drug reaction (ADR), as defined by the World Health Organization, is any noxious, unintended, and undesired effect that occurs at normal drug doses. ADRs can be mild (e.g., nausea, drowsiness) or severe (e.g., neutropenia, hypotension). ADRs are more likely to occur in very young or elderly patients as well as in those taking multiple medications. The following is a partial list of some cardiovascular ADRs and some of the classes of drugs that may cause them.

A REMINDER: Not all drugs in a particular class carry equivalent risk. This table may look frightening, but it is intended to instill caution in clinicians who prescribe or administer medications.

ADVERSE DRUG REACTION	POSSIBLE CAUSATIVE AGENTS
Cardiorespiratory arrest	Anxiolytics
Chest pain	Antidepressants Bronchodilators
Dysrhythmias	Antiepileptics Antipsychotics Anxiolytics Bronchodilators Central nervous system stimulants Oral contraceptives Tricyclic antidepressants
Hypertension	Antidepressants Central nervous system stimulants Oral contraceptives

continued

ADVERSE DRUG REACTION	POSSIBLE CAUSATIVE AGENTS
Hypotension	Antidepressants Antipsychotics Anxiolytics Bronchodilators Central nervous system stimulants Opioids
Orthostatic hypotension	Antidepressants
Palpitations	Antidepressants Bronchodilators Central nervous system stimulants
Prolongation of QT interval	Antibiotics Antidepressants Bronchodilators Decongestants
Syncope	Antidepressants Antipsychotics
Tachycardia	Antidepressants Antipsychotics Bronchodilators Central nervous system stimulants
Thrombotic disorders	Estrogen hormones Oral contraceptives Selective estrogen receptor modulators Tricyclic antidepressants

Index

Note: Page numbers followed by *f* indicate figures; *t*, tables; *b*, boxes.